SELF-CARE NURSING:
THEORY & PRACTICE

Nancy J. Steiger, R.N., M.S.
Clinical Nurse Specialist
Petaluma Valley Hospital
Petaluma, California
Assistant Clinical Professor
Department of Physiological Nursing
University of California, San Francisco

Juliene G. Lipson, R.N., Ph.D.
Associate Professor
Department of Mental Health and Community Nursing
University of California, San Francisco

BRADY COMMUNICATIONS COMPANY, INC. ● BOWIE, MARYLAND 20715
A Prentice-Hall Publishing Company

Publishing Director: David Culverwell
Acquisitions Editor: Richard A. Weimer
Production Editor/Text Designer: Janis K. Oppelt
Art Director: Don Sellers, AMI
Assistant Art Director: Bernard Vervin
Manufacturing Director: John A. Komsa

Indexer: Lea Kramer
Typesetter: Carver Photocomposition, Arlington, Virginia
Printer: R.R. Donnelley & Sons Company, Harrisonburg, Virginia
Typefaces: Franklin gothic book (text); Caledonia (display)

Self-Care Nursing: Theory & Practice

Library of Congress Cataloging in Publication Data
Steiger, Nancy J., 1952–
  Self-care nursing.

  Bibliography: p.
  Includes index.
  1. Self-care, Health. 2. Nursing—Study and teaching. I. Lipson, Juliene G., 1944– II. Title. [DNLM: 1. Self Care—methods-nurses' instruction. 2. Patient Education—methods—nurses' instruction. W 85 S818s]
  RA776.95.S74   1985   613'.07   84-14459
ISBN 0-89303-841-5

Prentice-Hall International, Inc., *London*
Prentice-Hall Canada, Inc., Scarborough, *Ontario*
Prentice-Hall of Australia, Pty., Ltd., *Sydney*
Prentice-Hall of India Private Limited, *New Delhi*
Prentice-Hall of Japan, Inc., *Tokyo*
Prentice-Hall of Southeast Asia Pte. Ltd., *Singapore*
Whitehall Books, Limited, Petone, *New Zealand*
Editora Prentice-Hall Do Brasil LTDA., *Rio de Janeiro*
Prentice-Hall Hispanamericana, S.A., *Mexico*

Printed in the United States of America

85 86 87 88 89 90 91 92 93 94 95   1 2 3 4 5 6 7 8 9 10

Contents

Foreword

Self-Care Nursing: Theory & Practice proceeds from the premise that self-care can be a powerful philosophical, biological, psychological, sociocultural, and economic basis for nursing practice in a variety of health care settings. The book's approach is theoretically based; a new conceptual model for self-care may be emerging in it from the amalgam of nursing, social and behavioral science theories cited. Concomitantly, the text is eminently practical, using the nursing process as a vehicle for analysis and presentation. Principles and practices are described; tools and techniques for encouraging self-care, case studies, and care plans are provided. Cultural sensitivity is demonstrated throughout. The very enlightening historical perspective developed in the beginning culminates in a discussion of the future of self-care nursing with implications for education, service, and research.

Such a unique blend has been achieved through the combined talents and interests of a clinical specialist and a nurse anthropologist. Their work has much to offer clinicians in all settings as well as faculty and students in all programs, all of whom are urged to serve as role models through their own health promotive behaviors.

Every nurse who is convinced, or needs to be convinced, that self-care is a powerful force in nursing practice should have a copy.

Margretta M. Styles, R.N., Ed.D.
Dean and Professor
School of Nursing
University of California
San Francisco, California

Preface

The basic premise of self-care is that individuals have the ability to influence their health and to participate in their health care. Self-care is defined here as those activities initiated or performed by an individual, family, or community to achieve, maintain, or promote maximum health potential.

Although individuals and families have always performed self-care, many health care consumers are taking increased interest in their health, as evidenced by demands for more information about health and more responsibility in their own care. This trend has its roots in the women's health movement and the consumerism that began in the 1960s. In actuality, at least 75% of health care is self-care and includes activities that substitute for professional intervention as well as those that supplement professional intervention (Williamson and Danaher 1978).

Since the 1960s, health care professionals have also become interested in self-care as an adjunct to professional medical care. The benefits of self-care are increasingly recognized as especially important in chronic and long-term care. The nursing profession has been in the forefront in its advocacy of client education. However, this book goes beyond patient education as it relates to disease and treatment. Our intent is to provide the reader with tools to teach clients how to systematically think through and decide how to take care of themselves, and when to seek professional care.

We view self-care in broad terms as a philosophy and approach to nursing care rather than a specific kind of intervention. Dorothea Orem's self-care deficit theory is used as a point of departure, and we address much of the same content, although we do not use her terminology. We include theoretical contributions of Martha Rogers and Madeleine Leininger, as well as relevant social science theories. Our intent is not to elaborate a new conceptual model or to differ from Orem but to focus on implementation of self-care concepts into clinical practice. Although the book is theoretically based, it is intended as a practical step-by-step approach through use of the nursing process.

This book is intended for nurses who work in a variety of contexts and at any educational level. The theory and techniques of self-care are the same, and the difference in the depth and expertise with which they are used depends on the sophistication of the nurse who uses the book.

Thus, practicing nurses, as well as students, who may be unfamiliar with the concepts of self-care, are provided simple guidelines for incorporating self-care principles into their clinical practice. Readers can personally benefit from using the assessment tools and suggestions we provide in their own health promotion.

Critics have claimed that the self-care movement is popular with and relevant to only well-educated and mainstream middle class people. We believe, however, that the philosophy and practices of self-care are valid for a range of socioeconomic and cultural groups, if the values of each group are taken into consideration. Cultural material is integrated throughout the book, and suggestions are provided for modifying the self-care approach for work with clients of varying socioeconomic and ethnic backgrounds.

The book is organized into four sections. The first focuses on historical, philosophical, and theoretical apsects of self-care. We trace the history of self-care from ancient Chinese and Greek medicine to the current self-care movement. Our own philosophical tenets include the idea that individuals have the potential to significantly influence their own health status and can be equal partners in planning and carrying out their own care; we also believe that the nurse should set an example of a healthy lifestyle.

Part Two focuses on the importance of self-care in the clinical context, using the nursing process. We distinguish between self-care in health and self-care in illness because we think that clients' perceptions of their health and their motivation to engage in self-care differ. Case studies illustrate implementation. A separate chapter presents specific strategies for teaching self-care. Such strategies include enhancing communication, helping clients to change unhealthy behaviors, mutual problem solving, nurses as models of health, use of self-assessment tools, and contracting.

The third section elaborates on the components of health presented in Chapter 4. Specific assessment tools and substantive content are described for the purpose of increasing the individual's self-care ability. This section is useful not only for clients but for nurses themselves. Each chapter includes current knowledge and issues, related research, and clinical application.

Part Four is one chapter that addresses the potential impact of self-care in nursing education, nursing practice, and nursing research. Self-care needs to be taught as an emphasis in nursing education before students are immersed in the medical model, in which there is an emphasis on disease and cure. Despite the ideal of emphasis on health promotion in nursing, the medical model often obscures concepts of prevention and health promotion in practice.

In this book, we use the designation "client" instead of "patient" throughout because "client" connotes a more active role in relationships with health care professionals. "Patient" connotes a horizontal, powerless person to whom health care interventions are done. Some case examples accompanying the chapters are true, while others are fictitious; some case examples include nursing care plans. Study questions are included in each chapter.

Acknowledgments

A number of people have helped to make this book possible. But without the love, support and patience of our families, we would have never completed it.

Special acknowledgments go to Toni Ayres, R.N., Ed.D. for writing the chapter on sexuality and also to Jackson Helsloot for original cover design and for the artwork he contributed.

Our great appreciation goes to Kathryn May, R.N., D.N.S., and Barbara McLain, R.N., M.S., whose excellent suggestions and helpful critiques strengthened the entire book.

We thank the following people who reviewed selected chapters and gave invaluable guidance: Susan Baldi, R.N., M.S.; Diane Branton, R.N., MS.; Barbara Burgel, R.N., M.S.; Merit Carnahan, R.N., B.S.; Joy Dobson, R.N., M.S.; David Duncombe, B.D., Ph.D.; Heidi Farmer, R.D.; Kathy Fitzgerald, R.N., M.S.; Yolanda Gutierrez, R.D., M.S.; Shirley Laffrey, R.N., Ph.D.; Charlotte Lane-McGraw, R.N., M.S.; Deborah Larson, R.N., B.S.; Norine Mugler, R.N., B.S.; Jane Norbeck, R.N., D.N.S.; Leslie Ray, R.N., M.A.; and Sharon Jeanne Smith, R.N., Ph.D.

Case studies were contributed by Barbara Burgel, R.N., M.S.; Parie Lambert, R.N., B.S.; Glenda Dickinson, R.N., M.S.; Kathy Fitzgerald, R.N., M.S.; Peggie Griffin, R.N., M.S.; and Cheryl Hubner, R.N., M.S.

We wish to thank Lillie Shortridge, R.N., Ed.D., who inspired Nancy Steiger to begin the book, and Priscilla Nunn and Barbara Mow who patiently typed and retyped the entire manuscript.

We thank Richard Weimer, Joanne Haworth, Janis Oppelt, and Edie Plunkett of Brady Communications Company for their support of this book.

Finally, we thank our students and colleagues who stimulated and taught us, and most importantly, our patients and clients to who this book is dedicated.

PART ONE

SELF-CARE
IN
NURSING
PRACTICE

1

History and Philosophy of Self-Care

During the past decade, there has been an enormous increase in public and professional interest in the significance of self-care in health. The casual observer cannot help but be aware of large numbers of health-related publications, classes, and groups currently available that are based on the self-care and self-help movements. During the past five years, we have seen burgeoning growth in the self-care theme. For example, participants at an international symposium on the role of individuals in primary health care, held in 1975, were unwilling to call the self-care trend a full-blown social movement (Levin, Katz, and Holst 1979). But by 1979, Levin stated, "We cannot be but astonished at the developments in self-care that have occurred since 1976. . .we have seen a bewildering variety of manifestations of interest and growth in self-care" (1979:80). Interest in self-care is increasingly evident in nursing as well.

Why is self-care now a topic of such great interest? It is not a new concept but a revived idea with roots in ancient history. Over the years, there has been a varying degree of interest in and recognition of the importance of the individual's, family's, and community's responsibility in health promotion and illness prevention. This changing emphasis is intricately related to society's view of humankind and its relationship to the world, as well as its view of illness and healing (Leder 1984). In addition, major health problems have shifted from acute conditions to chronic conditions, and new forms of care have not been incorporated into the traditional care mode. The cost of health care has risen to such an extent that care has become inaccessible to many people. Health care consumers, employers, third-party payers, and health care providers are making concerted efforts to contain health care costs while increasing the health care system's effectiveness (Zapka and Averill 1979; Roberts, Imrey, Turner, Hosokawa, and Alster 1983; Cadmann, Chambers, Feldman, and Sackett 1984). Further, disillusionment with traditional care has grown,

3

people have begun to demand more active participation in their care, and alternative treatment models have been sought.

We will now briefly describe some of the historical themes that underlie the current self-care movement in the United States. It is beyond the scope of this book to provide a complete history or to include the wealth of data available in medical anthropology on indigenous health care activities in small-scale societies. Our purpose is to mention a few key historical developments to provide a context for understanding the present-day, self-care movement.

HISTORY OF SELF-CARE

While animals tend to avoid or abandon their sick, human beings, for the most part, have attempted to cure their ailing group members from earliest history (Foster and Anderson 1978). Although we must assume that the majority of health care through the ages occurs in the context of the family, and health practices are passed down through the generations in all societies, specific self-care practices, especially in the area of health promotion, are not often described in ethnographic and historical documents. There is more data on what people do when they get sick. In addition, history tells us little about what most deeply concerned ordinary people and their ideas about health and healing. Thus, when discussing the history of self-care, we must depend on accounts of major indigenous medical systems. With the exception of Risse, Numbers, and Leavitt (1977) and Hand (1976), there is little published literature on the history of lay traditions in health care in the United States.

Ancient and Early European History

In reference to health philosophy and practices in ancient civilizations, perhaps the most is known about the ancient Chinese civilization. Ancient Chinese medicine emphasized balance and harmony with nature and the rhythms of the universe. The emphasis was on maintenance of health rather than treatment of illness (Veith 1949). Traditional Chinese medicine continues to be based on the same tenets today.

Leaping several centuries, we know that ancient Greek medicine was associated with the Goddess Hygeia, who was said to advocate living wisely and preserving health through hygienic living habits and proper nutrition. Illness was seen as a disruption in the equilibrium of the four humors of the body (blood, phlegm, black bile, and yellow bile) and of the harmony between the human body and the environment. Hippocrates, born in 406 B.C., advocated the importance of caring for one's own body through diet, exercise, rest, and baths. The work *Aphorisms*, attributed to Hippocrates, emphasized "the healing power of nature," which the physician should support rather than interfere with (Sigerist 1961). This holistic perspective continues to be present in the folk traditions of many cultures, as well as in many medical systems throughout the world. In contrast to an emphasis on individual health practices and habits of living, later physicians, such as Aesclediades, denied the healing power of nature and insisted that illness be treated quickly and aggressively.

In Europe, several centuries later, most social institutions were controlled by the church. Illness was regarded as punishment for sin, and prayer was, therefore, the only appropriate medicine, because Christ was believed to have healed without medicine or surgery. Following the development of medical schools and increasingly during the Renaissance (fourteenth to sixteenth centuries) and as knowledge of human anatomy grew, the human body came to be regarded as a machine. Engel describes the perspective of disease at this time as ". . .the breakdown of the machine and the doctor's task as the repair of the machine" (1977:131). Further, "the positivist view of disease as a deviation from a biochemical norm reached its heyday in nineteenth century Europe with the formulation of the germ theory of disease and with concomitant advances in immunology, pathology, and surgical techniques" (Ahmed, Kolker and Coelho 1979:8). This perspective, later to be known as "the medical model," gained strength as physicians were increasingly trained in universities, with church sanctions of medicine, and with improvements in sanitation which resulted in decreases in communicable disease.

Despite some successes in medicine as it was practiced in the nineteenth century, such antiquated practices as bloodletting and purging continued until the twentieth century. Most of the population had no access to formally trained physicians. Those who sought care beyond prayer or home remedies were treated by lay practitioners. Ehrenreich and English describe such healers as follows:

Women have always been healers. They were the unlicensed doctors and anatomists of Western History. They were abortionists, nurses, and counselors. They were pharmacists, cultivating healing herbs and exchanging the secrets of their uses. They were midwives, traveling from home to home and village to village. For centuries, women were doctors without degrees, barred from books and lectures, learning from each other, and passing on experience from neighbor to neighbor, and mother to daughter. They were called "wise women" by the people, witches or charlatans by the authorities (1973:1).

American History

Early American history of health care was similar to what was going on in Europe during the seventeenth to nineteenth centuries. Formally educated doctors were middle- or upper-class men, who treated mainly middle- and upper-class patients who could afford their services (Ehrenreich and English 1973). Most other people were served by midwives, lay practitioners, and "empiric" doctors who used herbal and other remedies. Such remedies were less strenuous than the bloodletting and purging used by "regular" doctors. At the same time, American philosophy began to emphasize the possibility of social change through individual responsibility, and the spirit of populism stimulated the development of what became known as the "popular health movement" (Risse 1977).

The era of Andrew Jackson was among the most self-care oriented periods in American history. A rising standard of living, scientific and technological progress, and the belief that human beings could control their own destinies (including no longer needing to tolerate sickness) were forces that stimulated the popular health movement. This movement, which was based on the belief that health was each person's own responsibility, peaked during the 1830s and 1840s. People wanted to learn more about the workings of their own bodies. For example, Ladies' Physiological Societies were formed to educate the public about anatomy and personal hygiene and were the backbone of the popular health movement (Ehrenreich and English 1973).

A number of different sects developed within the movement. One of the best known was the "botanical movement," founded by Samuel Thomson, a New Hampshire farmer, who learned his methods from a root and herb "doctoress." The Thomson family claimed that his book, *New Guide to Health*, sold more than 100,000 copies (Starr 1982). Thomson believed that the cause of disease was "cold" and that treatment should restore health by "steaming," "poking," and "peppering." He was adamantly opposed to the medical profession and its methods and urged Americans to regard themselves as equal to doctors in their medical knowledge. In a different sect, begun by Sylvester Graham, personal hygiene, fresh air, vegetarianism, and exercise were advocated to maintain health and prevent illness. Yet a different system, hydrotherapy, which advocated drinking mineral water and taking baths, began during this period and continued in popularity for many years. Although these seem like commonplace ideas today, they were in direct contradiction to the popular view of bodily dirt as being a sign of "honest toil, plain living, and good health."

A system that gained popularity among the privileged classes in the 1800s was homeopathy, which is based on the theory that extremely small dosages of chemical substances will stimulate the body's own healing powers. Samuel Hahnemann, who brought homeopathy to the United States from Germany, advocated the importance of fresh air, proper diet, public sanitation, and personal hygiene long before they were advocated by regular physicians. The purpose of *The Homeopathic Guidebook* was to help families in treating minor illnesses. Readers were urged to seek qualified medical assistance for serious illness. The focus on professional care as an adjunct to self-care had a curiously modern ring, and homeopathy is still a viable medical system today.

Another force that encouraged self-care in the 1800s was popular use of patent medicines, which proprietors touted as being more painless and "nicer-tasting" than the "lancet and mercury" used by "regular" doctors (Young 1977:100). Finally, a number of self-care books written by physicians were published in the nineteenth century (King 1967). An American version of Buchan's *Domestic Medicine*, entitled *The Family Physician*, was published by Anthony Benezet in 1926 and widely used all over the country (Lawrence 1975). It included descriptions of various illnesses and specific therapies for each, such as calomel and tartar emetic (purges), opium, and tonics such as Peruvian bark.

As the nineteenth century progressed, however, family medical guides changed from recommending specific treatments for major illnesses to merely describing such illnesses and suggesting first aid. The guides strongly urged readers to seek professional care. Likewise, the "popular health movement" began to decline toward the end of the nineteenth century, probably for several reasons. As the population grew, farmers who had been major supporters of the movement became less isolated and had easier access to professional medical care. Some of the movement sects became politically divided at a time when the American Medical Association, formed in 1848, was gaining power and influence. The AMA strongly discouraged popular use of sectarian doctors and women practitioners (Ehrenreich and English 1973).

During the early twentieth century, massive philanthropic programs such as the Carnegie and Rockefeller Foundations sponsored medical reform. In this way, they contributed to an increasingly scientific and respectable American medical profession. Following the Flexner Report in 1910, which strongly propounded the elitist and academic viewpoints (King 1984), the majority of "irregular" medical schools, sectarian schools, and schools for women and blacks closed, establishing medicine . . . "once and for all as a branch of 'higher' learning, accessible only through lengthy and expensive university training. . . . Medicine had become a white, male middle class occupation. . . ." (Ehrenreich and English 1973:31). Subsequent advancements in medical technology led to dramatic breakthroughs in control of some epidemic diseases and significantly reduced mortality rates. These advances captured the popular imagination—many people became convinced that only the formally educated medical doctor was qualified to determine the status of one's health and, further, that one needed to undergo a battery of tests to determine whether one was healthy or ill. As medical interventions came to be held in increasingly high regard, self-care became increasingly devalued, and people were not encouraged or taught to evaluate their own health status and to care for themselves and their families.

But the limitations of modern medical miracles, such as antibiotics and advances in diagnostic and surgical techniques, became apparent in the challenges of chronic and long-term illness. Ahmed, Kolker, and Coehlo (1979) suggest that we have now returned to the premodern conception of illness as a sociocultural phenomenon and that health is a process of many dimensions which involves the whole person in the context of the environment.

In summary, people's perceptions of health and illness and the locus of responsibility for health care have shifted through the ages and are intimately tied to the dominant philosophy of a society in any given historical period, as well as to the structure of the medical system of that society. History shows that self-care has not been limited to middle-class groups, as some suggest. Rather, self-care by indigenous healers was the norm, with only the elite receiving services by professional medical personnel. We will now turn to a discussion of how some of these historical themes influence our current philosophy of self-care and how the current self-care movement relates to nursing practice.

SELF-CARE TODAY

Foster and Anderson define a medical system as "embracing all the health-promoting beliefs and actions and scientific knowledge and skills of the members of the group that subscribes to that system" (1978:36). The medical system is an integral part of each culture and cannot be understood apart from the culture in which it is embedded. Health care systems have both professional and self-care components. Professional care is differentiated from self-care on the basis of such characteristics as specialized training and knowledge, responsibility for care, and expectation of payment for services.

Many professional health care providers regard self-care practices as "'vestigial' health functions to be avoided or deplored in the wake of 'modern medicine,' folk practices that contribute to the failure of laypersons to follow prescribed medical regimens" (Levin et al., 1979:9). In reality, however, perhaps 75% or more of health care is self-care (Williamson and Danaher 1978) and includes both activities that substitute for professional intervention and those that supplement professional care (see Figure 1–1.). Indeed, as Levin and his colleagues point out, "It may be historically more accurate to state the proposition in reverse: that professional health care procedures include those which supplement or substitute for self-care behavior" (1979:13). Williamson and Danaher (1978) suggest that self-care is the first level of health care and the largest part of the health care system. Fuchs suggests that while medical care can be made more accessible through institutional change, "the greatest potential for improving health lies in what we do and do not do for ourselves" (1974:151). Simonton (1978) believes that if people could mobilize their own resources and actively participate in maintaining their own health, they could exceed their life expectancies and significantly improve the qualities of their lives.

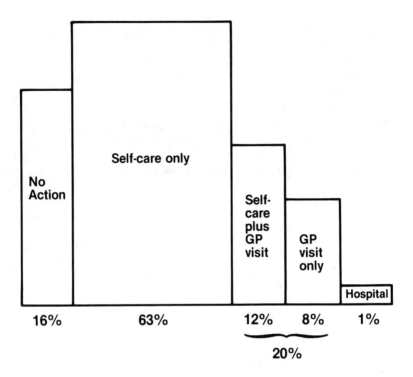

Figure 1–1. What people do about their symptoms. From Williamson JD, Danaher K: *Self-Care in Health.* Croom Helm, London, England, 1978 (reprinted with permission from the publisher).

The growing strength of the current American self-care movement is illustrated by a national preoccupation with exercise and nutrition, wide availability of self-care classes, holistic and wellness clinics, and health self-help groups. This movement can be traced to the women's health movement and consumer movements of the 1960s. Levin, Katz, and Holst (1979) suggest that the following social forces underlie the current self-care movement:

1. The demystification of primary medical care
2. Consumerism and popular demands for increased self-control related to anti-technology, anti-authority sentiments
3. Changes in life-style and rising educational levels
4. Lay concern with regard to perceived abuses in medical care
5. The lack of availability of professional services.

Economic issues are relevant to self-care, particularly the recent rapidly escalating costs of health care. Insurance companies are now viewing self-care as an important consideration in determining insurance premiums (Mosler, Rafter, and Gajewski 1984). The American health care system is currently experiencing another major turning point. During the 1960s, federal health insurance programs were developed to attempt to provide health care services for *all*. In light of recent funding cuts and prospective payment by the federal government, it appears that health care may once again be available only to those who can pay.

Although self-care has received considerable attention in the past decade, there is no commonly agreed-upon definition. Ferguson (1979) describes self-care as the power to take responsibility for one's own medical education according to individual need, as well as the ability to choose, understand, and evaluate professional health care services. Levin et al. (1979) suggest that self-care includes those processes that permit people and families to take initiative and responsibility for func-

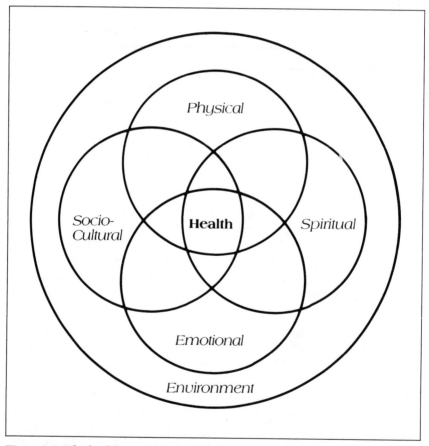

Figure 1–2. The health process—an integration and balance of a person's physical, emotional, sociocultural, and spiritual environment.

tioning effectively to develop and maintain their own health.

Semantic confusion prevails in the terms "self-care" and "self-help." We think that *self-help* refers more accurately to a group approach to a common problem or interest and can include such areas as cooperatives, social, grass roots, political, or community efforts, and self-help/mutual support groups, such as Alcoholics Anonymous or Ostomy groups. We use self-care to refer specifically to health-related activities that an individual, family, or community utilizes on a regular basis. Self-care activities are often taught and encouraged in self-help groups.

"Holistic health" and "high-level wellness" are also terms that may be encountered in relation to self-care. Holistic health refers to the integration and balance of the physical, emotional, and spiritual aspects of the individual to achieve total well-being. Some use the term holistic health to refer to "alternative" health practices that contrast with mainstream Western medical practices. High-level wellness, a term coined by Halbert Dunn in the late 1950s, views health as a way of functioning that maximizes the potential of the individual.

These concepts of health contrast with widespread definitions of health as "absence of disease" or "ability to function normally." The "absence of disease" definition, in particular, defines health by what it is *not*. In our view, health is a process in which physical, emotional, sociocultural, and spiritual aspects of the individual are integrated and functioning in harmony with the environment; health signifies the highest level of well-being obtainable for the individual at various points over time.

Health is a process, rather than a static state. It is different from disease or illness and should be considered separately. Thus, we discuss health and illness separately in Chapters 4 and 5.

THE SELF-CARE PERSPECTIVE
IN NURSING THEORY

Health promotion has long been a foundation of nursing practice. Henderson (1964) defined the practice of nursing as assisting clients, sick or well, in the performance of those activities that contribute to health, which would otherwise be performed unaided if the client had the necessary strength, will, and knowledge. Schlotfeldt (1972) defined the goals of nursing as helping clients to attain, retain, and regain health. She stated that nurses are concerned with their clients' health-seeking and coping behaviors in pursuit of health. The American Nurses' Association (1980) defines nursing as "the diagnosis and treatment of human responses to actual or potential health problems." These definitions consider health, rather than illness, the primary focus of nursing; the nurse's role is to support the client's adaptive coping mechanisms related to human responses to alterations in health.

Other nursing theorists suggest similar concepts in their discussion of nursing education, research, and practice. In reference to self-care, Orem's (1980) self-care deficit theory is probably best known. It explicitly defines the nurse's role as enhancing the client's ability to practice self-care. Although Rogers is not known as a self-care theorist, her nursing science theory defines the role of the nurse as assisting clients to achieve their maximum health potential. Rogers views the world in a truly holistic way; man and the environment are coextensive energy fields (Rogers 1970, 1980).

Other nurses incorporate many of these ideas in their own definitions of self-care and holistic health, which are translated into nursing practice. Pender's (1982) volume, *Health Promotion in Nursing Practice*, provides a conceptual framework for health promotion and disease prevention. Clark's (1981) approach to "enhancing wellness" is helping the person grow toward harmony and balance, the end result being that the person is helped, rather than the disease treated. In Clark's view, health is fundamentally related to life-style and environmental factors. Flynn's (1980) holistic health perspective views the person as a whole being who is greater than the sum of the parts; Flynn advocates individual responsibility for participation in care. Blattner (1981) describes holistic nursing as an integrated process-oriented approach to promoting health in a variety of settings and populations. We think that self-care is fundamental in health promotion and disease prevention.

Patient education, another vital component of nursing practice, is also important to consider in discussing self-care. Although the ideas of patient education and self-care are often used synonymously, they are not the same. Levin (1978) points out critical distinctions between patient education and self-care (see Table 1-1). We support patient education and encourage its expansion to include self-care and more active client participation.

PHILOSOPHY OF SELF-CARE

Self-care literature, related nursing theories and practice, knowledge and practice in holistic health and wellness, health promotion, and patient education all contribute important themes to *our* philosophy of self-care. Adapted from Orem and Rogers, we define self-care as **those activities initiated or performed by an individual, family, or community to achieve, maintain, or promote maximum health.** Maximum health refers to the highest level of health an individual can achieve at that specific point in time. The potential for health varies with the individual's developmental and situational stressors; thus, different individuals have different maximum health levels. The maximum level of health of one person should not be compared with that of another. Rather, the actual health status should

TABLE 1-1. A COMPARISON OF SELF-CARE AND PATIENT EDUCATION CONCEPTS

Self-Care	Patient Education
Personal responsibility for managing disease and achieving optimal level of wellness.	Professional responsibility to help patients achieve optimal compliance with *professionally prescribed health behavior.*
Clients select educational and behavioral goals based on personal needs and preferences, with professional consultation.	Professional initiates patient education goals in response to disease.
Clients take an active role in directing their own health care.	Patients assume passive "sick role."
Clients control decision-making process.	Professional control, which fosters "poor compliance."
Allows individualized strategies for changing health behaviors. (Health care system becomes resource which accommodates client needs.)	Promotes strategies which standardize and regulate health behavior. (Patient behavior to accommodate health care system.)
Fosters independence and initiative, with increased transfer of health care skills to clients and their families.	Fosters dependence and resistance, with less transfer of health care skills to clients and their families.

Adapted from Levin LS: Patient education and self-care: "How do they differ?" Nursing Outlook, Vol 26, No 3, pp 170–175, 1978

be compared to the individual's maximum health potential at that specific time.

Self-care activities in which people engage are those that will help them realize their maximum health potential. Such activities include personal or environmental hygiene, nutrition, preventive practices, and medications and medical treatments (both "folk" and "scientific") which are intended to heal or cure. Self-care activities can substitute for, or be used in conjunction with, professional care.

We see the major components of self-care as the following:

1. Health promotion
2. Health maintenance
3. Disease prevention
4. Disease detection
5. Disease management.

Health promotion refers to activities in which individuals actively engage to maximize their health. The motivation is to improve health, rather than to prevent disease. For example, individuals may exercise to use their bodies to the full potential and to help them feel their best.

Health maintenance refers to maintaining homeostasis or the status quo; it may be active or passive. Examples include getting adequate rest and eating regular meals.

Disease prevention activities are aimed at reducing or eliminating risks of specific diseases. Examples include immunizations and reducing dietary fat and salt.

Disease detection activities refer to increased awareness of bodily states and symptoms and use of diagnostic tools and techniques. Examples include breast self-examination and blood pressure screening.

Disease management includes carrying out and monitoring prescribed treatment regimens and incorporating the disease and treatment regimen into one's daily life.

Health promotion and disease prevention are often used interchangeably. However, in our perspective, they are not the same, nor are they mutually exclusive. For example, behaviors that are designed to prevent disease usually maintain or promote health, and health promotion should be incorporated into disease management.

Critical readers may notice an unresolved issue—who defines self-care activities, and what part does individual perception play? For example, is the individual who believes that drinking eight cups of coffee daily contributes to a high level of functioning wrong? Would you consider this a self-care activity? Both client and professional definitions are important, and we raise this issue only for consideration rather than to suggest answers. Health promotion and maintenance will be discussed at length in Chapter 4, and disease prevention, detection, and management will be discussed in Chapter 5. Our approach to self-care is based on the following assumptions.

People are ultimately responsible for their own health. In large part, health or illness is affected by what people do and do not do for themselves in terms of life-style choices, knowledge, and beliefs about health, and appropriate use of the health care system. This is not the same as "blaming the victim." Obviously, the factors that influence health and illness are complex and include those that are out of an individual's immediate control, such as genetic endowment and some environmental and situational factors. Individuals take responsibility for their health to different degrees at different times in their lives. Pursuing maximum health may not always be a priority and may be superseded by such other concerns as getting a job or maintaining a significant relationship. But we do believe that the extent to which individuals assume responsibility for their own health is critical to a positive health outcome. Health professionals have the responsibility to provide their clients with information in an objective manner so that informed choices can be made, if the client so chooses.

People have the right and ability to make choices about their health and health care. Health professionals must understand this right and support their clients' choices, even if the professional does not agree with the choice. Current legal precedent supports clients' rights to make health care decisions. This includes the right to refuse any, all, or part of interventions, with a few exceptions, such as minors and some individuals with impaired mental functioning.

Self-care knowledge and skills decrease the individual's or family's reliance on professional care and increase the ability to assess health status and need for intervention. Such knowledge and skills increase the ability to make informed choices. Thus, clients can utilize the health care system more effectively, seeking its services only when there is need for professional expertise.

The relationship between the client and health care professional should be a partnership. In the past few decades, American health care providers and consumers have operated under the unchallenged assumption that professional care is the universal and exclusive health care resource. In rejecting this concept, some critics have gone to the opposite extreme and suggested that "all care should be self-care" or, for example, that "religious faith is all that is necessary for healing." We believe that a partnership between professional and client is the ideal and that clients or families are responsible for caring for themselves to the best of their abilities, utilizing the professional only when needed.

Health care professionals need to be fully aware of their own health beliefs and practice. We believe that it is the professional's responsibility to be a model of good health practices and to work toward achieving the maximum health potential. We do not mean that the professionals should be a model of perfect health but only that the efforts in the direction of good health be obvious.

A self-care emphasis is relevant to people of a variety of socioeconomic and cultural backgrounds. However, the professional's approach must be modified to be congruent with the individual's or family's cultural values, health beliefs, and practices. In some cases, the nurse's approach to self-care must be modified to fit the expectations of individuals of some cultural groups. Such modifications may seem to contradict the tenets of self-responsibility and individual choice. For example, some Asian-Americans expect health care professionals to prescribe treatment with authority and respond to this approach rather than to expectations that the client make the decisions. In this case, nurses may need to use their authority to prescribe self-care. In the long run, the goal is to help clients to care for themselves and to make positive changes in their health behavior.

Self-care is an approach to nursing care, rather than a specific intervention. It is a perspective that permeates all aspects of care, guiding nurses to consider all the ways clients can care for themselves in illness and in health. Rather than a *type* of intervention, the self-care approach should specifically fit with the unique characteristics of individuals in their sociocultural context.

SUMMARY

We have illustrated that the tenets and practices of self-care are as old as recorded human history and that societal and individual attitudes about self-care are philosophically tied to cultural themes and medical systems through time. In the context of a recent and growing body of knowledge on self-care and health, we presented a philosophy and the assumptions that underlie the following chapters.

Discussion Questions

1. Discuss the relationship between holistic health, high-level wellness, and self-care.
2. Describe the differences between patient education and self-care.
3. Describe your own cultural background and how it influences your self-care practices.
4. Discuss the concept of choice as it relates to self-care.

REFERENCES

Ahmed PI, Kolker A, Coehlo GV: Toward a new definition of health: An overview. *In* Ahmed PI, Coehlo GV (eds): Toward a New Definition of Health, Plenum Press, New York, 1979

American Nurses' Association: Nursing: A social policy statement. NP-63, 35M, Kansas City, 1980

Blattner B: Holistic Nursing. Prentice-Hall, Inc., Englewood Cliffs, New Jersey, 1981

Cadmann P, Chambers L, Feldman W, Sackett D: Assessing the effectiveness of community screening programs. Journal of the American Medical Association, Vol 251, No 12, pp 1580–1585, 1984

Caplan AL, Englehardt HT, McCartney JJ (eds): Concepts of Health and Disease. Addison-Wesley Publishing Co., Reading, Massachusetts, 1981

Clark CC: Enhancing Wellness: A Guide for Self-Care. Springer Publishing Co., New York, 1981

Dunn HL: High-Level Wellness. R. W. Beally Co., Arlington, Virginia, 1961

Ehrenreich B, English D: Witches, Midwives and Nurses. Feminist Press, New York, 1973

Engel GE: The need for a new medical model: A challenge for biomedicine. Science, Vol 196, pp 129–136, 1977

Ferguson T: Statement of purpose, Editor's page. Medical Self-Care, No 6, Fall 1979

Flynn PAR: Holistic Health: The Art and Science of Care. Robert J. Brady Co., Bowie, Maryland, 1980

Foster GM, Anderson BG: Medical Anthropology. John Wiley and Sons, New York, 1978

Fuchs V: Who Shall Live? Basic Books, New York, 1974

Hand WD (ed): American Folk Medicine: A Symposium. University of California Press, Berkeley, California, 1976

Henderson V: The nature of nursing. AJN, Vol 64, No 6, pp 62–68, 1964

King LS: Do-it-yourself medicine. Journal of the American Medical Association, Vol 200, No 1, pp 129–135, 1967

King LS: The Flexner report of 1910. Journal of the American Medical Association, Vol 251, No 8, pp 1079–1086, 1984

Lawrence DJ: William Buchan: Medicine laid open. Medical History, Vol 19, No 1, pp 20–35, 1975

Leder D: Medicine paradigms of embodiment. The Journal of Medicine & Philosophy, Vol 9, pp 29–43, 1984

Lee PR, Brown N, Red I (eds): The Nation's Health. Boyd and Fraser Publishing Co., San Francisco, California, 1981

Levin LS: Patient education and self-care: How do they differ? Nursing Outlook, Vol 26, No 3, pp 170–175, 1978

Levin L, Katz A, Holst E: Self-Care: Lay Initiatives in Health. Provost, New York, 1979

Moser M, Rafter J, Gajewski J: Insurance premium reductions: A motivating factor in long-term hypertensive treatment. JAMA, Vol 251, No 6, pp 756–757, 1984

Norris CM: Self-Care. AJN, Vol 79, No 3, pp 486–489, 1979

Orem DE: Nursing: Concepts and Practice. McGraw-Hill, Inc., New York, 1971

Orem DE: Nursing: Concepts and Practice, 2nd ed. McGraw Hill, Inc., New York, 1980

Pender NJ: Health Promotion in Nursing Practice. Appleton-Century-Crofts, Norwalk, Connecticut, 1982

Risse GB, Numbers RL, Leavitt J: Medicine Without Doctors. Science History Publications, New York, 1977

Roberts CR, Imrey PB, Turner JD, Hosokawa MC, Alster JM: Reducing physician visits for colds through consumer education. Journal of the American Medical Association, Vol 250, No 15, pp 1986–1989, 1983

Rogers ME: An Introduction to the Theoretical Basis of Nursing. F. A. Davis, Philadelphia, Pennsylvania, 1970

Rogers ME: Nursing: A science of unitary man. In Riehl JP, Roy C: Conceptual Models for Nursing Practice, 2nd ed. Appleton-Century-Crofts, New York, 1980

Schlotfeldt R: This I believe: Nursing is health care. Nursing Outlook, Vol 20, No 4, pp 245–246, 1972

Starr P: The Social Transformation of American Medicine. Basic Books, New York, 1982

Sigerist HE: A History of Medicine, Vol II. Oxford University Press, New York, 1961

Simonton OC, Matthews-Simonton S, Creighton J: Getting Well Again. Tarcher, Inc., Los Angeles, California, 1978

Veith I: The Yellow Emperor's Classic of Internal Medicine. University of California Press, Berkeley, California, 1949

Williamson JD, Danaher K: Self-Care in Health. Croom Helm, London, 1978

Young JH: Patent medicines and the self-help syndrome. In Risse G (ed): Medicine

Without Doctors. Science History Publications, New York, 1977

Zapka J, Averill BW: Self care for colds: A cost effective alternative to upper respiratory infection management. American Journal of Public Health, Vol 69, No 8, pp 814–816, 1979

2

Theories Related to Self-Care

The purpose of theory is to explain, predict, and verify the scientist's speculations about phenomena in the real world (Stevens 1979). Nursing theories help to clarify the goals and purposes of nursing, to distinguish nursing from other major disciplines, and to provide a basis for nursing education, practice, and research. The purpose of this chapter is to summarize theories that underlie our approach to self-care in nursing practice. It is often difficult for nurses to derive applications from theoretical constructs in clinical settings; thus, our focus is to make some of the constructs usable in self-care. Although Dorothea Orem has been the pioneer in self-care theory in nursing, we also include constructs from other theoretical models to contribute to a holistic or eclectic approach. Among nursing theories, we focus on Orem's self-care theory, Rogers' science of unitary man, and Leininger's transcultural nursing theory. From the social and behavioral sciences, we include constructs from adult learning theory, symbolic interactionism, explanatory models of illness, and the health belief model.

NURSING THEORIES

Orem

Dorothea Orem's self-care model is used to organize the curricula in many schools of nursing. Orem defined self-care as ". . . the practice of activities that individuals initiate and perform on their own behalf in maintaining life, health and well-being" (1980:35). In relation to nursing, Orem said:

Nursing has its special concern for the individual's need for self-care action, and the provision and management of it on a continuous

*basis, in order to sustain life and health, recover from disease or
injury, and cope with its effects (1980:6).*

The phrase "sustain life and health" denotes the idea of health maintenance. However, health requires more than maintaining the status quo; a
positive approach to health *enhancement* is important enough to be
emphasized more strongly.

Orem describes three major theories in her model—the self-care deficit
theory, theory of self-care, and theory of nursing systems. **Self-care deficits** are health-related or health-derived limitations that render a person
incapable of effective or complete self-care. Such deficits are indicators
of when and why nursing is required. **The theory of self-care** states that
self-care and care of dependent family members are learned behaviors
that purposely regulate human structural integrity, functioning, and
human development (1980:28). **The theory of nursing system(s)** suggests
that the nursing system is the product of nursing practice through which
the patient's ability for self-care is regulated. It explains how persons can
be helped through nursing.

Central to Orem's theory is the concept of **agency,** referring to a set of
human abilities for meeting self-care requisites, such as acquiring knowledge, decision-making, and taking action for change. The term *"agent"* is
used in the sense of the person taking action (1980:35). Thus, the self-
care agent is defined as the provider of self-care, and the provider of
infant, child, or dependent care is called the *dependent care agent.* Orem
states that "nursing agency refers to the nurse's ability to provide care that
compensates for or aids in overcoming the health-derived or health-
related self-care or dependent-care deficits of others" (1980:87). The
nurse assesses the patient's self-care deficits, and either provides the
care that the patient needs or teaches the patient to do self-care. Orem
suggests that nurse and patient relationships are complementary and that
nurses help patients to assume responsibilities for self-care. With the
exception of the partly compensatory nursing system (1980:101), it might
appear to some readers that the nurse alone determines clients' self-care
needs. This emphasis might devalue the client's ability to do self-assessment and planning. The "patient" may be seen more as a receiver of care
than an active participant in determining the care, as one might expect in a
self-care framework. However, the client's responsibility and role are *as*
important as, if not *more* important than, the nurse's role. Thus, the
nurse's role is to support and encourage the client to participate actively in
planning and performing self-care in all phases of health care.

Orem describes three types of self-care requirements—universal, developmental, and health-deviation. **Universal self-care requisites** (1980:
42–47) are activities required by all people during all stages of the life
cycle to maintain health and life and include the following:

1. Maintenance of sufficient air

2. Maintenance of sufficient water
3. Maintenance of sufficient food
4. Provision of care associated with the elimination processes and excrement
5. Maintenance of a balance between activity and rest
6. Maintenance of a balance between solitude and social interaction
7. Prevention of hazards to human life, human functioning, and human well-being
8. Promotion of human functioning and development within social groups, in accord with human potential, known human relationships, and the human desire to be normal.

With the exception of the last requisite, Orem's self-care requisites primarily relate to health maintenance and disease prevention and management. We expand on these areas in the interest of health promotion and add such health components as stress management, spiritual and psychological well-being, sexuality, and environmental awareness.

Developmental self-care requisites (1980:47–48) are specialized requirements related to developmental processes, acquired conditions (e.g., pregnancy), or associated with an event (e.g., death of a family member). Orem describes two categories:

1. Maintenance of living conditions that support life processes and promote the processes of development, or human progress, toward higher levels of organization of human structure and toward maturation
2. Provision of care either to prevent the occurrence of deleterious effects of conditions that can affect human development or to mitigate or overcome these effects from various conditions.

Health deviation self-care requisites (1980: 48–51) relate to changes in self-care activities brought by illness, injury or disease. Orem describes six categories of health deviation requisites:

1. Seeking and securing appropriate medical assistance in the event of exposure to specific physical or biological agents or environmental conditions associated with human pathological events or states, or when there is evidence of genetic, physiological, or psychological conditions known to produce or be associated with human pathology
2. Being aware of, and attending to, the effects and results of pathological conditions and states
3. Effectively carrying out medically prescribed diagnostic, therapeutic, and rehabilitative measures directed to the prevention of specific types of pathology
4. Being aware of, and attending to or regulating, the discomforting or deleterious effects of medical care measures performed or prescribed by the physician

5. Modifying the self-concept (and self-image) in accepting oneself as being in a particular state of health and in need of specific forms of health care
6. Learning to live with the effects of pathological conditions and states and the effects of medical, diagnostic, and treatment measures in a life-style that promotes continued personal development.

In summary, Orem is the major nursing theorist to date whose approach to nursing is based on the concept of self-care. Her self-care requirements are an excellent way to assess health and self-care needs and organize nursing practice according to these needs. For example, Orem suggests the phrase "therapeutic self-care demand" to refer to sets of actions that need to be performed in self-care. Self-care agency, or ability to perform self-care actions, is determined through assessment of history, developmental status, social and familial characteristics, and health habits (basic conditioning factors). Orem's model has been utilized in different types of care settings, especially in the area of oncology and psychiatric nursing. For particularly good examples of its usefulness as a framework for organizing nursing care, we refer you to the work of those who have discussed Orem's model in this regard, such as Anna, Christensen, Hohon, Ord, and Wells 1980; Backscheider 1974; Bromley 1980; Goodwin 1979; and Underwood 1980.

Despite Orem's comprehensive and pioneering efforts, some limitations in her model are apparent. Orem's work is difficult for some readers to understand because of its organization and terminology. Although we hold many of the same beliefs and are guided by her work, we do not use Orem's terminology because of its tendency to confuse the reader. Although Orem refers to sociocultural aspects as a basic conditioning factor, her theory is confined mainly to Western professional medical practices; popular and folk health practices can be legitimately considered part of self-care. To supplement Orem's theory, we turn now to Rogers' more holistic view of humankind and Leininger's emphasis on culture, which are important bases of our approach to self-care.

Rogers

Martha Rogers is the *first* nursing theorist to propose a truly holistic approach, an approach that does not separate mind from body or human beings from their environment. Few nursing theories are as comprehensive. Further, Rogers advocated ideas in the 1960s that are still considered innovative today. Rogers' Science of Unitary Man is based on her conceptualization of "man as a unified whole," interacting with the environment. The concern of nursing is with human beings in their entirety and with assisting people to achieve their maximum health potential (1970:86). The theory is based on a number of assumptions from the natural and social sciences. These assumptions are as follows:

1. "Man is a unified whole" (1970:47). Human beings possess an integrity and manifest characteristics that are more than and different from the sum of the parts. Any change in a part reflects a change in the whole. This idea is based on general systems theory and is a basic assumption underlying our view of nursing.
2. "Man and the environment are continuously exchanging matter and energy with one another" (1970:54). Change in the environmental field can both cause, and be the result of, change in the human field; thus, human beings and the environment are complementary systems. This assumption underlies the belief that the actions of people can negatively or positively influence the environment, and that the environment affects human health. When the influence is negative (e.g., pollution), the results may be illness (e.g., asthma, COPD, or cancer).
3. "The life process evolves irreversibly and unidirectionally along the space-time continuum" (1970:59). The life process is always shaping, and being shaped by, the environment. Because time is unidirectional, nothing is reversible, including sequential stages of human development. As we understand this idea, people are constantly in the process of becoming. Thus, even if a person repeats the same pattern of behavior, there is a difference because of increased age and experience. In the context of self-care, no matter what the person's past health or behavior patterns have been, the configuration of patterns and experience at this point in time is different, and self-care behaviors can direct change in health towards a positive direction.
4. "Pattern and organization identify man and reflect his innovative wholeness" (1970:65). Pattern and organization maintain the order of the universe amidst constant change. Similarly, "man's capacity to maintain himself while undergoing continuous change is a remarkable characteristic" (1970:63)—commonly referred to as man's self-regulatory ability. Rogers suggests that man has the capacity to knowingly rearrange his environment and to exercise choices in fulfilling his potential. This idea is basic to self-care in nursing practice—the role of the nurse is to help people to *equip themselves* to exercise such choices.
5. "Man is characterized by the capacity for abstraction and imagery, language and thought, sensation and emotion" (1970:73). Human beings differ from animals in how we attempt to make sense of the world through these capacities, as well as the basic needs to know and discover. In the context of self-care, we relate such capacities to human beings' need for meaning in life (see Chapter 10).

In summary, a number of basic assumptions in Rogers' model support a self-care approach to nursing, although perhaps not explicitly. Such assumptions include the importance of the environment, the holistic view of human beings in the world, and the concept of ever present change. These concepts continue to evolve (Rogers 1980). From this perspective, the nurse and other health care providers are seen as part of the client's environment, and nurse and client are seen as interactive and complementary systems. As such, a change in one is related to a change in the other. For example, when an ill person recovers, the relationship with the nurse changes. Clients interact with nurses differently as their abilities to care for themselves change. Rogers' focus is primarily health promotion. Maximizing health is viewed as more dynamic and important than health maintenance or disease prevention. Disease management focuses mainly on the individual and family's response to the disease; therefore, health promotion is implicit in disease management.

The major criticism of Rogers' model is that it is so broad and abstract that it is difficult to understand and operationalize. Nurses who cannot view the real world of nursing as energy fields and resonating waves are the most resistant to the theory (Stevens 1979:34). However, there is great value in this breadth, scope, and holistic perspective, and its greatest contribution may be in broadening our perspectives as nurses. We turn now to the most specific of the three nursing theories covered here, the transcultural nursing model of Madeleine Leininger.

Leininger

Madeleine Leininger defines transcultural nursing as the subfield of nursing which focuses upon a comparative study and analysis of different cultures and subcultures in the world with respect to their caring behavior and health-illness values, beliefs, and patterns of behavior. The goal of transcultural nursing is to develop a scientific and humanistic body of knowledge in order to provide culture-specific and culture-universal care practices (1978).

Leininger suggests that a local culture's views, knowledge, and experiences are extremely important in planning and implementing nursing care; if the cultural component is not recognized, nursing care will be less effective and there will be unfavorable consequences to those served. Transcultural nursing theory refers to a set of interrelated cross-cultural concepts and hypotheses which take into account individual and group caring behaviors, values, and beliefs based on culture. The theory is based on the proposition that individuals representing different cultural groups have the ability to determine and request most of the care they desire or need from professional caregivers (1978).

Leininger states ten basic assumptions about transcultural nursing, three of which are particulary relevant to self-care:

1. "Nursing is essentially a transcultural phenomenon in that the context and process of helping involves at least two persons generally having different cultural orientations or intracultural lifestyles" (1978:35). It is vitally important for the nurse to be aware of professionally and culturally based values that he or she brings to the interaction, as well as values that the client holds.
2. "What constitutes efficacious or therapeutic nursing care is largely culturally determined, culturally-based, and can be culturally-validated" (1978:36).
3. "Cultures have their own naturalistic or familiar "built-in" modes of caring behavior which are generally known to the people, but are frequently unknown to nurses of other cultural backgrounds" (1978:36). We believe that the only way the nurse can encourage the client to undertake self-care is to learn about such modes and to utilize them in planning.

In addition to these assumptions, Leininger identifies a number of propositions, three of which specifically relate to self-care:

1. Identifiable differences in caring values and behaviors between and among cultures lead to differences in the nursing care expectations of careseekers (1978:37).
2. The greater the differences between indigenous (or folk) cultural caring behaviors and modern professional nursing care values, the greater the signs of cultural conflict and stresses in care-giving and care-receiving contexts (1978:37).
3. Self-care practices will be more readily espoused by cultures which value individualism; whereas group and family care practices will be espoused in cultures which place limited emphasis upon the individual and more on social or group ties (1978:37).

Leininger's theory of transcultural nursing is the first nursing theory that addresses the neglected area of culture as it relates to nursing practice. Leininger suggests that the goal of transcultural nursing is to "make professional nursing knowledge and practices culturally based, culturally conceptualized, culturally planned, and culturally operationalized. If the goal is achieved, one can predict greater client and population satisfaction than heretofore seen in nursing" (1978:12,13). Although her theoretical model is not yet fully developed, Leininger's pioneering work is important in nursing.

Leininger's work is useful for our approach to self-care. She expands the concepts of choice and self-determination to refer not only to individuals and families, but also to cultural and subcultural groups. Norms and values are important contexts within which the behavior of individuals and families can be understood; however, both individual and cultural frameworks need to be considered. There is wide individual variation in any cultural group, and human beings internalize different aspects of their cultures to different degrees. However, to a large extent, culture determines individual and group perceptions of health and illness, as well as proper modes of prevention and treatment, and must be carefully considered in relation to self-care.

Leininger's specific references to self-care need some explanation. She uses the term self-care to refer only to an individual's personal care and implies that individuals in family- or group-oriented cultures are not likely to be motivated to practice self-help. However, we define self-care more broadly and include the family or social group as appropriate self-care providers or agents. For example, interdependency among family members is more strongly valued than individual independence in many cultures. From our perspective, self-care would thus encompass health care provided by the family to an individual member. In this sense, we contrast self-care with professional care and would include folk and popular care as legitimate types of self-care, including what Leininger addresses as culture-specific caring practices. Figure 2-1 summarizes how three nursing models contribute to our perspective of self-care. Although the models are not congruent, we selected components from each model that are compatible with our philosophy.

SOCIAL AND BEHAVIORAL SCIENCE THEORIES

In addition to nursing theories, there are other theoretical frameworks which lend support to our approach to self-care, particularly in the application of self-care in nursing practice. Such theories describe and explain the conditions under which people are more or less likely to care for themselves, motivating factors that facilitate self-care, and ways that the nurse and other health care professionals can enhance the client's ability to care for self. We limit our description to brief summaries of four such selected areas—symbolic interactionism, the health belief model, explanatory models of illness, and adult learning theory.

Symbolic Interactionism

Symbolic interactionism is a theoretical perspective on human behavior developed by Herbert Blumer (1969), based on the work of G.H. Mead and other sociologists. The major premises of symbolic interactionism are:

1. Human beings act toward things (e.g., physical objects, institutions, other people, and their actions) on the basis of the meanings that these things have for them
2. The meaning of such things arises out of social interaction with fellow humans
3. These meanings are created, maintained, and modified through

Orem
Well-Developed
Self-Care
Nursing Theory

Rogers
Holistic
(environmental)
Approach

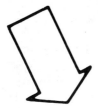 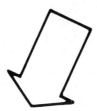

the
Process of Self-Care
in
Nursing Education,
Practice & Research

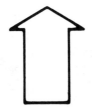

Leininger
Cultural Influences on Health,
Illness, & the Nurse-Client
Interaction

Figure 2-1. Selected nursing theories related to self-care.

an interpretive process used by the person in dealing with the things he encounters.

In short, individuals behave according to their perceptions of a given situation, another person, or even themselves, based on the *meaning* of the situation or person to the individual. In order to understand a client's health behavior, for example, the nurse should try to understand the client's perception of appropriate health behavior, of symptoms, of treatment, and indeed, of the world in general. Although the importance of this concept of meaning seems obvious, it is ignored by, or unknown to, many health professionals. This concept helps explain human behavior and is potentially very useful.

Symbolic interactionism explains the impact of people's views of themselves and their world on their behavior. In the context of self-care, it is vital for the nurse to learn how clients perceive themselves, health, and illness in order to plan an appropriate self-care regimen. The health belief model can be interpreted as a method by which symbolic interactionism can be operationalized within the context of health behavior.

Health Belief Model

Rosenstock's Health Belief Model (1966) links individual attitudes about health to health actions. The model proposes that before care-seeking behavior takes place, the individual must experience a cue or trigger for action. Such cues might be internal (e.g., a symptom or change in usual functioning) or external (e.g., pressure from family members to seek care, knowledge that another has contracted a particular illness, or the media). Thus, it is the individual's perception of the situation that leads to health action.

Four variables account for differences in how individuals use health services. These variables are the individual's:

1. Perception of susceptibility to illness
2. Perception of the seriousness of the illness
3. Perception of the benefits and barriers to taking action to reduce the threat
4. Beliefs about how beneficial the various alternatives would be.

Thus, the health belief model explains why some individuals are more likely than others to seek care for illness or to take actions to prevent illness. For example, a woman may be more likely to practice breast self-exam if she thinks that she is susceptible (e.g., her mother had breast cancer) and if she perceives breast cancer as serious. The nurse will be more effective in self-care teaching if she determines clients' beliefs about their susceptibility to illness, the seriousness of the illness, and benefits and barriers to taking action, and tailors the nursing approach to address these beliefs. Questions that elicit the client's beliefs in these areas are an important part of the assessment process in the self-care approach. However, communication between nurse and client about health beliefs and desirable action is often difficult when nurse and client are speaking from very different perspectives. Some differences may be based on cultural, ethnic, or socioeconomic backgrounds, while others may be based on whether health is considered from a professional, popular, or folk perspective. These differences and their effects on inter-actions about self-care are addressed by the concept of explanatory models.

Explanatory Models

Kleinman and his colleagues note that individuals' experiences of illness are shaped by culture. How people perceive, experience, and cope with sickness is based on a cultural group's explanations of sickness. Thus, they call these perspectives "explanatory models." Kleinman et al. (1978) propose that cultural groups have distinct explanatory models and that such differences in perspectives often cause conflict between the health care professional and the client.

One major difference in perspective described by Kleinman is that health care providers diagnose and treat *diseases* (abnormalities in the structure and systems) while patients suffer *illnesses* (the meaning and experience of sickness). Communication difficulties might arise, for ex-ample, when a health professional talks to a patient about physiological characteristics of a particular symptom and the patient talks to the physi-cian about how the symptom interferes with life—neither may understand that the other is talking from a different perspective.

One of Kleinman's major contributions is his translation of an-thropological and cross-cultural concepts into specific strategies useful in patient care. This work suggests that the health care provider should elicit the client's explanatory model of illness and communicate his/her own model to the client. Some clients will not be aware that they have an explanatory model of illness until such discussion occurs. (See Chapter 3, page 37, for suggested questions for eliciting the client's model.) Next, provider and client should discuss and compare their models and talk about differences. Finally, provider and client can negotiate with each other to develop shared models in which expectations and therapeutic goals are clear to both. In their description of a desirable provider-client relationship, Kleinman et al. reinforce an idea we consider important in our approach to self-care, that is, the process of active negotiation about treatment and expected outcomes, with the *patient as a therapeutic ally.* They state that this approach ". . . may well be the single most important step in engaging the patient's trust, preventing major discrepancies in the evaluation of therapeutic outcomes, promoting compliance, and reducing patient dissatisfaction" (1978:257). The theme of engaging the client as a partner and working with identified client needs appears as an important one in educational psychology, particularly theories about how adults learn.

Adult Learning Theory

Knowles' (1973) adult learning theory states that adults are motivated to learn as they experience needs and interests that learning will satisfy. Such needs may be related to health or illness and often are emotional, social or familial in nature. A basic assumption of Knowles' theory is that in order for learning to take place, the adult must be ready and willing to learn. That is, the individual must have experiential willingness (necessary knowledge and skills to learn) and emotional willingness (willingness to change through learning). In addition, adults have a stronger need to be active participants in the learning process as well as to be more self-directed than children. Knowles further suggests that adult learning differs from child learning in that it is problem-centered rather than subject-centered. For example, Tarnow (1979) contrasts a course in beginning Spanish at the high school level with a course entitled "Conversational Medical Spanish" as taught to a group of nurses who are having difficulty communicating with their Spanish-speaking clients. These factors, as well as the individual's readiness and ability to learn, will ultimately influence health and illness behavior and *should* affect the nurse's approach to self-care.

We think that some principles of adult learning theory may also apply to children in the context of learning about health and self-care. That is, teaching about health might be more effective if the teacher and learner assess the learner's readiness to learn and plan teaching sessions appropriately. The nurse should remember that health teaching must address the client's *specific* concern rather than dealing only with more general issues. Figure 2-2 summarizes how some social and behavioral science concepts contribute to our theoretical perspective of self-care.

SUMMARY

This chapter has summarized selected nursing and social science theories which provide a framework for our approach to self-care in nursing practice. Orem's theory defines self-care as a basis for nursing practice, and we use it as a basis for our approach. We include Rogers' theory because of its breadth and potential for explaining the interactional characteristics of human beings in their environment. It is an umbrella under which parts of Orem's and Leininger's postulates are embedded. Leininger's transcultural nursing focus is described because in our opinion other nursing theories neglect the importance of cultural aspects in nursing practice.

*Beliefs about susceptibility
   and seriousness of illness
Beliefs about benefits and
   barriers to actions
   and alternatives*

*Perceptions of self-
   health providers, and
   the meaning of the
   health*

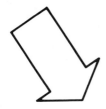 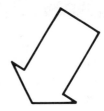

Motivation
for
Self-Care

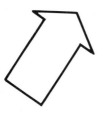 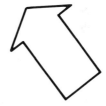

*Culturally based
   explanations of
   illness
Health-provider's and
clients' negotiations
   re: explanatory
models, treatment,
and expected outcomes*

*Willingness and
   readiness to learn*

Figure 2-2. Social science theories related to motivation for self-care.

Symbolic interactionism, the health belief model, and explanatory models of illness share an emphasis on perception of a situation, problem or person, and the meaning of it to the individual involved. This meaning arises through social interaction with others (e.g., family members, health care providers), previous experience or knowledge of a particular illness, one's cultural background, and the relevant health care domain. These factors also affect readiness and willingness to learn (adult learning theory).

We are not proposing a new conceptual model but have included several existing theories, taking from each what we consider most relevant to our perspective on self-care. Please keep these concepts and assumptions in mind as you read the following chapters. We will return to a discussion of relevant theory in Part IV when we suggest implications for the future of self-care in nursing education, practice, and research.

Discussion Questions

1. How does the client's role compare to the nurse's role in self-care?
2. How does culture influence perceptions of health and self-care?
3. List the variables outlined in the health belief model and discuss their importance.
4. What principles of adult learning theory are applicable to children?

REFERENCES

Anna DJ, Christensen DG, Hohon SA, Ord L, Wells SR: Implementing Orem's conceptual framework. Journal of Nursing Administration, Vol 8, No 11, pp 8–11, 1978

Backscheider JE: Self-care requirements, self-care capabilities, and nursing systems in the diabetic management clinic. American Journal of Public Health, Vol 64, No 12, pp 1138–1146, 1974

Blumer H: Symbolic Interaction: Perspective and Method. Prentice-Hall, Inc., Englewood Cliffs, New Jersey, 1969

Bromley B: Applying Orem's self-care theory in enterostomal therapy. American Journal of Nursing, Vol 80, No 2, pp 245–249, 1980

Dodd MI: Assessing patient self-care for side effects of cancer chemotherapy, Part I. Cancer Nursing, Vol 5, No 6, pp 447–451, 1982

Goodwin JO: Programmed instruction for self-care following pulmonary surgery. International Journal of Nursing, Vol 16, No 1, pp 29–38, 1979

Kearney BY, Fleischer BJ: Development of an instrument to measure exercise of self-care agency. Research in Nursing and Health, Vol 2, No 1, pp 25–34, 1979

Kleinman A: Concepts and a model for the comparison of medical systems as cultural systems. Social Science and Medicine, Vol 12, No 2, pp 85–93, 1978

Kleinman A, Eisenberg L, Good B: Culture, illness and care: Clinical lessons from anthropologic and cross-cultural research. Annals of Internal Medicine, Vol 88, No 2, pp 251–258, 1978

Knowles M: The Adult Learner: A Neglected Species, 2nd ed. Gulf Publishing Co., Houston, Texas, 1973

Leavitt F: The health belief model and utilization of ambulatory care services. Social Science and Medicine, Vol 13A, No 1, pp 105–112, 1979

Leininger M: Transcultural Nursing: Concepts, Theories, and Practices. John Wiley & Sons, Inc., New York, 1978

Orem DE: Nursing: Concepts of Practice, 2nd ed. McGraw-Hill Book Co., New York, 1980

Rogers M: Nursing: A science of unitary man. *In* Riehl J, Roy C: Conceptual Models for Nursing Practice, 2nd ed. Appleton-Century-Crofts, New York, 1980

Rogers M: An Introduction to the Theoretical Basis of Nursing. F. A. Davis, Philadelphia, Pennsylvania, 1970

Rosenstock I: Why people use health services. Millbank Memorial Fund Quarterly, Vol 44, No 3, pp 94–127, 1966

Stevens B: Nursing Theory. Little, Brown and Company, Boston, Massachusetts, 1979

Tarnow K: Working with adult learners. Nurse Educator, Vol 4, No 5, pp 34–40, 1979

Underwood P: Facilitating self-care. *In* Pothier P (ed): Psychiatric Nursing: A Basic Text. Little, Brown and Company, Boston, Massachusetts, 1980

3

Self-Care and the Nursing Process

The nursing process is a systematic way of organizing and providing nursing care. The nursing process consists of four phases:

- Assessment
- Planning
- Implementation
- Evaluation (Yura and Walsh 1983).

This model has been described for the purpose of analysis and explanation of the components of nursing care. However, in actual nursing care the phases do not occur in a linear fashion; rather, two or more components of the process are most likely enacted simultaneously. This ideal model is most useful in describing what the nurse actually does in providing care because it outlines basic problem-solving. We will focus this chapter specifically on how the nursing process is used in self-care.

ASSESSMENT

The assessment phase provides a data base from which client strengths, concerns, and problems can be identified. A data base contains information related to three components: the nursing history, the physical examination and clinical studies. The client's self-assessment supplements the information in the data base. Information collected in this data base (see sample on page 36) is essential for planning, implementing, and evaluating self-care.

How does the nurse collect information from which an assessment can be accomplished? Ideally, the nurse and client have enough time for an in-depth interview so that data can be gathered systematically. Reprinted questionnaires that clients can complete are used to gather information in some settings, to more actively involve the client, or to preserve more time to concentrate on the client's concerns.

Written questionnaires are limited in that they tend to provide only general categories and often do not elicit information on health beliefs and values that would emerge during an interview. They can be inappropriate for some clients, such as some immigrant populations who are unwilling to use written forms or whose English reading and writing skills are poor or nonexistent. If a questionnaire must be used, however, it should alert the nurse to specific questions for follow-up during the physical examination or a subsequent interview. However, self-assessment by questionnaire is a valuable way to gather data in self-care planning and is one way to raise client awareness of current health status. For example, an adolescent girl who is requesting birth control could be given a self-assessment tool that includes questions related to knowledge about prevention of pregnancy and sexually transmitted diseases and questions about current sexual practices.

In addition to assessment data provided by the client, information is sought from medical records, family members, or friends who accompany the client, and other members of the health team who have worked with the client.

Nursing Data Base

The nursing data base should include the reason for contact, usual source/pattern of health care, past health history, sociocultural data, sexual history, self-care behaviors, physical assessment, and clinical studies. The nursing history typically begins by asking clients why they have contacted the health care system, which is usually called a "chief complaint." Although a chief complaint is usually required to enter the health care system, this term implies a medical diagnosis and disease orientation. We prefer to use *reason for contact* to describe the client's motivation to seek care. There *is* a difference in attitude between asking questions in one way or another. "What is your chief complaint?" or "What is the matter with you?" versus "Why are you seeking care today?" or "How can we help you?" The reason for contact may be any of a number of possibilities, such as follow-up care, health promotion or maintenance, disease detection or prevention, or general support or counseling.

The reason for contact describes the *client's* reason for the visit, and perception of personal health needs. For example, a medical chart that lists "chronic renal failure" as chief complaint gives the medical and pathophysiological perspective but does not suggest major client concerns, such as the number of hours spent on the dialysis machine, dietary restrictions, and decreased libido. Because the client's and family's perceptions of the current situation and health needs are vitally important to self-care and health care, we suggest that the nurse include specific

NURSING DATA BASE

NAME _____

ADDRESS _____

AGE _____ SEX _____ MARITAL STATUS _____

REASON FOR CONTACT _____

USUAL SOURCE/PATTERN OF HEALTH CARE _____

RELATED HEALTH BELIEFS _____

Past Health History

Childhood illness: _____

Immunizations: _____

Allergies: _____

Hospitalizations and serious illnesses: _____

Accidents: _____

Obstetric history: _____

Medications: _____

Habits: _____

Sociocultural Data

Family relationships and friendships: _____

Ethnic identity: _____

Occupational history: _____

Educational history: _____

Economic status: _____

Living circumstances: _____

Sexual History

Satisfaction with current sexual activity: _____

Learning needs: _____

Usual Self-Care Behaviors

Nutrition: _____

Activity, rest, and exercise: _____

Stress management: _____

Psychological and spiritual health behaviors: _____

Sexual behavior: _____

Personal hygiene: _____

Safety: _____

Physical Assessment

Neurological system: _____

Gastrointestinal system: _____

Integumentary system: _____

Endocrine system: _____

Musculoskeletal system: _____

Respiratory system: _____

Cardiovascular system: _____

Genitourinary system: _____

Menstrual history: _____

Clinical Studies

Diagnostic procedures: _____

Laboratory findings: _____

---

questions in the history that will elicit this information. Kleinman, Eisenberg, and Good (1978) give examples that are useful with clients of most sociocultural backgrounds:

1. What do you think has caused your problem?
2. Why do you think it started when it did?
3. What do you think your sickness does to you? How does it work?
4. How severe is your sickness? Will it have a short or long course?
5. What kind of treatment do you think you should receive?
6. What are the most important results you hope to receive from this treatment?
7. What are the chief problems your sickness has caused for you?
8. What do you fear most about your sickness? (1978:256)

Questions related to the health belief model (Lousteau 1979) shown on page 39 are also useful in assessing a client's perception of susceptibility to illness and cost versus benefits of treatment. In addition to focusing the nurse on the client's perception of the problem, such questions are likely to yield important cultural themes and values which must be taken into consideration in self-care planning.

When the client has a specific complaint, e.g., "my stomach hurts," the nurse asks detailed questions about sequence and chronology, characteristics of pain (e.g., duration, frequency, location), associated symptoms, effects on other activities and bodily functions, aggravating and alleviating factors, and setting in which the problem occurs. It can be revealing to ask the client for a literal interpretation of a symptom. For example, you might ask a woman with muscle tension and neck pain, "What's really a pain in the neck for you?" Or a man who complains of nausea, as "*What makes you sick to your stomach?*" Of particular importance for self-care is the assessment of whether clients can link their symptoms to their life situations or daily behavior. For example, does a client perceive a relationship between a demanding work schedule and insomnia?

It is important to learn about the client's past sources and patterns of seeking health care. Have other clinicians been seen about this reason for contact, and is the client "shopping?" What information may be available from other sources of health care? Questions related to how the client sought care in the past can reveal some aspects of self-care motivation.

Past health history. In the past history, the nurse and client gather information about previous health and illness states and contacts with health professionals. Data should include developmental history, review of systems, and practices that restored or promoted health and prevented illness in the past. The review of systems is a method of obtaining information about past or present conditions, including accidents, injuries, serious illnesses, and hospitalizations, focusing on the major anatomical areas of the body. (See page 85.) In general, the review of systems is useful for helping the client and nurse group symptoms and health practices so that their relationships can be identified. However, mental/emotional health is neglected in most reviews; we encourage you to include specific questions in your assessment. Examples include: Do you generally feel relaxed or nervous and keyed up? Are you generally happy or frequently feel sad and discouraged? How much energy and pep do you have? Are you satisfied with how your life is going? The answers to such questions are important for planning self-care. Questions about previous health practices, such as immunizations, eye or dental examinations, provide information about clients' preventive or detection efforts, risk factors, and the clients' previous ability to carry out a treatment regimen.

Sociocultural data. A component of the nursing history which has particular importance for self-care is the *sociocultural data.* Because we view the family as a system, a change in the health of one member affects

---

HEALTH BELIEF MODEL SAMPLE QUESTIONS

Susceptibility

What kinds of things cause you to be ill?
When you become sick, what do you think has most frequently been the cause?
In comparison to other people your age, how would you rate your health—poor, average, or good?
How much do you worry about getting sick?

Severity

How severe do you think your present health problem is?
Could it cause other health problems?
If it could, what would these be?
If you were to get sick, what would the effects be on your work, responsibilities and others in your immediate environment (e.g., spouse, children)?

Benefit of Treatment

To what extent do you think treatment (medication, diet, change in life-style patterns, or keeping clinic appointments) will either cure or control your health problem?
How would you rate the safety of the treatment that has been prescribed?
How likely are health professionals to be able to cure or control your problem?
How able do you think health professionals are to prevent complications from occurring for people who have health problems like your health problem?

Cost of Treatment

How difficult is it for you to get transportation to keep your clinic or doctor appointments?
Do you have to take time off from work to keep your appointments?
Do you lose pay for that time?
How long did you wait to see the care provider today?
In your opinion, did you have to wait too long to see the care provider?
How much is the treatment (diet, activity changes, etc.) interfering with your normal routine?
Has the treatment meant that you have given up pleasurable activities?

Adapted from Lousteau A: Using the health belief model to predict patient compliance. Health Values: Achieving High-Level Wellness, Vol 13, No 5, pp 241–245, 1979

the health of other individual members, as well as the health of the family as a whole. In addition, hereditary factors are important in the causation and expression of certain conditions. The family affects health status through providing most individuals with their basic needs and with social support and through providing definitions of health and appropriate health practices.

It is critically important to learn who the client identifies as family, whether family of origin, family of procreation, or others. Family can be defined as two or more persons who share common goals and who may maintain the functions of rearing children, providing shelter, food, clothing, health care and safety, and socialization of members, allocating resources, dividing labor, and providing for emotional needs and social support (Mahoney, Verdisco, and Shortridge 1976). It is important to consider with whom clients live and if clients consider that person(s) their family, even if not biologically or legally related. It is important to know who the client calls on when sick or in need of help. Clients' feelings about family members are also important. Are they seen as sources of support? Do clients consider their families stable? Are there specific interruptions in family relationships? Consider the example of a homosexual man whose partner is his "family" and major source of support and whose biological family has "disowned" him. In reference to self-care, a stable family is a factor that positively influences the client's ability to carry out a therapeutic regimen (Sackett and Haynes 1976).

Detailed information on the family is important for assessment of all clients, but it is even more important when considering a client whose culture values family welfare and relationships more strongly than the welfare of the individual, such as in Middle Eastern cultural groups. See Family Assessment form below.

FAMILY ASSESSMENT

COMPOSITION OF THE FAMILY

Members of the immediate family—parents, siblings, spouse, and children _____

Members of the extended family—grandparents, grandchildren, aunts, uncles, and cousins _____

Significant others—heterosexual or homosexual partners, friends.

HEALTH STATUS OF FAMILY MEMBERS

General health status of each member _____

Other major family stressors _____

RELATIONSHIPS AMONG FAMILY MEMBERS

Interactions _____

Roles _____

- Who makes decisions about what? _____
- Who manages the household? _____

- Who cares for the children? _____
- Who disciplines the children? _____
- How do the children assist with household activities? _____
- Who is responsible for providing health care? _____

Genogram (include familial illnesses):

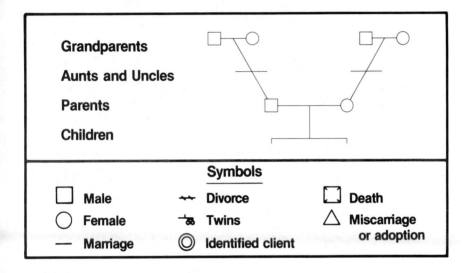

Grandparents

Aunts and Uncles

Parents

Children

Symbols

☐ Male   ⌒⌒ Divorce   ⌷ Death

○ Female   ⊸ Twins   △ Miscarriage

— Marriage   ◎ Identified client   or adoption

Adapted from Mahoney EA, Verdisco L, Shortridge L: How to Collect and Record a Health History, J. B. Lippincott Co., Philadelphia, 1976 and from Wright LM, Leahey M: Nurses and Families: A Guide to Family Assessment and Intervention, F. A. Davis Co., Philadelphia, 1984.

In addition to questions that assess the family in general, specific questions about self-care should be asked, e.g., what are the self-care practices of individual family members? How does the family as a unit help individual members with self-care? The nurse should ask herself how cultural beliefs influence individual and family self-care.

Sociocultural data also include socioeconomic, ethnic, and cultural factors. The nurse needs information about the client's occupation, education level, home environment (especially with regard to adequacy of space, exposure to pollutants, sanitation, water fluoridation), and adequacy of income for meeting basic needs. Questions about life-style might include how clients spend a typical day, recreation and interests, and with whom they spend time in work and recreation.

Ethnicity contributes to differences in disease rates, health maintenance and home treatment, variant forms of illness behavior, and variations in use of health resources, including use of folk healers (Harwood
1981; Orque, Bloch and Monrroy 1983). The concept of ethnicity is more
useful than the concept of culture in some ways in our pluralistic society.
Ethnic group can be defined as a *self-identified* group that has a distinct
language or dialect, customs, food, mode of dress, life-style, race, religion, and a sense of common ancestry. Ethnic identity is a subjective
sense of belonging to a particular group, and individuals choose how
strongly they identify with the group. Therefore, it is important for the nurse
to ask clients how they identify themselves, and if they view illness,
health, death, birth, and medical treatment in a similar way to others in
their ethnic group. Tripp-Reimer and colleagues (1984) provide a good
overview of cultural assessment.

Religion is particularly important in nursing assessment, as it can affect
birth and death rituals, diet, and views of health and illness. For example,
in some ethnic groups, intense religious faith is considered the most
appropriate form of self-care, and other self-care measures are acceptable only in this context.

Finally, if the client is an immigrant, the nurse needs to know how long
the client/family has been in this country, why they have come, degree of
English proficiency (spoken and written), and how much stress is being
experienced because of transition, culture shock, financial difficulties,
and/or legal problems associated with immigration.

Sexual history. The importance of obtaining a *sexual history* varies
with the individual's reason for contact and is not always necessary.
Nurses can use their own judgment but should *not* automatically avoid this
area of assessment.

Self-care behavior. This area of the data base provides the nurse and
the client with a general impression of the client's health activities. It
includes details of specific concerns, if any, and daily habits and activity
patterns in the areas of nutrition, activity, rest and exercise, stress management, psychological and spiritual health behaviors, sexual behavior,
personal hygiene, and safety. Additional questions related to habits (e.g.,
tobacco, alcohol) should be asked. Misconceptions about health and
health practices and lack of information can be identified as a health need
at this time. Self-care behavior questions also provide the nurse and client
with information about the client's past ability to promote health and
current motivational level, as well as identifying daily activities that contribute to poor health.

The physical assessment. The physical assessment is an important
time for gathering data and teaching self-care. First, when examining a
particular part of the client's body, the nurse can ask specific history
questions relating to the client's self-care practices. For example, when

examining the mouth, the nurse asks "Do you brush or floss your teeth?" When examining the breasts, "Do you do regular breast self-examination?" The physical examination is also a good time to teach clients how to examine their own bodies. Client self-examination skills can include taking a pulse, temperature, and blood pressure, breast examination, testicular self-examination, examination of the throat and lymph nodes, and examination of and description of the skin. In addition, parents can be taught to examine their children and how to interpret and report the findings. Learning physical examination skills can help clients understand when to enter the health care system, which is an important component of self-care.

Clinical studies. The last component of the data base is the clinical studies, which have an important implication for self-care. Clinical studies can alert the nurse to client needs for self-care and health teaching. If a blood glucose level is too high, the nurse might assess the client's need for diet and medication instruction. The results of lab values and other clinical studies can be used in teaching the client about health and illness. Such test results may be necessary to help clients accept the reality of health situations. For example, a young and otherwise healthy man who has just been diagnosed with idiopathic thrombocytopenia has been prescribed prednisone. The client is reluctant to take the medication because a friend got sick when he took the same medication. The client may not be convinced of his need for prednisone only on the basis of his easy bruising. If he is told that his platelet count is less than 10% of normal and the implications are explained, the client may be more willing to take the prescribed medication.

Another reason clinical studies are important in self-care is that clients can be taught to monitor many of their own tests. Examples include urine testing for sugar, ketones or protein, self-pap smears, home pregnancy tests, testing stool for guiac, and home strep tests. Recently, blood glucose monitoring devices have been successfully used for closely monitoring diabetic blood sugars and keeping blood glucose levels in a more narrow range.

In addition to questions on our data base, the nurse may want to identify risk of illness. A Health Risk Appraisal (Goetz 1980; Wagner, Berry, Schoenback, and Graham 1982) might be used, or an outline for determining risks such as Pender's (1982) scheme could be used (see example beginning on page 44). Note that many of the risk factors are potentially modifiable through self-care practices. For example, hypertension is potentially modifiable through dietary changes, relaxation, and exercise.

Nurses and other health care professionals are skilled in writing problem lists and, indeed, thinking about client problems in general. We are not as skilled at identifying a client's strengths. Devising a strengths list is an important component in the assessment phase. Such a list should

RISK APPRAISAL FORM—RISK FOR CARDIOVASCULAR DISEASE

In each row, place a check in the box that best describes your current life situation or behavior.

RISK FACTOR		INCREASING RISK				
Sex and age:	Female under 40	Female 40–50	Male 25–40	Female after menopause	Male 40–60	Male 61 or over
Family history (mother, father, brothers, sisters)						
High blood pressure	No relatives with condition	One relative		Two relatives	Three relatives	
Heart attack	No relatives with condition	One relative with condition after 60	Two relatives with condition after 60	One relative with condition before 60	Two relatives with condition before 60	
Diabetes	No relatives with condition		One or more relatives with maturity onset diabetes		One or more relatives with preadolescent or adolescent onset	
Blood pressure*						
Systolic	120 or below	121–140	141–160	161-180	181-200	above 200
Diastolic	70 or below	71–80	81–90	91–100	101–110	above 110
Diabetes*	No diagnosis	Maturity onset, controlled	Maturity onset, uncontrolled	Adolescent onset, controlled	Adolescent onset, controlled	Adolescent onset, uncontrolled

*Weight**	At or slightly below recommended weight		10% overweight	20% overweight	30% overweight	40% overweight	50% overweight
Cholesterol† level (mg/100 ml)*	Below 180	181–200	201–220	221–240	241–260	261–280	Above 280
Serum triglycerides (mg/100 ml) fasting*	150 or below		151–400		401–1000		Above 1000
*Percent of fat in diet**	20–30%		31–40%		41–50%		Above 50%
*Frequency of exercise** — Recreational	Intensive recreational exertion (35–45 min at least 4 times/wk)		Moderate recreational exertion		Minimal recreational exertion		No recreational exertion
Occupational	Intensive occupational exertion		Moderate occupational exertion		Minimal occupational exertion		Sedentary occupation
*Sleep patterns**	7 or 8 hr sleep/night		More than 8 hr sleep/night			4–6 hr sleep/night	
*Cigarette smoking** — No./day	Nonsmoker		1–10/day	11–20/day	21–30/day	31–40/day	Over 40/day
No. of yr smoked	Nonsmoker		Less than 10 yr	11–15 yr	16–20 yr	21–30 yr	31 yr or more

Continued

*Stress**	Domestic	Minimal	Moderate	High	Very High
	Occupational	Minimal	Moderate	High	Very high
*Behavior pattern** *(particularly males)*		*Type B* Relaxed, appropriately assertive, not time dependent, moderate to slow speech		*Type A* Excessively competitive, aggressive, striving, hyperalert, time dependent, loud, explosive speech	
*Air pollution**		Low	Moderate	High	
*Use of oral contraceptives** *(females)*		Do not use oral contraceptives	Under 40 and use oral contraceptives	Over 40 and use oral contraceptives	

*Indicates risk factors that can be fully or partially controlled.

†Serum lipid analysis is also recommended to determine low-density (beta) and high-density (alpha) lipoprotein levels. Evidence suggests that high-density lipoprotein (HDL) carries cholesterol from tissues for metabolism and excretion. An inverse correlation appears to exist between HDL and coronary artery disease.

RISK APPRAISAL FORM—RISK FOR SUICIDE

RISK FACTOR	INCREASING RISK				
Family history:	No history		One family member		Two or more family members
*Personal history**	Seldom experience depression	Periodically experience mild depression	Frequently experience mild depression	Periodically experience deep depression	Frequently experience deep depression
*Access to hypnotic medication**	No access		Access to small or limited dosages		Unlimited access to large dosages

*Indicates risk factors that can be fully or partially controlled.

Risk appraisal forms from Pender NJ: Health Promotion in Nursing Practice, Appleton-Century-Crofts, Norwalk, Connecticut, 1982 *(Used with permission of Appleton-Century-Crofts).*

include what the client does to contribute to good health, and personal and family strengths which potentially increase the client's confidence and willingness to make changes in behavior which will promote better health. Examples of strengths include past successes in changing health behaviors (e.g., decreasing smoking or increasing exercise), achievement in school or work, close social ties with family and friends, and a positive attitude. These strengths can be utilized to help the client change other life-style practices.

Self-Assessment

Self-assessment can be an invaluable way of completing the assessment phase of the nursing process. When clients are asked to assess their own health, they are asked to begin to take a responsibility and an active role in evaluation. In rating one's own health and health practices, individuals are encouraged to take a serious look at their health behavior and how their life-style affects health in an organized manner. The self-assessment process potentially increases awareness, which is the first step to changing behavior. Self-assessment involves the client in both self-care and professional care. It helps the client make associations between life-style and health and suggests ways in which clients can most effectively participate in professionally prescribed care. Because assessment is the first step in problem-solving, self-assessment encourages and teaches clients how to think through and find appropriate solutions to health problems. In addition, self-assessment potentially can help clients to increase their sense of self-control and power.

An important part of self-assessment is establishing a good base line or the usual practice or level of activity. For example, when planning a weight reduction program, one should find out exactly what, and how much, a person is eating normally. A daily log is useful in this regard. For example, some people who cannot understand why they do not lose weight in spite of "hardly eating anything" may be surprised to learn from such a log just how many calories they consume through frequent "healthy" snacks such as cheese or dried fruit.

The assessment phase of the nursing process is completed when a nursing diagnosis is made and goals for self-care are set. The nursing diagnosis is based on the assessment of client needs in such areas as health teaching, medical supervision, specific skills, or increased awareness of certain bodily functions.There is considerable controversy over what are acceptable nursing diagnoses. Kim, McFarland, and McLain (1984) list such diagnoses, e.g.:

- Alteration in nutrition—less than body requirements
- Variations in functional performance or self-care activities—alterations in ability to perform.

We suggest that such diagnoses be converted into a health needs list rather than a problem list of chief complaints. Such a needs list should be based on data obtained in the assessment and be written in cooperation with the client. When nursing diagnoses and self-care needs lists are developed, the planning stage of the nursing process begins.

PLANNING

While the assessment phase of the nursing process establishes clients' health needs, the planning phase establishes goals based on these needs and suggests specific interventions to meet these goals. The first step in planning is *assigning priority to health-related goals,* which involves deciding the order of importance and which goal must be addressed first. Clearly, there are times when a number of health needs and goals demand attention at the same time. For example, a diabetic may not be able to realistically decide whether to focus on insulin administration or dietary restrictions, which is most important and what should be done first. In contrast, the individual who is overweight, overworked, and sedentary has the luxury of deciding to manage work stress before beginning a weight reduction program. Individuals may choose to focus first on other areas of life, such as personal finances or finishing college, and not want to attend to health needs that the nurse considers a priority.

Before a goal is set, the nurse and client together must decide whether the goal is realistic and attainable. Nothing is worse for clients than unrealistic goals that set them up to fail before they begin. There are a number of ways the nurse and client can plan to avoid such an outcome. For example, brainstorming can be utilized to identify all the alternative possibilities to meet the goal, no matter how farfetched such possibilities may seem (Ferguson 1979). Reliable sources, such as books, other health professionals, or self-help groups might be used to help the nurse and client list alternative ways of meeting the goal.

When setting health goals, it is important to determine if the need is for knowledge, skill, or attitude or behavior changes, because the kinds of interventions will differ (See Chapter 6). We also recognize that there are different planning schemes based on how many and how serious the client's health needs are. Baldi and colleagues (1980) make several useful suggestions that are appropriate for health promotion. One suggestion is *choosing the right time to begin.* Although a newly diagnosed diabetic cannot decide to wait until next year to begin a diabetic diet, the individual who wishes to begin an exercise program or stop smoking should consider *when* that can be done most *successfully.* For example, a nursing student who wishes to reduce stress might begin a stress management program during vacation, rather than just before finals.

A second rule is *choosing one goal at a time,* whenever possible. Although clients with chronic problems may need to change several behaviors at once, we think that changing one behavior is difficult enough and clients should be encouraged to work on one goal at a time. Success in one area helps build the confidence to try another. According to Farquhar (1978), stress management is a good non-threatening way to begin a health program. The third rule is to allow *more* time to meet a health goal than one would anticipate. If inadequate time is allowed, clients may set themselves up for failure. It is also important to set time aside to carry out the activities designed to meet the goal.

Finally, Ferguson (1979) suggests that adding something rather than depriving oneself of something is helpful in meeting one's goal. For example, adding a walking program for weight reduction is more pleasant than just depriving oneself of excess food. If the client wants to stop smoking, the nurse could suggest adding some other kind of treat, such as using the money saved for some unnecessary, but delightful, splurge.

Criteria for evaluation should be determined in the planning phase. The more clearly the goals are delineated, the easier the evaluation process. The goals may need to be modified during the implementation phase, and the criteria should be modified as well. Evaluation criteria need to be as clear and as objective as possible so that the client and nurse can judge whether the goal has been met. For example, if the goal is stress reduction, the criteria should not be stated as "less stress." Rather, specific parameters should be outlined, such as systolic and diastolic blood pressure, amount of anti-anxiety medication taken, and what kinds and how often stress management techniques are used in a specific period of time. It is useful for the client to assess the amount of stress experienced each day using a self-reported record, such as rating stress on a scale of one to ten.

IMPLEMENTATION

The third phase of the nursing process is implementation or putting the plan into action. We must consider that the client's attitudes or behaviors, or other people, can sabotage the client's self-care plan through thoughts and actions that interfere with achievement of the designated goal. For example, a common attitude of dieters that sabotages their efforts is the statement, "Well, I blew it for today when I ate that cake; I might as well have the ice cream, too." Other rationalizations which sabotage self-care efforts are such statements as, "I'm too busy to practice stress management," or "I'm too tired to exercise." Actions can also sabotage implementation, such as grocery shopping when hungry or having a drink after work before one's intended time to exercise. Other people's "kindness" can also sabotage one's efforts. The classic example is "Let's go out to dinner; you can start your diet tomorrow," or "Why do you take all that trouble to meditate; wouldn't a pill be easier?"

Identifying saboteurs and planning ways to avoid or cope with them is essential for implementation. Similarly, the nurse and client should identify strengths, attitudes, or other people that will support implementing a self-care plan, who are important resources on which to rely during difficult moments. For example, Alcoholics Anonymous uses a "telephone buddy" system to help members resist drinking when they are tempted to do so.

Important to implementation are "records and reminders" (Baldi et al. 1980). One must rely on more than memory when implementing a self-care plan. The nurse and client can discuss the ways the client would prefer to keep records. Some people keep a journal; others would rather put a note on a calendar; still others like to cross items off a daily list. For some people, it is helpful to write reminders on cards to be posted in strategic locations. For example, a reminder to floss one's teeth can be put on the bathroom mirror, a note to wear seat belts on the steering wheel, or a picture of a model or an athlete on the refrigerator. Medication boxes with the days marked are useful.

EVALUATION

The final phase of the nursing process is evaluation. During this phase, the effectiveness in meeting goals of the self-care plan is appraised, as are changes in the client's needs or self-care abilities. The evaluation phase of the nursing process should examine not only the pre-determined criteria for evaluation but the entire process. Nursing process is circular and, therefore, the nurse and client must evaluate whether the assessment itself was appropriate and/or complete and, if not, what information is needed to complete the assessment. Next, goals should be reevaluated. Were they realistic and attainable? Did the client meet the goal? If not, what were the barriers? Were the plans appropriate to meet the goal? And finally, were the criteria for evaluation appropriate?

Most importantly, if a client has not met the goal, it is important to recognize and help the client understand that this is not a personal failure—*rather, the plan did not work.* Recognition of limitations of the plan and barriers to carrying it out are vital in evaluation and lead to revised plans that are more likely to be successful. There are several variations in evaluation outcomes (see below).

VARIATIONS IN OUTCOMES OF EVALUATION

1. Criteria met, problem resolved
2. Criteria met, problem partially resolved: look again at criteria or approach

3. Criteria met, problem not solved: modify criteria or intervention
4. Criteria not met: re-assess both problem and approach.

SUMMARY

The phases of the nursing process, despite the linear fashion in which they are described, often occur simultaneously and in a circular fashion in practice. However, it is useful to spell out each phase as a way of thinking about organization of care and self-care. In actuality, the nursing process is none other than basic problem-solving. In self-care, the client is an active participant in assessment, planning, implementation, and evaluation. The nurse's role is to encourage the client to use effective self-care strategies, and a good way of approaching self-care is through the problem-solving process. By encouraging the client to learn and use this process and apply it to health needs, the nurse can be more effective in helping clients to practice responsible self-care.

Discussion Questions

1. Choose an area of health on which you would like to work: do a self-assessment, set a goal, and determine criteria for evaluation.
2. Write a list of potential sabotages and supports for your plan.
3. Describe three criteria for evaluation in a weight reduction program.
4. Identify a needs list for a client with a gastric ulcer.

REFERENCES

Anna DJ, Christensen DG, Hohon SA, Ord L, Wells SR: Implementing Orem's conceptual framework. Journal of Nursing Administration, Vol 8, No 11, pp 8–11, 1978

Baldi S, Costell S, Hill L, Jasmin S, Smith N: For Your Health: A Model for Self-Care. Nurses Model Health, South Laguna, California, 1980

Block GJ, Nolan JW, Demsey MK: Health Assessment for Professional Nursing: A Developmental Approach. Appleton-Century-Crofts, New York, 1981

Farquhar JW: The American Way of Life Need Not Be Hazardous to Your Health. Stanford Alumni Association, Stanford, California, 1978

Ferguson T: On developing a personal self-care plan, Medical Self-Care, pp 11–14, Fall 1979

Goetz AA: Health risk appraisal: The estimation of risk. Public Health Reports, Vol 95, No 2, pp 119–126, 1980

Harwood A: Ethnicity and Medical Care. Harvard University Press, Cambridge, Massachusetts, 1981

Joseph LS: Self-care and the nursing process. Nursing Clinics of North America, Vol 15, No 1, pp 131–143, 1980

Kim MJ, McFarland CK, McLain AM (eds): Pocket Guide to Nursing Diagnoses. The C. V. Mosby Company, St. Louis, Missouri, 1984

Kleinman A, Eisenberg L, Good B: Culture, illness and care: Clinical lessons from anthropologic and cross-cultural research. Annals of Internal Medicine, Vol 88, No 2, 251–258, 1978

Leininger M: Culturological assessment domains for nursing practices. In Leininger M: Transcultural Nursing: Concepts, Theories, and Practice. John Wiley & Sons, Inc., New York, 1978

Lousteau A: Using the health belief model to predict patient compliance. Health Values: Achieving High-Level Wellness, Vol 13, No 5, pp 241–245, 1979

Mahoney EA, Verdisco L, Shortridge L: How to Collect and Record a Health History. J. B. Lippincott Co., Philadelphia, Pennsylvania, 1976

Murray RB, Zentner JP: Nursing Assessment and Health Promotion Through the Life Span, 2nd ed. Prentice-Hall, Inc., Englewood Cliffs, New Jersey, 1979

Orque M, Bloch B, Monrroy L: Ethnic Nursing Care: A Multicultural Approach, The C. V. Mosby Company, St. Louis, Missouri, 1983

Pender NJ: Health Promotion in Nursing Practice. Appleton-Century-Crofts, Norwalk, Connecticut, 1982

Sackett, DJ, Haynes RB: Compliance with Therapeutic Regimens. Johns Hopkins University Press, Baltimore, Maryland, 1976

Shortridge LM, Lee EF: Introduction to Nursing Practice. McGraw-Hill Book Co., New York, 1980

Tripp-Reimer T, Brink P, Saunders J: Cultural assessment: Content and process. Nursing Outlook, Vol 32, No 2, pp 78–82, 1984

Wagner EH, Berry WL, Schoenback VJ, Graham RM: An assessment of health hazard health risk appraisal. American Journal of Pediatric Health, Vol 4, pp 347–352, 1982

Wright LM, Leahey M: Nurses and Families: A Guide to Family Assessment and Intervention. F. A. Davis Co., Philadelphia, Pennsylvania, 1984

Yura H, Walsh MB: the Nursing Process: Assessing, Planning, Implementing, 3rd ed. Appleton-Century-Crofts, New York, 1983

PART TWO

SELF-CARE PRINCIPLES

4

Self-Care in Health

Self-care behaviors cover the entire spectrum—health promotion, health maintenance, disease prevention, disease detection, and disease management. In this chapter, we differentiate between health and illness behaviors and propose that health and illness be seen on two separate continua. We describe individual and cultural factors that influence the definitions of health by clients and their families. Using the nursing process, the chapter outlines components of health assessment and describes decision-making, setting goals, planning, and evaluating through the use of clinical examples.

One of the major problems in health care delivery is the lack of a universally accepted definition of health. Assessment and diagnosis of disease have become sophisticated; given a certain set of data, many health care practitioners will reach agreement. There is far less consensus about indices of health. There are a number of definitions of health, but they are inconsistent and vague and do not provide parameters that can be used as the basis for the development of assessment tools. Indeed, most current assessment tools for "health" are oriented toward detecting the presence, absence, or risks of disease. The annual physical examination is a good example—if test results are negative, one is pronounced "healthy" (Figure 4-1). For many people, the concept of health is only apparent when it is lost.

It is important to determine just which conception of health clients and nurses use. Health goals and actions differ, depending on whether health is perceived as "absence of disease" or "optimal well-being." When nurse and client hold different conceptions of health, communication suffers, and they may be working at cross-purposes.

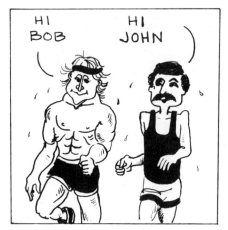
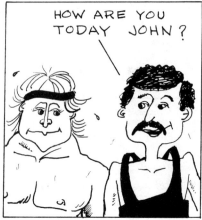
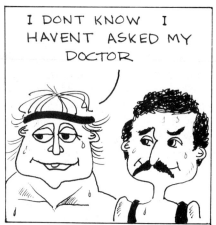

Figure 4-1. How do we define health?

Definitions of health can be grouped into categories. Smith (1981) uses four:

1. Clinical—health is seen as absence of disease
2. Role performance—health is seen as being able to do what is expected in one's own society in an adequate manner
3. Adaptive—health is seen as flexible adjustment to the environment
4. Eudaimonistic—health is seen as a state of optimal or positive well-being.

Laffrey's (1982) tool uses these categories to measure conceptions of health, by measuring agreement or disagreement with 28 statements that describe the meaning of health, Examples of statements are "I can fulfill my daily responsibilities," "not being under a doctor's care for illness," "facing each day with zest and enthusiasm," "not collapsing under ordinary stress," and "coping with changes in my surroundings." At this point, we will review some models of health and their relationship to models of illness.

As early as 1959, Halbert Dunn viewed health as more than the absence of disease and suggested that an individual's health status could range from death to peak wellness (see Figure 4-2). He coined the term "high-level wellness" to indicate a higher level of functioning than a stable state of relative homeostasis. He described wellness as an integrated way of functioning that maximizes the potential of the individual, the family, and the community.

Dunn's wellness concept has been recently popularized in the holistic health movement, in which health is determined by assessing the whole person within his environment. However, even within the holistic movement, health providers have difficulty reaching consensus about what health is, how to measure it, and how to help clients achieve it.

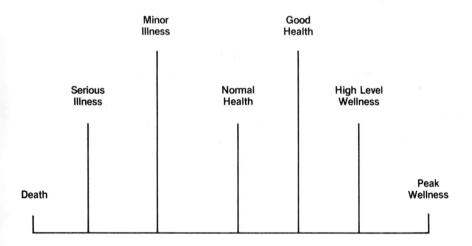

Figure 4-2. Dunn's health-illness continuum.

In contrast to the single continuum is a view of health and illness on two separate continua. In such a model, health and illness can co-exist. For example, Lamberton (1978) views the opposite of health as being no health, the opposite of illness as being no illness, and death as the natural end of the life process rather than as the ultimate illness (see Figure 4-3).

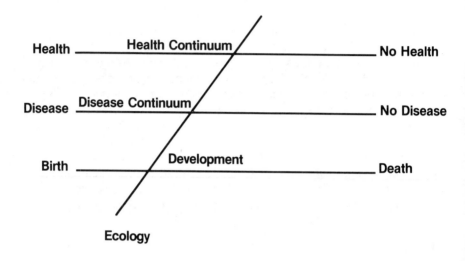

Figure 4-3. The Lamberton Model.

This model is a more productive way of viewing health and illness because it considers the individual's development within an environmental framework. To illustrate the utility of using separate continua for health and illness, consider a 39-year-old male smoker who has no desire to quit, who is 15 pounds overweight, who is a "chocolate addict," who uses television for relaxation when he gets home from a job he dislikes, and who has early morning insomnia related to work stress. He has no observable or measureable signs of disease, but would you judge him to be healthy? Then consider a 10-year-old girl who has well-controlled diabetes, excels in her studies and several hobbies, is popular with her friends, has a close and healthy family, and is generally a relaxed and happy child. Despite the presence of disease, we view her as having more areas of health than the 39-year-old man.

In actuality, however, it does not matter how health professionals define health and illness if they do not consider an individual's own personal definition, which has its roots in family and culture. Definitions of health and illness are intimately related to the way reality is perceived by each cultural group, and such "world views" differ to a great extent cross-culturally. For example, if maintaining a balance of yin and yang and harmony with the environment is the central concern in Chinese culture, then health is seen as the result of the individual's and family's attainment of balance, and illness a result of being out of harmony with nature or a disruption in energy flow. Some Fundamentalist Christians perceive illness as an indication of a person's having sinned or not having sufficient faith to ask for healing.

In addition, the importance of "good health" varies in accordance with the individual's socioeconomic status (Bullough and Bullough 1982). We have heard criticisms that the ideas and health practices advocated in the holistic health movement are relevant only to white, middle-class, urban Americans. This argument suggests that people who cannot afford adequate food, shelter, or clothing are unlikely to engage in such expensive therapeutic regimens as biofeedback, massage, exercise equipment, and vitamin supplements. Maslow's (1970) hierarchy of needs suggests that unless basic physiological needs are satisfied, it is difficult to consider cognitive or aesthetic needs.

To some individuals, regardless of the value of health in their cultural group, personal health is a less important goal than the pursuit of power or financial success. Ideas of individual progress and maximizing one's growth potential, so important in American white, middle-class culture, may be incomprehensible to people in a cultural group in which spiritual and physical harmony with nature and the importance of human *interde*pendence are guiding principles.

Thus, there may be great differences between the views of health and illness held by health care professionals trained in the Western medical model and the individuals with whom they work. It is important to ask clients how they perceive health and illness and to ascertain what they want out of life, in order to plan and implement appropriate self-care.

Among professionals, the definition of health continues to evolve. Defining health as maximizing one's potential has some limitations in the broader sociocultural context. We suggest, therefore, that health can be viewed as intimately related to life-style, which is defined by LaLonde (1974) as the personal decisions over which people have control. A useful way of assessing health is through assessing life-style, which is a concept that is broad enough to be valid cross-culturally. Thus, for the purposes of this book, we view health as more than the absence of disease, but a positive state of full functioning within one's capabilities and related to life-style. We suggest further that each individual's state of health and life-style must be understood in the context of individual circumstances, family, and cultural group.

NURSING INTERVENTIONS IN HEALTH

Along the health/no-health continuum, nursing interventions include promoting high-level wellness, maintaining wellness, preventing potential health alterations, detecting health alterations, and restoring health. Examples of these types of interventions will be described in the context of the nursing process as it relates to self-care in health. In addition to the nursing process of assessment, planning, implementation, and evaluation, we will discuss the importance of client responsibility for health.

Nurses and other health care professionals are usually considered to be "providers" of health and illness care services. This view implies a hierarchical relationship in which the professional has the power. This hierarchical relationship affects a client's health in a negative way. For example, if clients view care in the same way that they view other services, as something to be paid for, they will expect something to be done *for* them or *to* them; this stance conflicts with the idea of self-care.

Rather than a hierarchical relationship, a more equal relationship is desirable, a relationship in which the nurse and client work together to assess, plan, implement, and evaluate a self-care program. In such a relationship, the client is an active participant and the nurse functions as a facilitator. Clients make the final decision about whether to follow a suggested treatment regimen in any health care relationship. This is difficult for many health care professionals to accept. We suggest that the ideal goal is for clients to take responsibility not only for implementing a plan of care but for determining their own needs and planning a program, if they so choose.

In addition to difficulties in letting go of responsibility for clients' health, many nurses often underestimate the influence of the family in health choices. In many cultures, the individual does not have the power to make significant health decisions. Indeed, as Leininger (1978) suggests, "The greater the signs of group caring behavior espoused by a culture, the less evidence of a desire for self-care by the client of the designated culture." Self-care should be viewed in the context of the family as well as the individual, because the individual is an integral part of the family that shapes health values and behavior.

HEALTH ASSESSMENT

As mentioned earlier, most tools designed to assess health, such as the annual physical examination, actually assess disease or the absence of disease rather than health. For example, a normal blood pressure indicates that a person is not hypertensive but says nothing about the state of the cardiovascular system of a person in excellent physical condition. Another tool, the Health Hazard Appraisal, approaches health assessment through risk of illness. For example, questions deal with certain known risk factors including personal habits such as smoking or amount of alcohol intake. This approach suggests that one can assess health by assessing this risk of illness. Most of these tools suggest changes in life-style that may help to prevent illness, because it is in the area of risk factors for illness that most of the research has been done. In addition, some illnesses such as heart disease or cancer are so well-defined that there are categories or stages within which an individual can be placed. We need to define health with similar kinds of criteria and levels and to develop tools that suggest specific actions needed to promote good health.

There have been some recent innovative schemes developed which attempt to assess health. For example, Maslow's hierarchy of needs has been used in health assessment. Ardell (1977) suggests five areas of wellness assessment—self-responsibility, environmental sensitivity, stress management, physical fitness, and nutritional awareness. Breslow and Somers (1977) present a health monitoring program using a developmental framework, listing health goals for ten periods from gestation to old age.

It is difficult to discuss self-care in health in the absence of valid assessment tools. However, there are certain components of health that need to be included in any health assessment, some of which are included in the schemes mentioned above. Each component is important in and of itself, but the integration of these components and overall balance of activities that influence them are critical for the individual's health status. In planning self-care, each component must be assessed individually and in relation to the total (see Figure 4-4).

Nutrition and Elimination

To assess nutritional status, the nurse needs to ask about factors that influence the individual or family's diet. Such factors include individual food preferences, ethnic food practices, use of popular diets, perceptions about ideal body weight, and nutritional goals, such as weight gain or reduction or increased intake of fiber. Body weight and height should be measured and compared with the individual's ideal weight, as determined by an objective standard such as that provided by the Metropolitan Life Insurance Company (1983) and reproduced in Chapter 7 (see Table 7-2). The effect of obesity on overall health must be considered.

Elimination patterns vary considerably from individual to individual. Assessment begins with discussing past patterns of bowel and bladder functions and what the client perceives as having influenced these patterns. For example, do certain foods or stress influence elimination patterns? Is the client dissatisfied with past or current patterns? Does the client understand the relationship between fluids, fiber, and exercise and elimination? A full discussion of self-care techniques in nutrition and elimination is presented in Chapter 7.

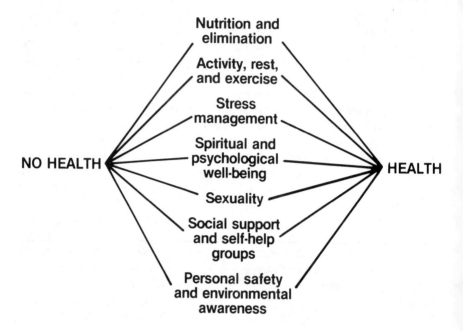

Figure 4-4. Components of health critical for individual's health status (Adapted from Shortridge LM: Conceptualization of the health continuum, 1978, unpublished).

Activity, Rest, and Exercise

A very important area for assessment is the client's awareness of the need for balance in rest and activity. The nurse and client determine together whether the client is in tune with his bodily cues for more rest, more activity, or a better balance. Some individuals have much more energy than others and more need for physical outlets; for others, intellectual activities take precedence over physical activities; both, however, need adequate rest.

The relationship between inadequate exercise and many health problems, such as depression, musculoskeletal problems, heart disease, and obesity (Bailey 1977) has received recent public and professional attention. To assess an individual's physical fitness potential, it is important to establish a baseline for activity patterns and exercise behavior. Such patterns include past exercise routines, beliefs and attitudes about exercise, and perceived needs for exercise. Before one can plan fitness activities, it is important to establish goals for which the individual needs to be fit, whether the goal is running a marathon or climbing a flight of stairs with comfort. Areas to assess include strength, endurance, cardiovascular functioning, flexibility, speed, balance, agility, coordination, level of energy, and reaction time. For a full discussion of these areas and specific self-care activities, see Chapter 8.

Stress Management

Although some level of stress is unavoidable, and in fact encourages adaptation, certain types of prolonged intense stress can lead to alterations in health and subsequent illness. Manifestations of stress include fatigue, malaise, muscle tension, elevated blood pressure and heart rate, and changes in hair, skin, weight, sleep patterns, and activity level. The client may describe feelings of anxiety and frustration and display nervous behavior. In assessing the level of stress, the client needs to become aware of the specific stressors in his environment and his individual responses to them. The nurse can facilitate such awareness as well as teach specific stress management techniques, such as those described in Chapter 9.

Psychological and Spiritual Well-Being

We regard this component in the broadest sense to include one's sense of purpose and meaning in life and a sense of fitting into one's world, however defined by one's cultural group. This component can include religious faith, such practices as meditation, or working for a cause one defines as meaningful. It also includes feelings of emotional well-being, emotional stability, satisfaction, and comfort, which for the most part predominate over negative or stressful emotions. The nurse and client assess this area for the purpose of helping the client find ways of increasing psychological well-being. Problems in this area often indicate problems in many other areas, such as inadequate social support or poor physical fitness. See Chapter 10 for a more detailed discussion.

Sexuality

Sexual self-care is an important component of health assessment and an area in which many nurses are not comfortable. Nurses can advocate sexual self-care in a number of areas including problems achieving sexual satisfaction, communication with partners, or birth control. Nurses can help clients to deal with changes in their sexual needs and expression during different developmental stages, such as adolescence, pregnancy, or aging. The most important asssessment factor in the area of sexuality is whether or not individuals are comfortable in the way they choose to express sexuality, whether the preference is heterosexual, bisexual, homosexual, or celibate. For a full discussion of sexuality, see Chapter 11.

Social Support

There is a recent emphasis on the importance of social support in maintaining health. Cobb (1976) defines social support as the reception of information that leads an individual to believe that he is cared for and loved, is esteemed and valued, and is a member of a network of mutual obligation. The quality of the client's relationships with close family members and friends has an influence on overall health status, as shown in several recent studies summarized by Cobb (1976). In addition, a strong social support system enhances a person's ability to cope with life changes. The nurse facilitates self-care by working with clients to assess their social support system and helping them to decide if and what changes are necessary. For a full discussion of social support and self-help groups, see Chapter 12.

Personal Safety and Environmental Awareness

Rogers (1970, 1980) views man and environment as interactive and integral systems in which a change in one system is related to a change in the other. Thus, for example, human industrial activities which pollute the environment influence human health, in Rogers' view. Self-care activities, such as recycling aluminum and glass, energy conservation, decreased use of the automobile for short trips, and not littering reflect a respect for the environment and a commitment to its health. Awareness of the environment also includes one's personal space; the nurse and client can discuss its characteristics, and effects on the client, and ways of increasing safety in the home, the road, and the workplace. See Chapter 13 for more detailed discussion.

Integral to the process of assessing specific health components listed above is assessing the individual's ability for self-care. This ability includes a motivation for taking responsibility, an ability to learn, a problem-solving ability, and the ability to make decisions and implement changes in life-style. The assessment process ends with a list of the client's needs and strengths in each area.

However, a very important part of the nurse's role in health assessment is facilitating clients' abilities to assess their own health. There are a number of benefits in the process of self-assessment. Clients become increasingly sensitive to subtle changes in their physical and emotional health. They relate more specific information to the nurse, which enhances the nurse-client partnership. Self-assessment is one of the major tools for health teaching. For example, in any nutritional assessment, clients evaluate their intake of substances such as salt, sugar, fiber, and caffeine, which then provides an arena for education. Self-assessment helps to increase clients' sense of power and control and reinforces their responsibility for their own health. Finally, increased awareness of one's own health is the first step for changing behavior.

PLANNING FOR SELF-CARE

Decision-making and health choices. As mentioned previously, health is intimately related to life-style, and life-style can be defined as the personal decisions over which people have control. Many life-style decisions are made in childhood or adolescence and are a product of a person's socialization. Thus, the individual may not be fully aware of the reasons some decisions were made. For example, a woman's choice of not engaging in strenuous physical activity may be based on her decision not to be physically strong, which she perceives as "unfeminine." Influences on life-style decision-making include sex, age, social status, traditional roles, and who is seen to be the decision-maker in the family.

The nurse and client need to discuss and understand past decisions and current choices, so that the client can consider making deliberate decisions to enhance health. In partnership with clients and/or their families, the nurse can facilitate conscious decisions which lead to goals for self-care in health.

Setting health goals. Health goals are based on the data collected by assessing current health status, health behaviors, and the client's baseline or usual mode of functioning. The most important part of setting health goals is choosing goals that are realistic. For example, on beginning an exercise program, a goal of running three miles a day sets up the client for failure if the client has not run previously. Goals are most effective when stated in terms of *long-term goals*, which establish a direction for change, and *short-term goals*, which can be accomplished in a short period of time. Goals will be most effectively acted on and met if they aim for *small* changes. If the client's long-term goal, for example, is to decrease stress, a short-term goal would be to increase awareness of the present stress level. The individual beginning an exercise program may set a short-term goal of running one half mile twice weekly and a long-term goal of three miles four times weekly.

Another important rule in setting goals is to work on changing only one behavior at a time. We are all aware of individuals who fail when they attempt to diet and to stop smoking at the same time. In contrast, working on only *one* behavior at a time may have a ripple effect that influences a person to gradually change others. For example, increasing physical activity may decrease a person's desire to smoke.

Goals should be chosen that can be attained with reasonable effort and within a short amount of time. When a goal is attained, it serves as positive reinforcement and encourages the client to continue in a healthy direction. On the other hand, failure to meet a goal can be discouraging and work against motivation to change behavior.

IMPLEMENTATION AND EVALUATION

The implementation of self-care plans is based on the health assessment as well as on health goals. When encouraging clients to use self-care, it is essential that the plan fit the client's own goals. If plans are based only on the nurse's goals, the client is less likely to act on such plans.

Self-care plans need to be based on answers to the following questions:

● What action is necessary to achieve each goal?
● How long should the action be carried out?
● Who are the people who will support or sabotage the plan, and how will they do so?
● What ideas expressed by the client will support or sabotage the plan?

An important part of planning is setting up a time for evaluation; no plan is complete without evaluation. Criteria for evaluating a self-care plan should be based on whether or not the client has met the short-term goals, and the response to that changed behavior. For example, a young woman who successfully met her goal of ending constipation through dietary changes was unhappy with a weight gain of five pounds. Through evaluation, she decided to change to low-calorie, high-fiber foods.

The evaluation may reveal that the plan has failed, and new goals must be set or new plans for the original goals must be set. Thus, the nursing process is ongoing.

SUMMARY

In this chapter, we explored universal, cultural, and individual definitions of health and their influence on the health assessment process. Although health and illness status coexist in the same individual, we separated them for the purpose of analysis and because such separation suggests different self-care interventions. In the next chapter, self-care assessment and intervention in acute and chronic illness will be described.

CASE EXAMPLE

Carlos is a 42-year-old, Mexican-American salesman who is married and has two children. His wife's family lives on the same block in a middle-class neighborhood. Carlos has a blood pressure of 146/92. His physician suggested a low sodium diet and referred him to the nurse to help him learn stress management. Together, the nurse and Carlos assess the stressors in his environment; he describes his physical response to stress—headaches and feelings of anxiety. The nurse gives Carlos a self-assessment tool so that he can learn the principles of self-assessment.

Having completed the self-assessment, Carlos informs the nurse that he has discovered that while he is driving in heavy traffic, he clenches his jaw and gets a stiff neck. He also notes that his heart rate increases and he feels quite uncomfortable during family gatherings when his mother-in-law brings up his financial state for discussion.

When the assessment is complete, the nurse and Carlos begin to set goals. Carlos states that his goal is to manage the stress, but the nurse suggests that such a general goal does not suggest specific actions. They agree that stress management is a long-term goal and decide to work with his response to one stressor, traffic, as a short-term goal. Carlos must decide whether his goal will be to eliminate, or avoid, the stressor in his environment or to alter his response. He might use a car pool or public transportation to decrease the stressor. On the other hand, he might decide to alter his physical response to the stress of driving in traffic through relaxation techniques such as autogenics, biofeedback, or deep breathing.

Carlos decides that car pooling or public transportation would be too inconvenient in his job and wants to alter his response to stress. The nurse provides Carlos with information about specific relaxation techniques, discussing their similarities and differences. He chooses deep breathing and progressive relaxation to help him decrease his jaw clenching and stiff neck. The nurse teaches him the techniques, and together they set up a self-care plan. He plans to do a full body progressive relaxation exercise for 15–20 minutes each morning upon arising and again every night before bed. He will also take his blood pressure twice a day. When he is driving in traffic, he will do neck and shoulder muscle tightening and releases at stop signals and will do deep slow breathing when he finds that he is clenching his jaw.

Carlos and the nurse identify the people and thoughts that might sabotage the plan. His wife wants him to help her with the children in the morning because she also works, and he wonders whether he will have the time and quiet in order to practice relaxation. He decides to ask her for her support and will get up earlier to do his exercises. He also verbalizes his thoughts about the plan. The nurse inquires about whether he believes that progressive relaxation will influence his response to stress. Does he verbalize doubts about the effectiveness of this technique?

The last part of the planning process is building in a method of evaluation. The nurse instructs Carlos to write down the number of times he does the exercises each day and to note the number of stress symptoms he experiences and the conditions under which they appear.

Carlos carries out his self-care plan for three weeks and makes a return visit to the nurse in order to evaluate the plan. He explains that he found it impossible to do the early A.M. exercises but was able to take the time to do them at lunch. He has had fewer headaches and reports that his jaw clenching has significantly decreased. He attributes this decrease to having become aware of when he begins to clench his jaw and relaxing it immediately. The progressive relaxation exercises and deep breathing have been effective in eliminating his stiff neck. His blood pressure at this visit is 130/84. Carlos and the nurse decide that he should continue the same program of self-care for another three weeks and will meet together to plan a new, short-term goal. To summarize, Carlos' self-care plan is shown on page 69.

SELF-CARE PLAN FOR CASE EXAMPLE

Assessment	Plan	Implementation	Evaluation
Inadequate stress management leading to jaw clenches and stiff neck when driving	Increase awareness of stress symptoms such as jaw clenching and stiff neck	Self-assessment of stress	*In two weeks:* Performance of relaxation exercises Client's attitude toward stress management Number of episodes of clenched jaw and stiff neck
Hypertension related to above.	Improve ability to relax	Learn Progressive Relaxation • Practice 15–20 minutes progressive relaxation exercises twice daily. • Practice shoulder and neck exercises in car. Practice deep breathing when jaw clenches.	Ability to carry out exercises. Number of times exercise carried out. Number of times shoulder and neck exercises carried out. Outcome of relaxation and deep breathing.
	Control blood pressure	Monitor blood pressure twice daily, in A.M. and h.s.	Blood pressure reading

CASE EXAMPLE*

Kate is a 32-year-old, white, married, primipara who is in her seventh month of pregnancy. She works full time as a recruiting officer for a bank. She describes herself as "a basically healthy person" and expresses a desire to participate in her own prenatal care. She and her husband are excited about the pregnancy and are beginning natural childbirth classes.

Kate and the nurse do a health assessment and identify three areas of concern—constipation, fatigue, and anxiety stemming from her concern about how her role will change when she delivers her baby. Together, Kate and the nurse set short-term goals that will address these concerns specifically and devise a general self-care plan consisting of the activities listed on pages 72 to 74.

Kate carried out the self-care plan for two weeks and met again with the nurse. They discussed Kate's three initial concerns and evaluated how the plan had worked. She had been able to increase her fluid intake and incorporate more roughage into her daily diet and found that her bowel movements had become more regular and softer. Fatigue had also been lessened through more sleep at night and more rest during the day. Once Kate tried the plan she realized that she really did need more rest at this time. Kate decided to continue these changed behaviors. Her anxiety about role change had not lessened significantly, despite attempts to talk with her husband about how their life would change once the baby arrived. Kate stated that part of her problem was that she did not have any friends who had babies or young children. The nurse suggested that she begin to attend La Leche League meetings, since she intended to breastfeed. Through this group she could meet other women with young infants and have the chance to participate in discussions of what it is like to have a first baby.

Following discussion of the three areas of concern, Kate and the nurse discussed the other parts of the self-care plan. Kate consistently drank five glasses of water, ate fresh fruit and vegetables daily, and practiced relaxation techniques regularly. The one activity she never attempted was daily prenatal exercises, rationalizing her aversion to a specific exercise routine by describing herself as lazy. In modifying the care plan, Kate agreed to substitute 15 minutes of walking daily for the exercises, an activity she enjoyed. In addition, she expressed difficulty in determining the correct food groups in which her food choices belonged. The nurse provided a different nutritional assessment tool for Kate, suggesting that she keep a three-day diary, and provided her with a list of foods with each grouping.

---

*Case contributed by Parrie Lambert, R.N., B.S., Staff R.N., Planned Parenthood, Oakland, California

A major limitation of Kate's self-care plan became obvious when the medical decision was made to perform a cesarean section. Although both Kate and her husband Parker had seen a childbirth film that covered cesarean birth, neither felt prepared when the decision was reached. Preparation for both vaginal and cesarean birth would have been very helpful in this regard.

A visit to the family one week following delivery of a nine pound, two ounce girl revealed that other aspects of the plan had been beneficial. Kate was breastfeeding successfully and effectively using support people for tasks that she was unable to do. The outcome of Kate and Parker's discussions about attitudes and feelings about parenting was a smooth beginning transition from a couple to a one-child family. Parker was actively involved in all aspects of baby care, and they both expressed pleasure with their new daughter. Their evaluation of the self-care plan was positive, and they noted benefits of increased knowledge, feelings of confidence, and less fear in an unknown situation.

SELF-CARE PLAN FOR CASE EXAMPLE

	Assessment	Planning	Implementation	Evaluation
Nutrition, Elimination	Constipation secondary to pregnancy and iron supplementation	Increase frequency of bowel movements	Kate will drink at least 5 glasses of water each day.	Number of glasses of water
		Decrease discomfort associated with constipation	Have at least 1 serving of bran, fresh fruit, or vegetables at each meal	Frequency of discomfort with bowel movements Number of bowel movements Number of servings of bran, fresh fruits, and vegetables
		Food intake, bowel pattern assessment	Kate will learn to keep a food diary and bowel pattern record and learn the purpose of each of the above interventions.	Evaluations of Kate's food and bowel patterns
Activity, Rest, and Exercise	Fatigue	Decrease fatigue	Kate will go to sleep an hour earlier and get at least eight hours of sleep each night.	Hour of bedtime for one week, Number of hours of sleep each night Subjective feelings of energy vs. fatigue
			Kate will elevate feet for 15 minutes at lunch and after work.	Number of times feet were elevated
			Kate will take afternoon naps on weekends	Number of naps taken Feeling of fatigue

Activity, Rest, and Exercise	Need for prenatal exercises	Achieve and maintain adequate exercise level	Kate will practice prenatal exercises with Parker	Number of days exercises were practiced
		Prepare for childbirth	Kate and Parker will participate in childbirth preparation classes	Number of childbirth preparation classes attended
				Feeling of preparedness for childbirth
Spiritual and Psychological Well-being	Anxiety about pregnancy and childbirth	Increase positive feelings about self and parenting	Kate and Parker will discuss new feelings about pregnancy and parenting	Number, length and quality of discussions
				Outcomes of discussions
				Subjective feelings about parenting
		Answer questions related to parenting	Get together with friends to discuss feelings	Number of get togethers and outcomes.
			Kate will practice exercises visualizing self as a good mother	Number of times visualization and relaxation exercises practiced
			Kate will practice relaxation exercises	Outcome of exercises
				Feeling of anxiety

SELF-CARE PLAN FOR CASE EXAMPLE (CONTINUED)

Assessment	Planning	Implementation	Evaluation
		In two weeks:	
Spiritual and Psycho-logical Well-Being	Anxiety about new mother role	Increase positive feelings about self and parenting	Kate will attend La Leche League or other prenatal support group	Number of meetings attended Number of contacts/friendships formed Subjective feelings of anxiety about new mother role
Nutrition and Elimination	Inability to determine the correct food groups in which her food choices belonged	Increase knowledge of food groups Increase ability to determine the correct food groups in which her food choices belong	Kate will use assessment tools for nutrition Kate will learn to keep a three-day food diary Kate and the nurse will review the four food groups and prenatal diet	Ability to determine the food groups in which her food choices Ability to assess her own nutrition

CASE EXAMPLE

Terry is a 58-year-old, Irish-American woman who has a history of alcoholism and fibrocystic breast disease. Through the help of Alchoholics Anonymous, she has not consumed alcohol in 15 years. She came to the outpatient clinic of the university hospital for "a checkup," stating that she had not seen a doctor in 10 years. The medical resident examined Terry and clinical studies were completed, determining that Terry had no major health problems at the current time. However, because she should have been examining her breasts on a regular basis, she was referred to the nurse for health teaching.

The nurse completed the nursing data base and asked Terry to complete several self-assessment questionnaires. They reviewed the information together. The nurse learned that Terry is a widow who lives alone and takes the bus to the office in which she is employed as a secretary. Terry described her work as "very stressful," although she "sits most of the day." She also described skipping lunch several days a week, substituting a cup of coffee, when work pressure was high. Terry has smoked for 28 years and has tried to stop several times. She expressed a desire to stop now but is afraid that she will fail again.

The nurse and Terry list the following self-care needs:

1. Need for exercise
2. Need for relaxation
3. Need to perform regular breast self-examination
4. Need for a balanced diet and regular meals
5. Need to stop smoking.

The nurse and Terry decided to begin the self-care plan with breast self-exam and relaxation. The nurse taught Terry to do a thorough breast examination and gave her written materials to take home. They also discussed how Terry might best incorporate regular relaxation sessions into her day. Terry expressed an interest in learning to meditate and stated that she wanted to take an evening class at the local high school. The nurse also taught Terry to do progressive muscle relaxation for the purpose of taking a rest in the women's lounge after lunch, particularly when her work day was hectic.

Although Terry wanted to stop smoking, the nurse explained that smoking cessation would probably be easier after Terry had incorporated regular relaxation routines into her usual daily activities. Breast self-examination and relaxation were chosen because they could be utilized immediately. The positive effects of these self-care activities, and the confidence Terry would gain by taking steps to improve her health, would provide a basis for more difficult subsequent life-style changes such as increasing exercise, improving her diet, and smoking cessation.

Discussion Questions

1. Give two examples of alterations in health.
2. A 15-year-old Samoan-American girl, who appears to be of ideal body weight, complains that she is "too skinny" and seeks information from you about how to gain weight. List five questions that you would ask her.
3. Set up a self-care plan for a 33-year-old salesman who complains of chronic constipation.
4. What would you say to a 65-year-old man who describes himself as healthy, but who has smoked for 40 years?
5. A 32-year-old mother of two children has just moved from another state and complains of early morning insomnia. On which components of health assessment would you focus initially?

REFERENCES

Ardell DB: High-Level Wellness, An Alternative to Doctors, Drugs, and Disease. Rodale Press, Emmaus, Pennsylvania, 1977

Bailey C: Fit or Fat? Houghton Mifflin Company, Boston, Massachusetts, 1977

Breslow L, Somers, A: The life-time health-monitoring program: A practical approach to preventive medicine. New England Journal of Medicine. Vol 296, No 11, pp 601–608, 1977

Bullough VL, Bullough B: Health Care for the Other Americans, Appleton-Century-Crofts, New York, 1982

Cobb S: Social support as a moderator of life stress. Psychosomatic Medicine, Vol 68, No 5, pp 300–304, 1976

Dunn HL: High-level wellness for man and society. American Journal of Public Health, Vol 49, No 6, pp 786–792, 1959

Gragg SH, Rees OM: Scientific Principles of Nursing, 7th ed., The C.V. Mosby Company, St. Louis, Missouri, 1976

Ineser CW: Ineser's Cyclopedic Medical Dictionary, 9th ed. F.A. Davis, Philadelphia, Pennsylvania, 1962

LaLonde M: Guest editorial, The Canadian Nurse, Vol 70, No 1, pp 19–20, 1974

Laffrey SC: Health Behavior Choice as Related to Self-Actualization, Body Weight, and Health Conception. Unpublished doctoral dissertation, Wayne State University, 1982

Lamberton MM: Health-Illness: A Conceptual Model Based on Coexistence Hypothesis. Unpublished paper, Denver, Colorado, 1978

Leininger MM: Transcultural Nursing: Concepts, Theories, and Practices. John Wiley & Sons, Inc., New York, 1978

Maslow AH: Motivation and Personality, 2nd ed. Harper and Row, New York, 1970

Metropolitan Insurance Companies: 1983 Metropolitan Height and Weight Tables, New York, 1983

Murray RB, Zentner JP: Nursing Concepts for Health Promotion. Prentice-Hall, Inc., Englewood Cliffs, New Jersey, 1979

Noble E: Essential Exercises for the Childbearing Years. Houghton Mifflin, Boston, Massachusetts, 1976

Norbeck JS, Lindsey AM, Carrieri BL: The development of an instrument to measure social support. Nursing Research, Vol 30, No 5, pp 264–269, 1981
Orem DE: Nursing Concepts of Practice. McGraw-Hill Book Company, New York, 1971
Rogers M: An Introduction to the Theoretical Basis of Nursing. F.A. Davis Company, Philadelphia, Pennsylvania, 1970
Rogers M: Nursing: A science of unitary man. In Riehl J, Roy C: Conceptual Models for Nursing Practice, 2nd ed. Appleton-Century-Crofts, New York, 1980
Shortridge LM: Conceptualization of the Health Continuum. Unpublished, 1978
Shortridge LM, Lee EJ: Introduction to Nursing Practice. McGraw-Hill Book Company, New York, 1980
Smith JA: The idea of health: A philosophical inquiry. Advances in Nursing Science, Vol 3, No 3, pp 43–50, 1981

5

Self-Care in Illness

The process of self-care in illness covers the whole spectrum from disease prevention to detection and management. Most people find it easy to visualize self-care behaviors that promote health, such as balanced nutrition and stress management but find it more difficult to envision self-care behaviors in illness, especially in such settings as critical care units. However, the acute phase in a client's illness can be a productive time to begin teaching self-care behaviors and techniques. This chapter focuses on the self-care process as it relates to three categories of illness—acute self-limiting or minor illness, major acute illness, and chronic illness.

Disease patterns in the United States have shifted over the past 40 years from a prevalence of acute infectious diseases to a prevalence of chronic illness. In spite of this shift, medical care is still oriented toward acute illness. Although popular belief holds that people who have chronic illness are cared for in such special facilities as nursing homes or clinics, most people with chronic illness are hospitalized in cure-oriented settings for acute phases of their illnesses. Specific self-care strategies for managing chronic illness are not usually taught in academic curricula nor are they advocated in acute care settings.

COMPONENTS OF SELF-CARE IN ILLNESS

Self-care behaviors in illness can be described in terms of three categories—prevention, detection, and management (see Figure 5-1). An important consideration in each of these components is the client's knowledge of when and for what reasons to seek professional care and appropriate use of the health care system.

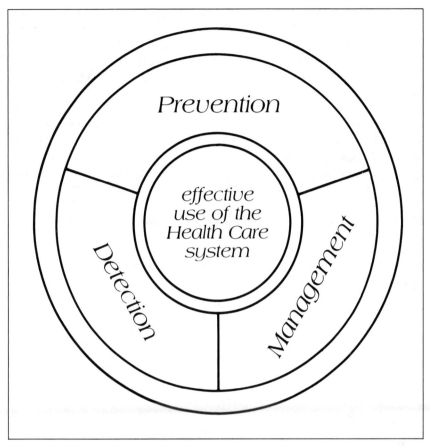

Figure 5-1. Three categories of self-care behaviors in illness.

Prevention

The first component of self-care in illness is preventing the occurrence of an illness or accident. An individual's awareness of the risk for illness or accidents, as well as this individual's susceptibility to a particular illness, is a key factor in prevention. The Health Hazard Appraisal (Goetz 1980, Wagner, Berry, Schoenbach, and Graham 1982) is an excellent tool for increasing awareness of how personal habits such as smoking, overeating, or excessive stress can lead to illness.

Motivation to engage in preventive behaviors is influenced by the individual's perception of the severity and susceptibility to an injury or illness (Becker, Drachman and Kirscht 1972; Haefner and Kirscht 1970; Rosenstock 1966; Suchman 1967). Most people are less concerned about preventing a cold than they are about preventing cancer or heart disease. In addition, the meaning individuals attach to a particular illness varies with their life situations. For example, an adolescent might be less concerned about a cold interfering with school attendance than with attendance at a football game. The Health Belief Model outlines such variations (see Chapters 2 and 3).

Examples of self-care behaviors to prevent acute self-limiting or minor illness include dental flossing and brushing to prevent tooth decay and gum disease, handwashing, avoiding close contact with others who have colds, and adequate rest. Prevention of major acute illness includes smoking cessation, receipt of immunizations, reduction of dietary cholesterol and fats, maintenance of ideal weight, use of seat belts, and avoidance of exposure to radiation.

In chronic illness, prevention is geared toward preventing slow deterioration and potential crises associated with chronic illness, such as cardiac arrests, epileptic seizures, or insulin shock. Prevention also relates to other conditions that might complicate the primary illness. For example, diabetics who regulate their diet and insulin correctly can minimize such complications as peripheral neuropathy, diabetic retinopathy, infection, or heart disease. (See Table 5-1 for examples of self-care behaviors for prevention.)

TABLE 5-1. PREVENTION

Illness or Injury	Self-Care Behavior
Burns	Sunscreen, potholders, smoke alarms
Accidents	Home safety, seat belts
Gum disease	Dental flossing
Tooth decay	Brushing, flouride
Colds	Adequate diet, rest
Communicable diseases	Immunizations
Cardiovascular disease	Decrease smoking
Cancer of lung, throat, mouth, esophagus	Decrease smoking
Irritability, insomnia, anxiety, cardiac arrhythmias	Decrease caffeine, increase exercise
Arteriosclerotic disease	Decrease cholesterol
Cirrhosis	Decrease alcohol
Obesity, diabetes, hypertension	Weight control
Crisis associated with diabetes, hypertension	Regulation of diet
Seizures	Adherence to medication regimen
Acute asthma	Avoidance of allergens
Aversion of crisis	Awareness of subtle changes
Social isolation	Social support
Social stigma	Self-help groups

Detection

Early detection of an illness can make a significant difference in its outcome. This is an area in which what a client does or does not do is very important. For example, early detection of breast cancer through breast self-examinations may modify the surgical procedure, alter or eliminate the need for chemotherapy, and significantly improve the prognosis.

Detection of minor or self-limiting illness, such as upper respiratory infections or backaches, allows the individual to take actions that will minimize more severe problems. Also, some self-limiting illnesses can be precursors to major acute illnesses, such as stress-related hypertension possibly leading to heart or kidney disease. Sensitivity to changes in one's body (such as pain, elimination, or appetite patterns) or psyche (excessive sleeping, irritability, confusion) can be crucial in detecting early signs of acute illness. Diagnostic tests, most of which are professionally administered, are other important means of detection. Some tests, such as blood pressure and pulse, throat cultures, urine tests for protein, sugar and acetone, and tests for presence of blood in feces are used increasingly in self-care.

The detection techniques listed below have been used to a greater extent in recent years for chronic illness. Individuals who have a chronic illness need to closely monitor their daily functioning to recognize signs and symptoms of a downward progression of the disease or a potential crisis associated with the disease. See Table 5-2 for examples of self-care behaviors for detection.

TABLE 5-2. DETECTION OF ILLNESS

Illness/Injury	*Self-Care Behavior*
	Tools and Techniques
Strep Throat	Throat Culture
Gastrointestinal Disease	Hemocult Test
Hypertension	Blood Pressure Screening
Cervical Cancer	Pap Smear
Breast Cancer	Breast Self-exam
Testicular Cancer	Testicular Self-exam
Diabetes	Urine Testing
Stress, Depression, Major Illness	*Awareness of Usual Functioning*
	Weight Changes
	Appetite Change
	Sleep Pattern Changes
	Pain
	Elimination Changes

Management

Although we usually associate the management of disease with professional care, we must not underestimate the client's capabilities to manage illness. A number of studies document the fact that most people successfully manage acute self-limiting illnesses without professional consultation (Dunnell and Cartwright 1972; Elliott-Bins 1973; Freer 1980). Although self-care is universal, specific self-care practices vary considerably with various cultural and family backgrounds. It is important, however, for the individual and family to recognize at what point in an illness professional help should be sought. Current self-care books, such as *Take Care of Yourself: A Consumer's Guide to Medical Care* (Vickery and Fries 1978) and *How to be Your Own Doctor (Sometimes)* (Sehnert 1975) can be helpful in this regard.

Although self-care in minor or acute self-limiting illnesses is generally well-accepted, many people will argue that there is little place for self-care in major illnesses, especially in the acute care setting. Clearly, when the client is being wheeled into the cardiac care unit, self-care is not a high priority in the minds of client, family, or staff. As soon as clients are stable, however, the client and the client's family should be included in the care, even in the cardiac care unit. While providing physical care for the client, the nurse can explain what is being done and why and encourage the client and family to participate progressively as the client improves. Examples of self-care activities include deep breathing, range-of-motion exercises, bathing, planning diet, bringing in special foods, keeping track of intake and output, and managing medication.

Among the barriers to self-care in major illness are the client's fear and discomfort in the hospital environment, as well as the stress associated with the illness and limitations imposed by the client's condition. Family members may also be uncomfortable and either avoid the hospital or refuse to leave the client alone in what they perceive as a hostile or dangerous environment. The nurse can be instrumental in helping to decrease the client's and family's fears by involving them to the best of their ability in the client's care, from asking questions to participating in treatments. By so doing, the nurse can help to demystify the experience and to give the client and family a sense of control in what may appear to be an uncontrollable situation.

Management of chronic illness involves a number of tasks which the individual must accomplish to maintain an altered level of health and to prevent crises and deterioration (see Table 5-4). Such tasks include carrying out a prescribed treatment regimen as well as making appropriate choices available within the regimen. For example, individuals with diabetes could possibly increase or decrease the insulin dosage they take depending on variations in activity or the amount of stress in their current social settings. Another part of management involves life-style changes in such areas as nutrition, activity, and rest, and others described in Chapter

4. Life-style changes include informing co-workers and acquaintances of how they can help in the event of a crisis and carrying necessary equipment and instructions on one's person.

TABLE 5-3. MANAGEMENT OF ILLNESS

Illness	Self-Care Behavior
Colds, Flu	Increase rest Increase fluids
Upper Respiratory Infections	Gargle Voice rest (Antibiotics, if prescribed) Increase humidity/vaporizer Aspirin
Diarrhea	Increase fluids Decrease dairy products Decrease fiber/roughage
Myocardial Infarction	Diet: decrease cholesterol decrease fat decrease salt Exercise: balance activity and rest cardiac rehabilitation program Medications Take pulse and blood pressure Stress management
Breast Cancer	Medication Prothesis purchase Diet (popular/experimental) Self-help groups

Finally, a major and difficult aspect of management of chronic illness is retaining an identity apart from the illness. For example, we can all think of people who identify themselves as "heart patients" and "cancer patients" instead of unique individuals who have heart disease or cancer. In the interest of health, it is critically important for the client to develop and maintain a sense of control over the disease rather than feeling that the disease has control of him. Table 5-3 contains examples of self-care management in minor, major, and chronic illness.

TABLE 5-4. COPING WITH CHRONIC ILLNESS

Necessary Tasks	Learning Needs
• Coping with life-style changes • Acceptance of the illness and treatment • Retaining one's identity apart from the illness • Redefining health and maximum health potential • Redefining family relationships and social support • Coping with discomfort • Coping with stigma	• Anatomy, physiology, pathophysiology of affected systems • Strategies for controlling symptoms • Techniques for organizing time for the treatment regimen

THE NURSING PROCESS

The assumption of responsibility and the process of assessment, decision-making, goal setting, planning, implementation, and evaluation are as useful for self-care in illness as they are for self-care in health.

In addition to the meaning the professional attaches to the client's illness, it is imperative to elicit the individual's and family's perception of the illness; it is this meaning that determines the decisions clients make and the extent to which they initiate and utilize self-care. The meaning attached to a set of symptoms is based on the individual's personality, lifestyle, family, values, and culture. For example, a 21-year-old college student who has pre-end-stage renal disease attributes his fatigue to his heavy course load and the winter months rather than to his anemia. Thus, he does not view his fatigue as illness-related and is not willing to participate in self-care. As another example, in some tribal societies in Africa, intestinal parasites are endemic and so universal that they are viewed not as illness at all, but as necessary for digestion. Thus, such people do not view treatment for worms as necessary.

Decision-Making and Responsibility

Based on the meaning the individuals and their families attribute to a set of symptoms, decisions are made to act or not to act. Individuals and their significant others decide what is treatable without professional consultation and when professional attention is necessary. People also make decisions about what kind of professional care to seek. For example, a Mexican-American folk illness is "mal ojo," or "evil eye," a disorder of children characterized by fitful sleep, crying with no apparent reason, fever, vomiting, and diarrhea, which occurs when another person admires a child without actually touching. Mal ojo is perceived as not being curable by conventional medicine, so a curandero (folk healer) is sought to perform a cure. Table 5-5 depicts the kinds of choices people can make between self-care and professional care, as well as between different types of professional care that are available.

TABLE 5-5. CHOICES FOR CARE

	Western Scientific Medicine		Indigenous or Popular Medicine	
Professional Care	Nurse Physician Physical Therapist Psychologist Nutritionist Social Worker		Curandero Espiritista Homeopath Masseuse Rolfer Acupuncturist	Touch Healer Rootworker Herbalist Minister
Self-Care	Home Throat Culture Blood Pressure Urine Testing Taking Temperature Increasing Fluids Insulin		Meditation Acupressure Prayer Herbs Pendulum Diet Therapy (e.g., hot and cold foods)	

*Adapted from Ferguson T: Self-Care and Alternative Medicine. Medical Self-Care, Summit Books, New York, 1980

The number, kinds, and seriousness of the decisions that face the client vary depending on the severity of the illness. Decisions exist in such areas as diagnostic procedures and medical and surgical therapies as well as life-style decisions. In many situations, the client must make such decisions in circumstances of uncertainty and stress. The nurse can play an important role in providing detailed information and emotional support so that the individual can make appropriate decisions; we repeat that no matter what the nurse thinks that the client should do, the decisions are ultimately the client's own.

Assessment

Assessment of illness covers two important areas—a professional emphasis on pathology and the perception of a changed bodily or mental state and the meaning attached to it. Because most medical care focuses on assessment of pathology, we suggest that the reader consult the literature on review of systems and physical and psychological assessment. As Figure 5-2 illustrates, illness assessment by health professionals is usually related to specific diseases or systems in the body, such as the respiratory system or the gastrointestinal system.

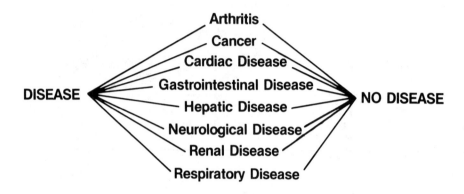

Figure 5-2. Assessment of illness.

In the acute care setting, assessment can serve as an excellent tool for teaching clients, especially in linking life-style behaviors with the current illness. For example, a man who is about to have coronary bypass surgery can link the role of dietary fat and cholesterol to heart disease and begin to see that his diet will need to change following surgery. Suggestions for dietary change should not be given judgmentally; helping the client become aware of the relationship between prior health behaviors and current illness is not the same as blaming the victim. In addition to the health components described in Chapter 4, the nurse and client should assess any limitations on self-care imposed by the particular disease and its treatment, as well as specific tasks associated with the disease and treatment.

Setting Goals

The overall purpose of setting goals for self-care in illness is to involve patients in participating effectively in their own care. Realistic goals for self-care are determined by the tasks required for treatment as well as the limitations imposed by the illness and the behavioral changes described in Chapter 4.

It may be unrealistic to expect major behavioral changes during a short hospital stay or self-limiting minor illness. A more appropriate goal is encouraging clients to examine their values and attitudes for the purpose of seeing how they influence their health-related behavior. Rather than blaming or lecturing a client hospitalized for a fractured femur and abdominal injuries following an automobile accident, the nurse can help the client examine the importance of driving within the speed limits, the relationship of alcohol and altered reaction times, and the importance of seat belts.

In the acute care setting or acute phase of a self-limiting illness, another realistic goal is ensuring that the client and family have a basic understanding of the relationship between the illness and its treatment, as well as some indication of the life-style changes that may be necessary. For example, a five-year-old boy is hospitalized for an acute asthma attack. His mother stated that she stopped his prescribed bronchodilators because the medication kept him awake all night and that he had no appetite. The goal was to help the mother and boy understand how the medication works to alleviate the symptoms and to have the boy take his medication regularly. Together the nurse and the mother discuss ways of decreasing his nausea (such as small frequent meals) and helping him to sleep (such as using guided fantasy). Equipped with this knowledge, the mother and boy decide to try the prescribed regimen once again.

Self-Care Planning, Implementation, and Evaluation

It is important to devise plans that are as specific and explicit as possible. Plans should help clients incorporate the treatment regimen into their life-style in a comfortable way that encourages adherence. For example, when a diuretic is prescribed, the nurse should suggest that the client take the medication on arising rather than before going to sleep. Life-style behaviors are often difficult to change. It is also important to consider whether the change involves adding certain behaviors (e.g., taking medication, irrigating a colostomy) or eliminating certain behaviors (e.g., avoiding certain foods or eliminating cigarettes). As described previously, the client should be a partner in devising the self-care plan. The plans should be acceptable and help clients achieve their own goals.

Criteria for evaluation should be built into every self-care plan. The criteria should be measurable. For example, a woman with diabetes was told by her physician to follow an 1800 calorie A.D.A. diet, to test her urine, and to take care of her feet. In a week's time, how would you evaluate her ability to carry out these instructions? Instead, we suggest that the nurse and client should spend some time together planning a diet that includes the number and size of servings of each food group daily, taking into consideration the woman's usual food preferences. If the woman keeps a food diary for three days, bringing it in for evaluation for the following week, criteria are built in. Did she maintain 1800 calories on a daily basis?

Similarly, the nurse needs to *demonstrate* urine testing and ask the woman to give a return demonstration to discuss when to test the urine, how to keep accurate records, and explain why these are important. These records can be used to evaluate the self-care plan. Lastly, the nurse and client talk about diabetic foot care and why it is important. If the client is encouraged to think of ways she can protect her feet, she might decide to stop wearing constrictive shoes. A week later, the criterion to evaluate the self-care plan is whether or not the woman made such changes.

The importance of including evaluation criteria in a self-care plan is that the evaluation points out specifically what parts of the plan did not work. Together, the nurse and client use these data to devise an alternate plan or set new goals. We want to emphasize that when a goal is not achieved, it is the *plan,* and *not* the client, that has failed.

SUMMARY

This chapter described the components of self-care in the face of minor, major and chronic illness, using a framework of prevention, detection, and management. Some general examples of self-care are provided using the framework of the nursing process. Chapters 4 and 5, self-care in health and self-care in illness, focus on what to do, while Chapter 6 focuses on how to do it. We will describe specific strategies on how to teach self-care.

CASE EXAMPLE

Ken is a 33-year-old, white, single man who has been hospitalized for acute episodes of schizophrenia several times since his discharge from the service 10 years ago. Prior to each hospitalization, Ken becomes extremely disorganized in his thinking and either voluntarily admits himself to the hospital or is brought in by the police by virtue of being unable to care for himself or disruptive behavior. He lives with his family of origin and is the oldest of five children. He is closest with his father, his relationships with his mother and brother are strained, and he has never felt close to his sisters, who are significantly younger than he is.

The nurse met Ken the day of his current psychiatric admission. He was brought to the hospital by the police because he was considered gravely disabled (unable to provide self with food, shelter, and clothing). His symptomatology included loose associations, confusion, and delusional ideas involving sexual matters and religion. When asked what brought him back to the hospital, Ken replied, "I'm a paranoid schizophrenic and I took the bus," demonstrating his concrete thinking.

An initial assessment with Ken was difficult to accomplish at this time because his thoughts were too disorganized to relate information in a manner understandable to the nurse. After two weeks of psychotropic medications, however, Ken was significantly more organized and expressed the desire to participate in his own care planning. Ken's assessment indicates that he has a number of psychological and social needs that are being initially addressed by psychotropic medications, supportive psychotherapy, and a structured ward milieu which includes recreational activities and a medication group. He has no significant problems in the physical arena, except that he feels restless, possibly as a side effect of his medications; he is having difficulty getting to meals on time (because of his disorganization) and complains of being frequently hungry.

Ken and the nurse begin self-care planning at this stage in his hospitalization. Short-term goals involve helping him deal with his restlessness and helping him to get to meals on time. The nurse assists him to identify the type of exercise he most enjoys, and they establish a realistic schedule of exercise one to three times a week. Because Ken enjoys golf, arrangements are made for him to go to the driving range Monday and Thursday afternoons. Ken also decides that he wants to begin walking every day after lunch. In reference to meals, the nurse assists Ken in determining ways of functioning more independently (e.g., using his watch) and asking other patients and staff to remind him of meal time. The rest of the staff are alerted to Ken's plans and agree to support them.

Ken implements his plan for a week and is reinforced by the staff with positive feedback. He and the nurse get together again to evaluate the plan. Ken reports that he feels more relaxed and less restless following his golf or daily walks. In addition, he states that he is sleeping better at night. He has missed only one meal during the week, has been late to only two meals, and is not as hungry.

Based on the success of his initial self-care plan, Ken and the nurse begin to formulate long-term goals that will direct his activities following discharge but which he will begin to work toward with short-term goals now. The particular areas on which Ken and the nurse focus are maintenance of a medication schedule and prevention of decompensation.

Ken initially experienced difficulty identifying his own behavior patterns that lead to hospitalization, although he expresses a strong desire to stay out of the hospital. Ken and the nurse discussed the feelings and behaviors that precede decompensation, such as the fact that he stops taking his maintenance medication. He decided that attending a medication group on a long-term basis would be helpful in this regard. In addition, he agreed to keep a journal in which he will record a brief assessment of his mood and the degree of organization of his thinking on a scale of one to ten on a daily basis. When Ken notes problems, such as neglecting to write in his journal or beginning to feel more confused, he will call the leader of his medication group.

Ken is discharged in one more week. He has been writing in his journal daily and states that it is very helpful to him to recognize how he reacts to stressful interactions with other people. He plans to continue his daily journal writing, as well as attending his medication group on a weekly outpatient basis. He is quite pleased at his feelings of being able to have more control in his care. Ken and the nurse plan to meet in a week to re-evaluate the plans.

SELF-CARE PLAN FOR CASE EXAMPLE

Assessment	Planning	Intervention	Evaluation
Week 1			
Loose associations	Decrease or eliminate loose associations	Psychotropic drugs and supportive therapy for two weeks	Extent of: • loose associations • confusion • delusional ideas
Confusion	Decrease or eliminate confusion		
Delusional ideas	Decrease or eliminate delusional ideas		
Week 2			
Disorganization leading to difficulty getting to meals on time	Increase organization Get to meals on time	Ask other patients and staff to remind him of mealtimes Use watch	Use of other patients and staff Use of watch
Hunger	Eat all meals		Number of meals he missed, or was late to
Restlessness	Decrease restlessness	Identify exercise he likes Establish realistic exercise plan 1–3 times a week Walk every day after lunch	Extent of restlessness Exercise 1–3 times a week Daily walking

Case contributed by Peggie Griffin, R.N, M.S. Clinical Nurse Specialist, Veteran's Administration Hospital, Albany, New York.

CASE EXAMPLE

Cardiac Rehabilitation

Daryl is a 42-year-old, black plant supervisor admitted to the coronary care unit for acute substernal chest pain. He is accompanied by his wife and two teenage sons. His wife is crying.

Daryl complains of crushing pain which radiates up his neck to his jaw and down his left arm. He appears anxious and frightened. The nurse places Daryl in a private room. He is connected to the cardiac monitor. Blood gases, cardiac enzymes, and admission serum studies are sent to the laboratory. His vital signs are temperature, oral, 37.7°C; apical pulse, 120 beats per minute with 15 premature ventricular contractions; respiratory rate is 30 per minute, shallow and regular. Blood pressure is 100/50 in both arms. He is cool and diaphoretic. Admission electrocardiogram findings are consistent with the diagnosis of anterolateral myocardial infarction.

Oxygen is administered via nasal cannula. Morphine sulfate is given intravenously to control pain and anxiety. A lidocaine bolus is given and a lidocaine drip is started at 2 mgm/min.

As Daryl's condition stabilizes and he feels more comfortable, the cardiologist explains to Daryl what has happened to his heart, what treatments the health team has completed, and what the therapeutic plans are for the next 24 hours. She encourages Daryl to express his feelings. She emphasizes that the health team will provide his care now, while his heart needs rest; but that as he regains his strength, he will take an active part in planning and carrying out his care. The health team will remain available to guide and support him.

As Daryl rests comfortably, the admitting nurse comforts Naomi, his wife, and completes Daryl's history. This is Daryl's first cardiac event. His history is significant for multiple atherosclerotic risk factors including hypertension × 10 years, high dietary salt and animal fat intake, cigarette smoking (2 pack/day × 23 years), stress, and a family history of cardiovascular disease. His mother died, age 72, of a stroke; his father died at age 54 of a myocardial infarction; his two brothers, ages 36 and 38, are hypertensive.

Daryl enjoys all sports. He is captain of the company basketball team and works out by lifting weights twice a week with his sons. He also enjoys backpacking, white-water rafting, and tennis. Daryl maintains his weight within normal limits. He has attempted to stop smoking twice (alone, not in a smoking cessation group) but started smoking again within one or two weeks.

His wife states his blood pressure is usually 150/90 when he takes his medication. However, she states, "There are so many pills; he always forgets at least one or two doses every day. Sometimes he doesn't take them for a week but starts again when he becomes dizzy." His wife is unaware of the effects of salt on blood pressure or the effect of skipping drugs.

Naomi states that lately her husband has seemed preoccupied with work. He is irritable, smokes more, and doesn't sleep well at night. She thinks it is related to the negotiations for the union contract.

During patient care rounds, the health team agrees that Daryl is a candidate for the Cardiac Rehabilitation Program. (See Chapter 8, page 179, Case Example). Daryl and Naomi agree to participate. Classes are scheduled so that the entire family can attend.

After a few days, Daryl's condition is stable. He has no chest pain, no arrhythmias, and his blood pressure is 130/80. His activity prescription is re-assessed, and he is allowed to perform more activities. He is taught to monitor his own pulse rate and to stop activities when his pulse increases 20 beats/minute over his baseline. At first Daryl is frustrated that he tires so easily. As he gains an understanding of why he becomes tired and how to balance his activities with rest, his spirits improve.

Naomi has been attending dietary classes. She is able to choose foods low in saturated fats from a list of foods. She also can list several salt-free condiments to substitute for salt in her cooking. She and her sons have been experimenting with new recipes at home.

Daryl has agreed to meet daily with the staff psychiatric nurse. He made a list of the major stressors in his life and is beginning to develop plans to minimize these stressors. He will join a stress-reduction group when his activity level permits.

Daryl agrees that he "loves" his cigarettes and that quitting will be difficult. Now that he has been transferred from the coronary care unit to the observation unit, he is focusing his attention on smoking. He has viewed the available learning modules on the effects of nicotine and carbon monoxide on his heart. Daryl and his primary nurse review available community smoking cessation groups. They choose three that are considered safe for cardiac patients, and Daryl calls each one. Since he has not smoked at all during his hospitalization, he hopes he will not need to join a smoking cessation group. However, he wants the security of knowing they are there, if he needs them once he goes back to work.

Two days prior to Daryl's discharge, the nurse notes that Daryl is irritable and depressed. He is angry that he will not be able to play basketball or continue weight lifting when he goes home. The nurse explains that weight lifting is an isometric exercise and will strain his heart right now. Basketball involves "arms overhead" movements and bursts of energy. He needs to recondition his heart before continuing such a strenuous sport. Together Daryl and the nurse review Phase II of the Cardiac Rehabilitation Program. They discuss the benefits of isotonic exercise, such as walking, jogging, cycling, and swimming. Daryl repeats back to the nurse the purpose for warm-up and cool-down exercises. He is relieved to know he is not a "cardiac cripple."

Prior to Daryl's discharge, Daryl and Naomi are able to describe signs and symptoms of cardiac ischemia, what to do if they suspect Daryl is having another heart attack, when to resume sexual activities, what risk factors they need to focus on individually and as a family, and where to get support for the many changes they are making. Daryl is also able to describe a safe home exercise program based on his low level treadmill stress test. The pharmacist discusses with Daryl the purpose, side effects, and dosage of his medications, especially nitroglycerin.

As Daryl and Naomi gather Daryl's belongings to go home, they are surprised by their two sons. The boys wheel a new 10-speed bicycle into the room—a coming home present for a dad they are proud of. Even though Daryl will not be ready for bicycling for several weeks, he feels better knowing it is there.

SELF-CARE PLAN FOR CASE EXAMPLE

Assessment	Planning	Intervention	Evaluation
A. Pain and discomfort due to myocardial ischemia and fever.	Control pain	Administer analgesics	Daryl states he has no chest pain and feels comfortable
	Prevent extension of infarction	Explain to Daryl cause of pain and effects of treatment	Daryl verbalizes understanding of pain and treatment
			EKG abnormalities stabilize
	Eliminate fever	Antipyretic drugs, as needed	Afebrile
B. Arrhythmias	Control ectopic beats	Anti-arrhythmic drugs	Normal sinus rhythm with no ectopic beats
		Record hourly the number of ectopic beats per minute	Number of ectopic beats per minute
		Explain to Daryl the presence of ectopic beats, effects of therapy, and possible side effects of the medication	Daryl verbalizes understanding of ectopic beats, therapy & side effects of medication
C. Anxiety due to life-threatening event	Decrease anxiety	Encourage Daryl and family to express their feelings	Able to state that he has had an MI
			Able to discuss his fears and concerns.

D. Limited activities, diminished independence	(see Chapter 8 for continuation)	
E. Personal strengths: Family support	Support and praise strengths	Discuss common emotional reactions to life threatening events—anger, depression
		Verbalize understanding of common emotional reactions
		Able to acknowledge feelings of anger and depression, and channel those feelings into constructive actions.
		Daryl continues to enjoy supportive, caring relationship with family.
Acceptance of diagnosis, willingness to participate in care	Provide educational content about disease and treatment	Provide cardiac rehab notebook for Daryl's reading
		Daryl reads cardiac rehab notebook
		Daryl's family to read notebook. Be available for questions
		Daryl's family reads cardiac rehab notebook
		Structure educational courses so that family can attend.
		Family attend classes, ask questions and express feelings.
		Reinforce strengths: use as example for other behavior changes.
		Daryl builds on strengths to change behavior

Active in sports	Identify sports and activities safe for his myocardial function.	Daryl outlines activities, including sexual activities, for a 7-day period, and stays within activity limitations after discharge. Daryl outlines a week of activities including time, duration and intensity, that are within his activity limits, including sexual activities.
Maintains ideal body weight	Discuss the benefits of maintaining ideal body weight and his prior strategies to do so.	Daryl can identify his strategies for weight maintenance and describe cardiovascular benefits of maintaining an ideal body weight.
	Referral to aerobic and reconditioning exercise program—cardiac rehabilitation program.	Participation in cardiac rehabilitation program.
F. *Atherogenic Risk Factors*		
Eliminate risk factors as best as possible	Provide adequate information and community resources to help Daryl control risk factors	
Smoking		
Smoking cessation	• Smoking cessation Modules (effects of smoking, methods to quit, common barriers to quitting smoking)	Daryl states that he has stopped smoking • Daryl describes the physiological effects of smoking

Poorly controlled hypertension (HTN)	HTN medications taken appropriately	• Help Daryl identify own supports and barriers to quitting smoking	• Daryl lists own supports and barriers to smoking cessation
		• Support and reinforce decision to abstain from cigarettes	• Daryl chooses a smoking cessation groups in the community
		• Provide Daryl with a list of smoking cessation groups considered safe for individuals with cardiovascular disease	
		Instruction on medication: therapeutic effects, side effects, importance of maintaining serum drug level	Daryl can state the name, dose, therapeutic effects, and side effects of his hypertensive drugs;
		Provide ideas on how to chart and monitor medication	Daryl modifies a pocket notebook to chart his daily medication times with daily activities to better recall when to take his medications
High salt and animal fat intake		Consultation with dietician about effects of salt on blood pressure and effects of fat on atherogenesis	Daryl can state effects of salt and fat intake
		Include Naomi and their sons when instructing how to plan seven-day menu	Daryl and Naomi can plan a seven day menu of low salt/low fat foods;

Stress	Stress management	Provide information on salt-free condiments	Daryl and Naomi can list salt-free condiments that can be substituted for salt in cooking
		Reinforce reduced salt intake	Daryl states relationship between blood pressure and sodium.
		Consultation with the staff psychiatric nurse regarding life stressors and management techniques	Daryl is able to identify major stressors in his daily life.
			Daryl can demonstrate several methods of stress reduction
		Provide a list of community resources for stress reduction classes	Daryl can identify community resource groups if he needs them.
G. *Discharge teaching about:* Medications: nitroglycerin s.l. (NTG)	Learn dose, effects, and side effects of NTG	Pharmacist to instruct Daryl on the use of NTG	Daryl states use of NTG, effects, side effects, how to tell if it is still potent.
Symptoms of angina vs. myocardial infarction	Differentiate angina from myocardial infarction	Discuss symptoms of angina vs. myocardial infarction	Daryl states symptoms of angina and myocardial infarction.
When to seek health care for chest pain and other cardiac symptoms	Identify reasons and symptoms to seek health care.	View slide/tape: "Signals for Action" from American Heart Association	Daryl states whan signs and symptoms should be reported.
		Reinforce material on tape	

Case example contributed by Cheryl Hubner, R.N., M.S., Vascular Nurse Specialist, Lecturer, Department of Physiological Nursing, University of California, San Francisco

Discussion Questions

1. Discuss the concept of prevention as it relates to minor, major, and chronic illness.
2. What are the criteria you use to detect illness in yourself or your family members?
3. List three self-care behaviors that would be appropriate for a client with psoriasis.
4. List three factors that might interfere with a client's attempt to carry out a self-care plan.
5. How would you and your diabetic client evaluate the effectiveness of medication, nutrition, and exercise plan?

REFERENCES

Becker MN: The health belief model and sick role behavior. Health Education Monographs, Vol 2, No 4, pp 407–419, 1974

Becker MH: Drachman RH, Kirscht JP: Motivations and predictors of health behavior. Health Services Rep, Vol 87, pp 856–861, 1972

Dunnell K, Cartwright A: Medicine Takers, Prescribers and Hoarders. Routledge and Kegan Paul, London, 1972

Elliot-Binnes CP: An analysis of lay medicine. Journal of the Royal College of General Practitioners, Vol 23, No 129, pp 255–264, 1973

Ferguson T: Self-care and alternative medicine. Medical Self-Care. Summit Books, New York, 1980

Freer CB: Self-care: A health diary study. Medical Care, Vol 18, No 8, pp 853–861, 1980

Goetz AA: Health Risk appraisal: The estimation of risk. Public Health Reports, Vol 92, No 2, pp 119–126, 1980

Haefner DP, Kerscht JP: Motivational and behavioral effects of modifying health beliefs. Public Health Rep, Vol 85, pp 484–487, 1970

Rosenstock I: The health belief model and preventive health behavior. Health Education Monographs, Vol 2, No 4, pp 354–385, 1974

Rosenstock I: Why people use health services. Milbank Memorial Fund Quarterly, Vol 44, No 2, 94–127, 1966

Suchman EA: Preventive health behavior, a model for research on community health campaigns. Journal of Health Social Behavior, Vol 8, No. 3, pp 197–205, 1967

Sehnert K: How to Be Your Own Doctor (Sometimes). Grosset and Dunlap, New York, 1975

Vickery DM, Fries JF: Take Care of Yourself: A Consumer's Guide to Medical Care. Addison-Wesley Publishing Co., Reading, Massachusetts, 1978

Wagner EH, Berry WL, Schoenbach VJ, Graham RM; An assessment of health hazard health risk appraisal. American Journal of Pediatric Health, Vol 4, pp 347–352, 1982

6

Teaching Strategies

A major concern of nursing is teaching clients about health, illness, and treatment, so that they may understand and improve ways in which they cope with health problems. Teaching about health and illness almost invariably involves helping clients change behavior or life-style patterns. However, increasing knowledge in and of itself does not necessarily lead to needed changes. Numerous factors must be taken into account for health teaching to be effective. The Health Belief Model and adult learning theory address many of these factors. The purpose of this chapter is to make the reader aware of knowledge and techniques for effectively teaching self-care. The informed health care consumer is better able to participate in both self-care and professional care. In this chapter, we discuss goals of health teaching and problems that interfere with teaching and learning.

Why are teaching and learning important to self-care? Self-care is a deliberate attempt to enhance health and/or ameliorate discomfort or inconvenience of illness. Most individuals want and need facts on which self-care practices are based. Individuals also need the opportunity to learn and practice self-care skills with supervision. In addition, as clients become more knowledgeable and skilled in self-care practices, they often teach self-care to family and friends.

Historically, patient education has been part of nursing practice. Frequently this took place in the hospital, where patients were taught about their diseases and treatments in preparation for discharge. However, the area of health teaching has expanded so that many professionals are involved; in fact, professional health educators are health care specialists who define their mission exclusively as teaching people about health and health-related problems. Despite this growth, health education is often poorly coordinated with no one group or individual taking primary responsibility. Health teaching is best conducted as a team effort. Nurses may be in the best position to coordinate this effort because of their comprehensive focus and the amount of time spent in direct contact with clients.

GOALS OF HEALTH TEACHING

The term "patient education" is often used interchangeably with patient teaching and health education. Many people do not distinguish self-care from patient education or health education. Patient education refers to the teaching activities designed to help people cope with illness, in hospital, clinic, office, or community settings. In this book, the words health education or health teaching are used because our focus is not merely teaching related to illness, or the view of "patient" as a passive recipient of care. Health education includes teaching and learning activities designed to prevent illness and maintain and promote health.

What are the goals of health teaching? What can it accomplish? Some people think that the only goal of health teaching is to cure disease or to change behavior. Such goals can be unrealistic and may set the stage for failure. Consider four less ambitious goals. The first goal is to **impart information so that the client can make rational decisions** with regard to health or illness. In the case of a specific disease, the client needs information about the disease itself, prescribed and alternative treatments, risks, benefits, cost of treatment, long-term implications, and expected outcomes. In health maintenance and promotion, the client needs to understand the ways in which life-style and behavior can prevent disease and/or promote health.

The second goal of health teaching is to **help clients participate effectively in care and cure.** This requires teaching specific self-care skills necessary for a prescribed treatment regimen or health promotion program. It also means helping clients to distinguish when they can handle problems themselves and when they need professional consultation.

The third goal of health teaching is to **help the client adjust to the realities of an illness and its treatment.** Teaching can help clients improve their coping mechanisms, acquire specific skills for debilitating conditions, and seek additional social support. The fourth goal of health teaching is to **help clients experience the satisfaction of seeing their own efforts contribute toward better health.**

Specific goals for health teaching should be derived from the client's needs and preferences as he/she identifies them, rather than determined solely by a health professional's view of what the disease demands. Ideally, health teaching should increase the client's or family's skills and promote independence and effective decision-making.

THE TEACHING-LEARNING PROCESS

Teaching is a process that facilitates learning. Teaching can be defined as imparting knowledge, assisting the learner to develop motivation to change, or guiding or interpreting the learner's experience. Learning can be defined as the acquisition of knowledge, the initiation of behavioral, attitudinal or perceptual change, or integration of knowledge, new behaviors, or attitudes. There are three areas of learning—cognitive (intellectual), affective (feelings, beliefs and values), and psychomotor (manipulative and motor skills). Learning is a process that requires the complete involvement of the learner and is usually influenced by the interaction with the teacher. Teaching and learning are interactive processes. As the learner learns, so does the teacher; thus, teacher and learner influence each other.

Recall that adult learning theory (Knowles 1973) assumes that adults learn most effectively when they are ready and willing to learn. At this time, they actively participate in the learning process, and the learning task is problem-centered rather than subject-centered.

The teaching-learning process is similar to the nursing process in that it can be analyzed using the same component parts of assessment, planning, implementation, and evaluation. As with nursing process, the steps or components of the teaching-learning process are separated for explanation only. In actual teaching and learning, the components often occur simultaneously and interchangeably and are difficult to separate. However, discussing teaching-learning activities in this way may help the teacher and learner determine the effectiveness of teaching.

Assessment

There are two major areas which should be assessed in relation to education—assessment of the **need for information** and assessment of **readiness to learn.** In the Western orthodox medical system, clients' learning needs are usually derived from the perceptions of the physician, nurse, or other health team member. The client should take a major role in this assessment. Many clients approach a health care professional with a list of questions, while others need to help in identifying their needs for learning. One important part of the nurse's role is helping clients identify their learning needs. However, if the client does not perceive such a need, regardless of how sure the professional is that the need exists, the success of any teaching intervention may be questionable.

A self-assessment tool is often a good way of encouraging clients to identify health-related questions and concerns. For example, some women will not request information about breast self-exam unless confronted with a self-assessment questionnaire which asks, "Do you examine your breasts regularly?" In addition to self-assessment, a thorough nursing history can identify client learning needs, such as inadequate knowledge about a specific health condition. For example, when asking a hypertensive client about his "low-sodium diet," one nurse asked about usual foods and was told that the client eats plain rice with fresh steamed vegetables and adds "just a little soy sauce." This illustrates the client's misunderstanding of what a low sodium diet entails and the lack of knowledge of the sodium content of soy sauce.

In addition to information obtained in the nursing history, observation can offer valuable clues to client learning needs. For example, a nurse may observe that a diabetic is wearing constrictive shoes or that a client taking anticoagulants has bruises. The physical examination also provides an excellent opportunity for observation. For example, when examining a woman with a colostomy, a nurse observes inflammation around the stoma site. This condition could indicate that the client lacks adequate information. Does the client know the signs and symptoms of infection? Does she perform stoma care properly? The medical record may provide other valuable information. In the case of the woman with the colostomy, does she have a high white blood cell count? Does the diabetic have a high blood sugar or ketones in the urine? Does the patient on anticoagulants have a markedly prolonged clotting time? Does the record indicate that a woman who seeks information about breast self-exam has been taught this procedure in the past?

Whether or not a client has had previous teaching about a particular subject is also important information to obtain in the assessment process. Is the client familiar with self-care or popular health literature? What particular techniques have been taught in the past? Does the client use these practices regularly? What specifically was the client taught? For example, in breast self-exam, has the client been taught "spokes of the wheel" or "circular" exam?

Once a learning need has been identified, the nurse and client need to assess readiness to learn. Critical to readiness is the client's perception of the need to learn. There are two types of readiness—*emotional readiness*, which encompasses the motivational aspects of learning (discussed as part of implementation) and *experiential readiness*, which includes adequacy of background knowledge, mastery of specific needed skills, attitudes related to learning, physical/emotional ability to learn, and values and beliefs related to health and learning (see below). Such

ASSESSMENT OF READINESS FOR LEARNING

- Awareness of medical diagnosis or health need
- Previous knowledge and experience
- Intellectual ability
- Motivational level
- Physical condition
- Psychological state
- Perceived need to learn

physiological conditions as fever, pain, metabolic disturbances, or lack of sleep can affect a client's ability to learn and can interfere with the learning process.

It is useful to actively involve adults in assessing their own readiness to learn. It is important to address the client's most pressing concerns first. Until these concerns are addressed, the client may not be able to make use of any other information you offer. Assessment ends with the client's and nurse's mutual decision that there is a specific learning need or that the client wants to learn. This suggests that teaching (filling the learning need) will produce some desirable outcome, which may in fact be a change in behavior.

EDUCATIONAL NEEDS RELATED TO PRESCRIBED TREATMENT

- Why is it done?
- How is it done?
- Who does it?
- When is it done?
- What does it feel like?

- How long does it take?
- Where is it done?
- What is the cost?
- What does the patient need to do?

From Chatham MA, Knapp BL: Patient Education Handbook, Brady Communications Company, Bowie, Maryland, 1982 (Used with permission from Brady Communications Company)

Planning and Implementation

A "desirable outcome" as mentioned above can be specified in the form of goals and objectives of the teaching-learning process. Goals are most effectively written in terms of overall long-term goals and short-term goals. Achieving the short-term goals should help the client achieve the long-term goal. For example, if the overall self-care goal is losing 20 pounds in six months, short-term *learning* goals might be learning about caloric needs, problems in past eating patterns, and the effects of exercise on metabolism. Learning goals must be realistic and attainable and will differ depending on whether the learning need is cognitive, affective, or psychomotor.

Once the client and nurse determine realistic short- and long-term goals, they can devise a teaching plan. A teaching plan communicates to all concerned the goals, the content to be taught, how it will be taught, and how and when the teaching will be evaluated. Such a plan helps to coordinate interdisciplinary teaching efforts and integrate teaching into the care plan (Strodtman 1984). Teaching plans can be standard or individualized. (See sample teaching plan on pages 106 to 108.)

EXAMPLE OF TEACHING PLAN

Hickman Catheter Educational Pamphlet

The Hickman Catheter is a soft plastic tube that provides long-term access to the venous blood system. The catheter is tunneled beneath the skin and placed in a large vein near the entrance of the heart. The purpose of the Hickman Catheter is to give you medication and to withdraw blood samples. This is done by inserting a needle into the catheter rather than into your vein. With proper care of the catheter, it can remain in place for up to one year or longer.

This instructional pamphlet is meant to assist you in learning how to take care of your Hickman Catheter. The nurses will teach and assist you in performing the catheter care tasks. It is recommended that a family member or a friend learn how to care for the catheter with you.

The following items are what you need to learn:

- How to change the Hickman Catheter dressing
- How to change the Hickman Catheter injection cap
- How to flush the Hickman Catheter
- How to recognize possible problems with the Hickman Catheter and what to do about them
- How to keep a record of Hickman Catheter care.

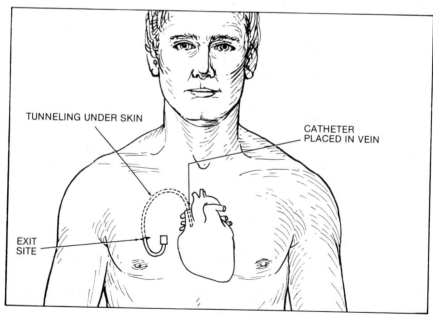

Figure 6-1. Hickman Catheter placement.

You will be given opportunities to learn with the help of the nurses. Please feel free to ask questions at any time.

HICKMAN CATHETER DRESSING CHANGE

Why do I change the catheter dressing?

After your catheter is inserted, you will need a dressing to protect the incision so it can heal. Once the incision is well healed, you may choose not to wear a dressing.

What are the supplies I will need?
- Sterile 2 × 2 gauze pads
- Sterile cotton tipped applicators (Q-tips®)
- Betadine wipes
- Betadine ointment
- One inch tape.

What are the steps I should follow?
1. Wash hands thoroughly.
2. Assemble all the supplies together on a clean surface.
3. Open supplies but leave in the package.
4. Remove the old dressing and discard.
5. Look at the site for signs of infection—tenderness, pus, warmth, swelling, redness
6. Clean exit site with a Betadine wipe beginning at the catheter and moving outward in a circular motion for 3 inches.
7. Take a second Betadine wipe and clean the catheter from the skin toward the plug. Do not pull on the catheter.
8. Apply a small dab of Betadine ointment at the exit site using the sterile Q-Tip.
9. Place one sterile 2 × 2 pad under the catheter and one over the catheter. Secure it with tape.
10. Place the catheter in a loop onto the chest and secure it with tape. This is done to prevent tension on the catheter.

If you notice any of the above signs of infection or have a fever or chills, contact your doctor.

HICKMAN CATHETER EDUCATIONAL RECORD

Use the sample teaching record on page 109 to document teaching interventions, the patient/helper ability to understand the concepts of Hickman

Catheter care, and the patient/helper ability to demonstrate care functions.

Use the comments column to describe the patient/helper actual performance and what intervention was provided to correct any difficulties the patient/helper is having. The comments column is intended as a day to day narrative. Please date all entries and initial note. Place signature at bottom of the sheet.

Use the patient performance column to record patient's ability to meet the learning objectives. Following a teaching interaction, use one square to record date, appropriate rating code(s), and your initials.

0 = Patient has no experience or knowledge
1 = Instruction provided
2 = Patient demonstrates task or verbalizes knowledge with guidance
3 = Patient demonstrates task or verbalizes knowledge independently

Note that in one interaction you may have two codes (i.e., you assess patient having no knowledge about signs of exit site infection (code = 0) and you proceed to teach this information (code = 1). If the patient needs to demonstrate knowledge or a skill at least three times, code 3 must appear three times in the patient performance column before that learning objective is complete.

For questions or concerns, please contact the Patient Education Coordinator or the Clinical Nurse Specialist.

Prepared by: Deborah Larson, R.N., B.S.N., Patient Education Coordinator, Petaluma Valley Hospital, Petaluma, California

Objectives. An effective teaching plan includes written objectives that will help clients achieve their learning goals. Learning objectives refer to observable actions that are expected of learners at the end of the teaching segment—what clients have to *do* to show they have learned what is needed (see pages 109 to 110). Because teaching content is covered in Part Three, this section will focus on other aspects of objectives. How does one write clear learning objectives? Mager (1975) suggests that a useful objective has the following characteristics:

1. Performance or behavior (what the learner will do)
2. Conditions under which the performance is expected to occur
3. Criteria, or level of performance, that will be considered acceptable.

Objectives are best written using verbs that describe a specific behavior that a client will perform, which are not open to a variety of different interpretations. Action verbs, which are observable to the teacher, include

Hickman Catheter Educational Record

PATIENT/HELPER PERFORMANCE

LEARNING OBJECTIVES

The patient/helper is able to do the following with 100% accuracy.

LEARNING OBJECTIVES	DATE/INITIAL/CODE					COMMENTS
1. Verbalize the purpose of the H.C. and describe its location in relation to the anatomy of the chest.						
2. Explain the procedure for changing the H.C. dressing.						
3. Demonstrate correct procedure for H.C. dressing change at least 3 times.						
4. Explain procedure for, and frequency of, irrigating H.C. with heparin-saline solution.						
5. Demonstrate correct procedure for irrigating H.C. with heparin-saline solution at least 3 times.						

6. State concentration of heparin-saline solution to use to flush the H.C.											
7. Explain procedure for, and frequency of, changing the H.C. injection cap.											
8. Demonstrate procedure for changing H.C. injection cap at least 3 times.											
9. Record H.C. dressing changes, flushes and cap changes on H.C. Care Calendar.											
10. Describe possible H.C. problems and appropriate action to take. —Inability to flush catheter —Drainage from catheter exit site —Oral temperature above 100° —Catheter break or tear											
11. Verbally acknowledges comfort and ability to perform H.C. self care.				YES		NO					
12. Receives H.C. discharge supply kit.				YES		NO					

SIGNATURES: _____

Prepared by: Deborah Larson, R.N., B.S.N., Patient Education Coordinator, Petaluma Valley Hospital, Petaluma, California write, list, state, name, identify, describe, compare, apply, demonstrate, define, select, record, explain, calculate, differentiate, and prepare. "Know," "understand," and "appreciate" are examples of descriptive processes that occur inside the client and cannot be observed.

In order to write appropriate objectives, the nurse needs to be aware of different kinds of learning, such as the well-known domains of learning described by Bloom (1956):

1. Cognitive domain—learning that involves thinking, recall of information, analysis, synthesis, and evaluation
2. Affective domain—learning that involves attitudes, values, beliefs, and emotions
3. Psychomotor domain—learning that involves psychomotor skills and practice.

Consider the different levels of thinking involved in the cognitive domain and the verbs that would be needed to write a clear objective.

Learning to write effective learning objectives takes time and practice. Most clients may have no idea of what an objective is or why it is important. However, the client and the nurse can discuss what must be learned and how it can be learned in a manner that makes sense to the client. The mother who has a child with an allergy to eggs has a number of learning needs. In the cognitive domain, she needs to be able to identify which foods contain eggs and to evaluate the severity of the reaction when eggs are ingested by mistake. Through discussion, the nurse and the client conclude that it is realistic for her to carefully *read food labels*, but that she cannot *evaluate severity* until she can *describe* basic types of allergic symptoms. If the client and teacher both understand where they are going with the teaching process, they can work in tandem toward that outcome.

Categorizing teaching goals and learning objectives into the general areas of cognitive, affective, and psychomotor learning will help the nurse decide on the specific content and most effective teaching method. When

---

THE COGNITIVE DOMAIN

- *Knowledge*—Ability to recall information (define, list, name, label, record)
- *Comprehension*—Ability to make use of knowledge (describe, explain, identify, discuss)
- *Application*—Ability to apply an abstract concept to a new situation which shows a higher level of understanding (translate, practice, interpret, demonstrate)
- *Analysis*—Ability to break down the information into separate parts and to understand the relationship between the parts (differentiate, debate, calculate, examine)
- *Synthesis*—Ability to bring together different parts of knowledge in new relationships to form a unique whole (plan, design, arrange, organize, prepare)
- *Evaluation*—Ability to make judgments on the basis of given criteria (evaluate, compare, choose, estimate, predict, select, assess, measure).

teaching the client to take a pulse, cognitive objectives include *defining pulse*, *describing* how to take one, and *naming* three places the pulse can be palpated. Affective objectives might include *describing why* pulse-taking is *important*, and a psychomotor objective would be *demonstrating* how to take a pulse. Most effective methods for teaching in the cognitive domain are discussions, lectures, pamphlets, dialogues, questions and answers, and audiovisual aids. In the affective domain, most effective methods include role-playing, case examples, sharing experiences in a group, problem solving, and simulations. And in the psychomotor domain, most effective methods include demonstrations, guided practice, step-by-step self-instruction, guides, audiovisual demonstrations, drills, and behavioral contracting.

The individual client. Tailoring the teaching to the individual client may be more important than selecting the most appropriate method for the learning objective. No matter how well-designed, printed and self-instructional teaching materials are obviously useless for illiterate or non-English-reading clients. Other clients may read poorly or may be "turned off" by being given material to read. Individuals learn differently. Some learn best by hearing, others by seeing, and still others, by doing. The nurse and client should discuss how the client prefers to learn and what has been most successful in the past. Using a combination of strategies is usually the most effective. A minimum of three strategies is recommended (see below).

LEARNING*

People remember:
- 15% of what they read
- 20% of what they see
- 30% of what they hear
- 50% of what they see and hear
- 70% of what they see, hear, and personally experience
- 90% of what they see, hear, personally experience and practice.

---

*From the Workshop in Intercultural Training sponsored by the Washington Association of Professional Anthropologists, given by Connie Ojile, at the Society for Applied Anthropology Annual Meeting, San Diego, CA, 1983 (March)

Using a combination of teaching strategies is particularly important when working with clients of varying ethnic and socioeconomic backgrounds. Middle-class health professionals tend to rely too extensively on written and verbal methods of teaching and may miss the fact that they are not communicating with some clients. For such clients, focusing primarily on *doing* is probably most effective. It has been found that acceptance of new health beliefs and practices depends on how well they fit with existing cultural values and assumptions and whether these new beliefs serve a useful purpose. People more easily accept new *practices* in medicine than the *ideas* which accompany such innovations, particularly if the new practices produce immediate positive results, few negative outcomes, and are consistent with cultural beliefs.

The more involved the client becomes in the learning process, the more effective the teaching becomes. Consider again that teaching-learning is a process for solving problems and that the goal of self-care teaching is to increase the effectiveness of the client's problem-solving skills and decision-making. Thus, the client plans the direction for learning and the nurse facilitates the planning and learning process. The better the planning, the more clearly objectives are written, the easier it is to identify the content which should be taught. Most importantly, clear objectives make it easy to document and evaluate the results of the teaching and learning endeavor.

Documentation and Evaluation

The teaching process is completed with documentation and evaluation. Documentation communicates that teaching has taken place, what has been taught, and the client's response. Anecdotal records or checklists can be used, as in the examples in Figure 6-2.

Clearly written objectives contain criteria for evaluation. An objective might say "by post-op, day three, the client will demonstrate the correct procedure for Hickman catheter dressing change." Various methods of evaluation can be used; these will depend on how the objective was to be met and the domain of learning. Cognitive learning might be evaluated by questionnaires or written tests, while psychomotor learning requires a demonstration of the newly acquired skills.

If the objective was not met or was incompletely met, the nurse and client discuss what is needed to achieve the goal or whether or not the objective was realistic. If the goal was realistic, what barriers to learning occurred? A plan or strategy fails; the client does not fail. Teachers do not fail either. The responsibility of the teacher is not to assure that the client learns but rather to continue to be available so that when the client does want to learn, the information is available. At this point, we will turn to some barriers that interfere with learning and will discuss some teaching strategies that are specific to self-care.

CHANGING HEALTH BEHAVIORS: PROBLEMS AND STRATEGIES

A number of barriers potentially interfere with learning and with self-care—communication barriers, lack of motivation, and structural constraints. Recall that the Health Belief Model (Rosenstock 1966) provides a

Patient Name: _____ **Date:** _____
Diagnosis: _____

Learning objectives	Teaching strategies and resources	Criteria and means for evaluating	Date objective accomplished and educator's initials	Comments

Figure 6-2. Example of anecdotal records or checklist from Chatham MA, Knapp BL: Patient Education Handbook, Brady Communications Company, Bowie, Maryland (*Used with permission of Brady Communications Company*)

framework for explaining why some individuals are more likely than others to seek illness care or engage in preventive health behaviors. Motivating factors include perceptions of illness susceptibility, seriousness of illness threat, or perceptions of benefits of taking action.

Motivation

When nurses plan to help clients change health behaviors, they assume that people want to learn and change. This may not always be true. Motivation is defined as the force that moves a person to action or inaction. There are two types of motivation—intrinsic and extrinsic. **Intrinsic motivation** comes from within the individual and is stimulated by past socialization, values, beliefs, attitudes, perceptions, unmet needs, and anxiety and fears. **Extrinsic motivations** are forces outside the individual which are stimulated by such factors as changes in health or life-style needs, interactions with peers, family or professionals, external rewards and punishments, and environmental factors. Individuals can be stimulated to change their health behavior by either intrinsic or extrinsic motivators. Changes stimulated by external factors may not be lasting because once the reinforcement is removed, the source of the motivation disappears. Thus, if the nurse helps the client to recognize and use intrinsic motivators, longer-lasting change may be more likely. However, the individual's personality and sociocultural background determine whether intrinsic or extrinsic motivators are more effective; the nurse and client should discuss what reasons are most meaningful to the client.

Many aspects of adult learning theory relate to motivation. We think that the principles of adult learning apply to children as well when the subject is self-care in health and illness. Children are motivated to learn about health as a personal need. Unfortunately, children are usually not interested in the benefits of healthy behaviors to reduce risks or reap rewards 20 years in the future. However, by using their own personal experiences with health and illness, the nurse can teach and reinforce healthy behavior. For children and adults, the factors in Table 6-1 are important influences. It is also important to identify the "why bother to learn?" In particular, children are greatly influenced by their parents and peers as role models. Children can also be great motivators for their parents.

A powerful strategy for teaching about changing health behavior is the practice of modeling positive health behavior. It is especially important for nurses and other health professionals to "practice what they preach." There is nothing less motivating than a health care provider who encourages the client to stop smoking or lose weight yet is overweight and smells of tobacco. As a group, many nurses are unhealthy and do not take responsibility for their own health. Many are overweight, under-exercised, over-stressed, and unaware of the unhealthy environments in which they live and work. If nurses want to motivate their clients, it behooves them to take their own advice.

TABLE 6-1. FACTORS INFLUENCING LEARNING*

Positive	Negative
• Clear, concise objectives/expectations	• Punishment
• Realistic goals/activities to meet goals	• Frustration
	• Boredom
• Reinforcement/praise/support	• Humiliation/embarrassment
• Knowledge of the results/progress reports	• Fear and anxiety
• Use of simple to complex examples, relevant to experience relating to the principles.	• Physical discomfort

*Adapted from de Tornay R: Strategies for Teaching Nursing, John Wiley & Sons, Inc., New York, 1971

In the context of self-care, other specific strategies can increase a client's motivation. In addition to the use of behavior modeling, the health behavior contract is an effective means of teaching and encouraging self-care (Farquhar 1978; Baldi et al. 1980; Steckel 1980, 1982; Janz, Becker, and Hartman 1984). The behavior contract incorporates the principles of self-directed change by shifting responsibility to the client and thus increasing his/her participation. It defines who will take what action for what results over a manageable time period. Social support and reinforcement are implied in the use of the contract, both of which are motivating factors. See Figure 6-3 for an example of a contract.

Communication

Communication is the exchange of information accomplished by sending and receiving messages. It is successful when both the sender and receiver understand the message in the same way. There are several kinds of communication. In addition to oral and written communication, one must be aware of messages conveyed by nonverbal communication (e.g., gestures, body movements, posture, voice tones, facial expressions). Also important is the context in which communication occurs. Context imparts its own message, and may be determined by the setting, the purposes of the communication, and the communicators' perceptions of roles, time and personal space. How the message is sent and received is based, to a large extent, on past experiences, sociocultural backgrounds, attitudes, communication skills, and knowledge of the subject matter under discussion.

SELF CONTRACT

MY GOALS:

Short term — by the end of *six weeks* I will . . . _____

Long term — by the end of *six months* I will. . . _____

ENVIRONMENTAL PLANNING: (all the steps I will take to reach my goal)

THOUGHTS AND ACTIONS

Helpful thoughts:	Helpful actions:
Non-helpful thoughts:	Non-helpful actions:

MY REWARD: (if I meet my goal)

THE COST: (if I fail to meet my goal)

RE-EVALUATION DATE:

I agree to help with this project: I agree to strive towards this goal:

_____   _____
Support person   *Your signature*   *Date*

Figure 6-3. Example of behavior contract (reprinted with permission of Nurse Model Health).

Without a basis for clear communication, it is difficult for the nurse and client to work together effectively. Clear messages in both directions are essential to the teaching-learning process. Blocks in communication arise from numerous sources, such as conflicts in role expectations, values, language barriers, and differing conceptions of health and illness.

Some role conflicts are illustrated by the following situations. Imagine the role conflict between the defensive health professional and the assertive client. The client's message to the professional is "Tell me so *I* can make the decision," which is in conflict with the professionals' message of "You don't need to know that. That's my job." A similar role conflict which can block communication arises when the nurse who advocates self-care works with the client who insists that health care is the professional's responsibility: "It's something I pay for. You take care of me." Finally, nurses who attempt to teach self-care may face conflicts in role expectations with an adolescent's mother insisting that it is *her* responsibility to care for her child.

Values are enduring beliefs that individuals hold in reference to how people should behave and what is most desirable in life. Examples of values about human conduct are honesty, hospitality, responsibility, and loyalty. Examples of life goals/preferences are freedom, self-respect, health, financial security, and social recognition. Values determine how individuals behave toward others, what they expect of others, and what they do to work toward what they consider most important in life.

Differences in values are frequent sources of communication problems between clients and nurses, particularly in reference to health and health behavior. Consider a middle-aged, Arab-American woman who is hypertensive and overweight. The nurse's priorities are likely to relate to health and prevention. The nurse may make suggestions intended to encourage the client to reduce her salt intake and lose weight, such as keeping fattening and high salt foods out of the house. However, while the client may agree and verbalize the importance of health, her behavior may reflect the equally strong value in her culture—hospitality—which is demonstrated by offering tea and pastries or by preparing exquisite meals for numerous family members and friends who drop in on a frequent basis.

Values clarification is useful for problem-solving in the health arena in that it helps clients increase their awareness of personal priorities, if and how value/behavior conflicts exist, and promotes behavior consistent with health-related values (Pender 1982). Further, it is useful for nurses to examine their own values about interpersonal behavior and life goals. Such examination facilitates awareness of situations in which the nurse acts toward clients on the basis of personal values rather than the client's values and either misses the client's concerns or offends him in some way. A number of tools for values clarification exist (Pender 1982).

Language barriers pose the most obvious communication problems. Everyone is familiar with the feelings of frustration that arise when nurse and client do not speak the same language. Even when an interpreter is available, there can be significant communication blocks. Family members, who are most often pressed into service as interpreters, often do a poor job because of role conflicts. Not only do they use their own perception of the situation to interpret both the health providers' and clients' responses, but they may withhold vital information from one or the other. A Mexican-American adolescent who is asked to interpret for her chronically ill father may feel that her first priority is to protect her father's dignity and self-image as protector of the family, even if it means not telling the nurse about potentially embarrassing symptoms.

Even when nurse and client speak the same language, difficulties can arise if the language is the second language for one or the other. Language determines to a large extent how any culture "cuts the pie of the universe" by naming what is important in the culture and not naming or screening out of perception what is not important. Thus, individuals who have grown up in different language communities will have subtly different perceptions of reality, even if competent in the second language. Dialects within a language can so differ that they are almost different languages. Consider Harlem, black dialect, "proper" Bostonian, and rural Oklahoma speech. Finally, communication difficulties arise among those who share the same cultural background, because of the meaning of the context in which the communication occurs. Consider the recovery room nurse who greets the waking patient with a cheerful, "It's all over." The patient may think he is dead! Children and clients who are highly anxious often take the professionals' words quite literally.

In addition to potential communication blocks due to language, role conflicts, and effects of the setting, non-verbal styles vary between subcultural groups and may hinder communiction. A white nurse may consider black or Native American clients evasive because they avert their eyes when talking with the nurse. To some of these clients, direct eye contact may mean confrontation, rudeness, or invasion of privacy, and clients show respect by averting their eyes. The same nurse may be highly uncomfortable with the Arab-American client who appears to be "intensely staring" or intruding on personal space. Remember, the client may experience similar discomfort with the nurse's nonverbal behavior. The work of Edward T. Hall (1959, 1966) is an excellent discussion of how culture determines conceptions of personal space, nonverbal gestures, and conceptions of time.

There may be communication problems that arise when nurse and client use different explanatory models for illness (see Chapter 2). The folk syndrome "high blood" among southern blacks, southern whites and Haitians means too much blood, which is thought to result from eating too much rich food. It may be confused with hypertension, and strokes are believed to be caused by excess blood backing up into the brain (Snow 1974).

Finally, communication blocks can exist between nurse and client because of mistrust based on their ethnic or cultural backgrounds. Some authors suggest that the optimal therapeutic relationship occurs between helping person and client who are most similar to each other in socioeconomic class, ethnicity, and sex (Carkhuff and Pierce 1967), and when counselor and client share the same world view and attitudes/beliefs (Sue 1981). Some differences between nurse and client always exist, but when the gap is too great, there is no basis for understanding. However, part of the teaching-learning process is increasing awareness of differences and negotiating between client and nurse to design a "cultural fit." Asian clients expect a directive and nurturant approach and practical results from therapy (Higginbotham 1977). Native American clients are more likely to be passive and non-verbal, to listen and absorb, preferring to use advice to solve problems themselves. They need to make their own decisions and may resist being pushed in a particular direction by people seeking to motivate them (Dinges, Trimble, Manson, and Pasquale 1981). Nurses can enhance effectiveness by being open-minded, willing to learn about the client's culture, and by adjusting their approaches in congruence with the client's expectation (see below).

THE CULTURALLY SKILLED NURSE*

- The culturally skilled nurse is aware of his/her own biases, values, and "cultural baggage" and how they may affect clients who differ from him/herself.
- The culturally skilled nurse can work comfortably with clients who differ from him/her in terms of race, ethnicity, or beliefs.
- The culturally skilled nurse is sensitive to personal biases, ethnic identity, or sociopolitical influences that may dictate referral of the minority to a health professional of his/her own race or ethnicity.
- The culturally skilled nurse has a good understanding of the nation's sociopolitical system with respect to its treatment of minorities.
- The culturally skilled nurse possesses specific knowledge about the culture and circumstances of the particular group(s) with whom he/she works.
- The culturally skilled nurse can send and receive a variety of verbal and nonverbal messages appropriately and in a flexible manner to be congruent with the interactional style of the client.

*Adapted from Sue DW: Counseling the Culturally Different, John Wiley & Sons, Inc., New York, 1981.

There are many potential communication barriers between nurse and client, and the teaching-learning process is impaired when such barriers exist. This discussion is intended to raise awareness of potential problems, and we suggest that a flexible approach will be more effective. The approach to each individual should be in the spirit of inquiry. One must remain aware that problems in teaching self-care may be created by a lack of cultural fit between the nurse's and client's communication styles, cultural backgrounds, and role expectations. One does not need extensive knowledge of every cultural group to work successfully with clients of different backgrounds. It is wise to learn as much as one can about cultures of those clients most frequently taught. But when a blank stare is encountered or a bland agreement is given to something the nurse suspects will never be carried out, it is important to stop and spend some time exploring communication. Find out from the client now he or she wants to learn. Try different approaches until the nurse and client can communicate more effectively. Finally, increase your own cultural awareness, and recognize that you cannot work effectively with every person; as a professional, you must refer or request consultation when it becomes clear that the teacher and the learner are not getting through to each other.

Compliance

Compliance is the extent to which a client's behavior coincides with a prescribed therapeutic plan. The term compliance is troublesome in the context of self-care because it presents the client as a passive follower of orders. Noncompliance, the term used when a client does not follow the "good advice" of the professional, is also an inappropriate term in a discussion of self-care. If clients choose not to follow the professionals' advice, they are exercising their rights. There is a legitimate question of the professional's responsibility when the client makes this choice. The man who is insulin-dependent and does not take insulin as prescribed will suffer serious consequences. Rather than simply labeling this client as non-compliant, it is important to determine the reasons underlying irregular use of insulin. Does the client understand the actions and his physiological need for insulin? Does he have enough insulin? Can he pay for it? Does he know how to inject it? Does he think it's useless? Does he think he will die anyway? What if a client chooses not to participate in a self-care regimen? Clients have the right to make choices about their health, their health care, and their own participation in care. But nurses and health educators have the responsibility of making sure that the client has the knowledge and skills to make informed decisions. Nurses have a responsibility to support clients in the decisions they make.

Additional Constraints

Despite the fact that nurses, health educators, physicians and other professionals on the health care team provide health education, patient teaching is often disorganized, ineffective, and sometimes conflictual. There may be confusion about who is teaching what and whose responsibility it is to coordinate the teaching efforts. There may be a lack of structural administrative support for providing the time and resources for health teaching. In acute care settings, there is often not enough time to provide health teaching, which is neglected in favor of physical care needs and paperwork.

Other problems that interfere with client health teaching exist within the professionals themselves. Many nurses have not been taught how to teach patients. Some nurses give lip service to the importance of teaching but do not actually perform it. Others are threatened by active health care consumers who have extensive knowledge. Such clients may be perceived as demanding by some health care professionals and, as a result, receive less sensitive care.

SUMMARY

A number of factors have been addressed that affect teaching and learning self-care. In order to help clients incorporate new self-care practices, it is important that the nurse understand the teaching-learning process. It is useful to analyze the process in terms of problem-solving—assessment, planning, implementation, and evaluation. Constructing careful learning objectives will give direction and structure to the learning process. Other factors that influence the success of learning include motivation, modeling, and contracting, as well as the most basic factor of communication. This chapter concludes Part II. With this general background, we turn to specific self-care practices in Part III.

CASE EXAMPLE

Teaching Example

Billy is an eight-year-old boy who has leukemia. Billy's primary nurse was assessing Billy's needs during the chemotherapy regimen and began to recognize that Billy wanted to participate in his treatment. Billy's mother was very protective of him and interfered with his attempts to be independent. Billy had been angry and sullen, acting out at times. The nurse realized that because Billy had cancer, a disease usually viewed as the body going out of control, he probably wanted to gain control in some area of his life, especially in light of his mother's overprotectiveness.

Billy's nurse had initial difficulty figuring out a way for Billy to participate in his own care. When he asked Billy what he was most worried about, Billy said "getting sicker again." The nurse used his answer to talk about Billy's increased risk of infection because of the chemotherapy and asked Billy to take responsibility for monitoring some signs and symptoms of infection.

SELF-CARE PLAN FOR CASE EXAMPLE

Assessment	Planning	Implementation	Evaluation
Need to learn how to read a thermometer	Billy will be able to identify the parts of a thermometer.	Demonstrate all the steps in taking a temperature. Explain rationale (in language he understands).	Billy verbalizes rationale for taking a temperature.
	Billy will be able to correctly read and shake down a thermometer.	With thermometer in hand, name parts of thermometer.	Billy accurately names parts of thermometer.
		Ask Billy to draw a picture of a thermometer.	Billy draws an accurate picture and studies it at home.
		Demonstrate how to read a thermometer.	Billy watches demonstration on reading a thermometer, how to record temperature, and clean thermometer.
	Billy will accurately and regularly record his temperature.	Demonstrate how to record temperature.	
	Billy will clean thermometer regularly.	Demonstrate how to clean thermometer.	
	In three weeks	Ask Billy to demonstrate how to take a temperature, record temperature, and clean thermometer.	Billy can accurately take temperature, record temperature, and clean thermometer.

Then the nurse developed a teaching plan for Billy to learn to take his own temperature. The teaching plan, described below, worked well. Billy proudly demonstrated his ability to take his own temperature and asked the nurse what he could learn next.

CASE EXAMPLE

Leah is a 42-year-old woman who has been a paraplegic for six years and has an indwelling foley catheter. Because of recurrent urinary tract infections, her urologist requested that the Clinical Nurse Specialist (CNS) teach Leah clean-technique, self-catheterization. The urologist had attempted to teach Leah self-catheterization on two previous occasions but was unsuccessful.

Leah was admitted to the hospital for diagnostic studies which included a cystogram and intravenous pyelogram. Prior to these procedures, the CNS verbally reviewed with Leah what the procedure would entail. She explained that following the diagnostic procedures she would perform catheterization for Leah and would then ask Leah to attempt self-catheterization every three to four hours after that under the supervision of the nursing staff.

Following the diagnostic procedures, the CNS gave Leah a mirror and carefully explained the technique while she inserted the catheter. Leah said, "Are you sure that *I* can do it?" The CNS replied, "No, I'm not *sure*, but I *do think* you can." Leah said she would do her best. Three hours later, the CNS observed Leah catheterize herself correctly on her first attempt. The CNS provided support and encouragement. Leah was surprised at how easy it really was. "You told me that it wasn't hard and that I could do it, but I guess I just wasn't sure." She catheterized herself correctly thereafter without difficulty.

Later, the urologist asked the CNS, "What did you do? I've tried twice to teach her." The CNS replied, "Her fear of kidney disease may have helped motivate her. In addition, I gave her very careful instructions including a written procedure. Most importantly, I told her that she *could* do it."

This is a true example.

REFERENCES

American Hospital Association: American Media Handbook. American Hospital Association; Chicago, Illinois, 1978

Baldi S, Costell S, Hill L, Jasmin S, Smith N: For Your Health: A Model for Self-Care. Nurses Model Health, South Laguna, California, 1980

Becker MH, Drachman RH, Kirscht JP: Motivations and predictors of health behavior. Health Services Report, Vol 87, No 9, pp 852–856, 1972

Bloom BS (ed): Taxonomy of Educational Objectives Handbook: Cognitive Domain. David McKay, New York, 1956

Chatham MA, Knapp BL: Patient Education Handbook. Robert J. Brady Co., Bowie, Maryland, 1982

Carkhuff RR, Pierce R: Differential effects of therapist race and social class upon patient depth of self-exploration in the initial clinical interview. Journal of Consulting Psychology, Vol 31, No 6, pp 632–634, 1967

de Tornay R: Strategies for Teaching Nursing. John Wiley & Sons, Inc., New York, 1971

Dinges N, Trimble JE, Manson SM, Pasquale FL: The social ecology of counseling and psychotherapy with American Indians and Alaskan natives. In Marsella AJ, Pedersen P (eds): Cross-Cultural Counseling and Psychotherapy: Foundations, Evaluation, and Ethnocultural Considerations. Pergamon Press, Elmsford, New York, 1981

Farquhar J: The American Way of Life Need Not Be Hazardous to Your Health. Stanford Alumni Association, Stanford, California, 1978

Hall ET: The Hidden Dimension. Doubleday, Garden City, New York, 1966

Hall ET: the Silent Language. Doubleday, Garden City, New York, 1959

Haefner DP, Kirscht JP: Motivational and behavioral effects of modifying health beliefs. Public Health Reports, Vol 85, pp 478–484, 1970

Hayes WS, Davis LL: What is in a health care contract? Health Values: Achieving High Level Wellness, Vol 4, No 2, pp 82–89, 1980

Higginbotham HN: Culture and the role of client expectancy. Topics in Culture Learning, Vol 5, pp 107–204, 1977

Hogue CC: Nursing and compliance. In Haynes RB, Taylor DW, Sackett D (eds): Compliance in Health Care. Johns Hopkins University Press, Baltimore, Maryland, 1979

Janz NK, Becker MH, Hartman PE: Contingency contracting to enhance patient compliance: A review. Patient Education and Counseling, Vol 4, No 5, pp 165–178, 1984

Knowles M: The Adult Learner: A Neglected Species, 2nd ed. Gulf Publishing Company, Houston, Texas, 1973

Lazes PM (ed): The Health Education Handbook. Aspen Systems Corporation, Germantown, Maryland, 1979

Lousteau A: Using the health belief model to predict patient compliance. Health Values: Achieving High Level Wellness, Vol 13, No 5, pp 241–244, 1979

Mager RF: Preparing Instructional Objectives, 2nd ed. Pitman Management and Training, A Division of Pitman Learning, Inc., Belmont, California, 1975

Ojile C: Learning. Presented during a workshop in intercultural training, Washington Association of Professional Anthropologists, San Diego, California, March 1983

Pender NJ: Health Promotion in Nursing Practice. Appleton-Century-Crofts, Norwalk, Connecticut, 1982

Reilly DE: Behavioral Objectives in Nursing: Evaluation of Learner Attainment. Appleton-Century-Crofts, New York, 1980

Rosenstock I: Why people use health services. Milbank Memorial Fund Quarterly, Vol 44, No 2, pp 94–127, 1966

Sackett DL, Haynes RB (eds): Compliance with Therapeutic Regimens. Johns Hopkins University Press, Baltimore, Maryland, 1976

Sackett DL, Haynes RB, Gibson ES, Taylor DW, Roberts RS, Jahnson AL: Patient compliance with antihypertensive regimens. Patient Counseling and Health Education, pp 18–21, First Quarter 1978

Snow LF: Folk medical beliefs and their implications for care of patients. Annals of Internal Medicine, Vol 81, No 1, pp 82–96, 1974

Steckel S: Contracting with patient-selected reinforcer. American Journal of Nursing, Vol 80, No. 9, pp 1596–1599, 1980
Steckel S: Patient Contracting. Appleton-Century-Crofts, Norwalk, Connecticut, 1982
Strodtman LK: A decision-making process for planning patient education. Patient Education & Counseling, Vol 5, No 4, pp 189–200, 1984
Suchman EA: Preventive health behavior: A model for research in community health campaigns. Journal of Health and Social Behavior, Vol 8, pp 197–209, 1967
Sue DW: Counseling the Culturally Different. John Wiley & Sons, Inc., New York, 1981
Tarnow KG: Working with adult learners. Nurse Educator, pp 34–40, September–October 1979
Wohl J: Intercultural psychotherapy: Issues, questions, and reflections. In Pedersen P, Draguns J, Lonnar W, Trimble J (eds): Counseling across Cultures. The East West Center, University Press of Hawaii, Honolulu, Hawaii, 1981

PART THREE

SELF-CARE PRACTICES

7

Nutrition

Adequate nutrition and elimination are critical for good health and essential in any discussion of health promotion, health maintenance, and disease prevention and treatment. Balance and moderation are the keys. While good nutrition enhances the health of every body system and organ, poor nutrition (including overnutrition) has potentially harmful physical and psychological consequences.

Increasing evidence relates dietary factors to health and disease. Many of the leading causes of death, such as heart disease, cerebral vascular disease, diabetes, and certain cancers are associated with nutrition and elimination problems. Dental caries and, recently, behavior problems (e.g., hyperactivity and juvenile delinquency, Lerner 1982) have been associated with use of particular foods or additives. Obesity, or overnutrition, is a major health problem in the United States and has clear implications for prevention of some of the diseases mentioned above.

In addition to an increasing clinical and research interest in the influence of nutrition on health, the public is demanding more information about diet. People want to know about cholesterol, sugar, alcohol, caffeine, food additives, and vitamins. More people are making informed choices about what to eat and what not to eat. This chapter emphasizes some current trends in nutrition and makes recommendations for changes in the American diet. In addition, discussion of overnutrition and consumption of potentially harmful substances are included. We suggest that readers consult general nutrition texts for a more detailed discussion (Brody 1982, Caliendo 1981, Williams 1982). How can nurses best counsel their clients for more effective self-care in nutrition and elimination? How can they help their clients deal with new information that is available almost daily?

Nutrition is a foundation on which many other self-care practices rest. Improved self-care in this area often leads to changes in health practices in many other areas. Techniques in counseling and tools of assessment and planning are covered beginning on page 139 of this chapter.

THE MEANING OF FOOD

The meaning of food and food practices are products of the cultural context. What is defined as food in one culture is not necessarily defined as food in another. A nutritionally acceptable diet could consist of foods most Americans never eat. For example, some nutritious items highly esteemed by members of other cultures include horse meat, dog meat, small birds, sea urchins, acorns, armadillos, rattlesnake meat, dragonflies, ants, grubs, and grasshoppers (Foster and Anderson 1978).

The concepts of the components of a meal, when it is eaten, and the etiquette of eating are also culturally defined, as well as what should be eaten cooked or raw, served hot or cold, or served appropriately together. For example, a Taiwanese student expressed her surprise at how many raw vegetables Americans eat. Hispanics and Middle Easterners identify certain foods as hot or cold, but with no relationship to the temperature of the foods. Hot-cold theory derives from humoral theory and specifies whether hot or cold foods are harmful or beneficial in various types of illnesses. In another example, Iranians consider walnuts and honey "hot," while cucumbers and yogurt are "cold." Too much "cold" or too much "hot" food at the same time is perceived to cause illness.

Foods are also classified into "high status" and "low status" ones. An example is the widespread use of infant formula in developing countries because it is considered better than mother's milk, although its improper use can result in infant illness or death. Another example of negative consequences of the perception of the status of food is the high intake of white bread and American junk food—and neglect of fresh foods—among some immigrants and teenagers.

Food has a psychological meaning too. Food is symbolic and associated with nurturing; it expresses affection or friendship in every society. For example, offering and accepting food is a gesture of trust among Middle Eastern people. A nurse who cared for an Arab child was not accepted by the family unit until it was suggested that she accept a meal at the family's house (Lipson and Meleis 1983). Food also expresses ethnic identity; for example, lamb in the Middle East, couscous in North Africa, chicken soup among Jews, and guacamole among Mexican-Americans. Food beliefs may be so strongly held that it is extremely difficult to persuade people to modify their traditional diets in the interest of improved health.

In addition to different perceptions of food are varying perceptions of health and illness in terms of body size. What is considered ideal weight or body size varies considerably throughout the world. "Thinness" means attractiveness among many Americans and Europeans but may be considered sickliness or unattractiveness among Hawaiians or Samoans.

COMPOSITION OF THE NORTH AMERICAN DIET

Farquhar (1978) states that the American diet is decidedly hazardous to one's health. It predisposes individuals to risks of cardiovascular disease and other obesity-related diseases such as diabetes, gout, osteoarthritis, gallbladder disease, and hypertension. Americans have heard for too long that more is better and that abundant food reflects prosperity and health. Fast foods have become part of the American way of life. Such attitudes need to change to correspond with current knowledge about food consumption and its relationship to health.

The major components of one's diet are proteins, fats, and carbohydrates. Proteins are the building blocks of the human body, comprising the fundamental structures of every cell. Adults can manufacture all but nine of the essential amino acids needed, and infants can manufacture all but ten; the others must be obtained from food. Meat and other animal proteins contain the full complement of amino acids, while plant proteins tend to lack, or be low in, one or more essential amino acids. Soybean protein is also essentially a complete protein. Its amino acid pattern conforms closely to that of milk. Two or more plant protein sources can be combined to form a complete protein, a process called protein complementing (Lappe 1975) (e.g., grains plus milk products, seeds plus legumes, grains plus legumes). Nutritious combinations include pasta with milk or cheese, cereal and milk, rice and bean casseroles, peas or beans on rice, pea soups and bread, and nuts or seeds in casseroles. Knowledge of protein complementarity is especially useful for vegetarians and low income families, since the cost of foods containing complete protein is often high.

The average per capita consumption of grams of protein has not changed significantly since the turn of the century, although the ratio of animal-to-vegetable protein has almost doubled, raising the level of consumption of fat and cholesterol. Recent studies indicate that many Americans consume far more protein than their bodies need for growth and repair.

Fats provide stored energy, carry fat-soluble vitamins, decrease gastric motility, and take longer to be digested. They are required for bile secretion from the gallbladder. Approximately 40% of the calories in the typical American diet are provided by fat. As a result of increased consumption of dairy products, shortening, margarine, and red meats and ingestion of saturated fat is significantly higher than levels recommended by the American Heart Association (1974).

Carbohydrates are the most immediate source of energy in the non-fasting state. One of the most important functions of carbohydrates is "sparing" protein so that protein can be used for tissue building instead of energy. In the United States, carbohydrates comprise approximately 40–50% of the calories in the normal diet, a major portion being contributed by simple carbohydrates. American dietary patterns have changed from consumption of primarily complex carbohydrates (such as rice, flour, beans, grains) to consumption of predominantly simple sugar carbohydrates, such as those found in milk, fruit, and sweeteners, such as refined sugar or honey. Sugar consumption now accounts for approximately 32% of the total carbohydrate consumption (Caliendo 1981) or 18% of total calories (Brewster 1978), which is inefficient. Although human beings have no physical need for refined sugar, the average American consumes 128 pounds of sugar a year (Liebman 1980) and 140–150 pounds annually for those aged 6–20 (Caliendo 1981).

Recommended Changes

National recommendations for change in the American diet are listed below. We describe some of these recommendations in detail. A more thorough discussion of obesity and use of the self-care approach begins on page 134.

GUIDELINES FOR HEALTHY EATING*

---

1. Eat only sufficient calories to meet body needs and maintain desirable weight (eat fewer calories if overweight).
2. Eat less saturated fat and cholesterol.
3. Eat less salt.
4. Eat less sugar.
5. Eat more complex carbohydrates such as whole grains, cereals, fruits, and vegetables.
6. Eat relatively more fish, poultry, legumes, and less red meat.

---

*United States Surgeon General's Report, September 1979, *Healthy People*

Decrease intake of fats and cholesterol. In 1974, the American Heart Association (1974) recommended reducing total fat calories from 40–45% of the diet to no more than 35%. Of this amount, saturated fats should be decreased to less than 10% and polyunsaturated fats should be increased to 10%; fats should be consumed throughout the day rather than at one time.

A diet high in saturated fats, calories, and refined sugar, and low in polyunsaturated fats, fiber, and certain trace minerals is hypothesized to lead to elevated levels of cholesterol and triglycerides, low density lipoprotein, and reduced high-density lipoproteins in the blood. These are thought to lead to lipid accumulation in the coronary arteries and atherosclerotic heart disease (Krehl 1977). It is recommended that cholesterol be decreased, especially for people with a family history of heart disease or who smoke. There is some evidence linking high fat diets to risk of breast and large bowel cancer (Pariza 1984; Willett and MacMahon 1984). Cholesterol can be reduced by substituting complex carbohydrate foods for fatty meats and dairy products, eliminating organ meats, reducing egg yolks to four a week, and substituting soft margarine and natural peanut butter for products containing saturated fats. Decreasing fat can be accomplished by reducing consumption of red fatty meats (beef, lamb, bacon, pork), substituting fish and poultry, trimming fat or skin from meat and poultry, broiling or roasting rather than frying foods, and substituting skim milk products for whole milk products (Farquhar 1978).

Decrease intake of salt. Salt has become America's number one food fear because of its contribution to hypertension, which contributes to half of the death rate in the United States annually (Wallis 1982). Hypertension is virtually unknown in such areas as New Guinea, the Amazon Basin, and the highlands of Malaysia and Uganda, where little salt is consumed. In contrast, in countries in which the salt intake is high (e.g., Japan), hypertension rates are also high (Wallis 1982). Despite some epidemiological evidence, the relationship between high sodium intake and hypertension is not as clear as is commonly thought. It is difficult to predict who is sensitive to salt and at risk for hypertension; therefore, reducing salt intake is recommended for everyone. Public pressure has led to recent industrial removal of salt from infant foods (thought to lead to developing a taste for salt later in life) and introduction of many low-sodium foods. Lowering salt intake from 11 to 5 grams a day seems to reduce hypertension, as demonstrated in the Stanford Heart Disease Program (Farquhar 1978). This may be difficult if the client's diet includes fast foods or prepackaged foods, which have a high salt content.

Decrease intake of sugar. Eating large amounts of refined sugar can be worse than eating nothing at all because sugar is only empty calories containing no protein, fat, vitamins, or minerals; sugar can deplete the body of nutrients (Fillip 1981). It is difficult to avoid sugar because it is added to so many processed foods, such as canned products and peanut butter. Approximately 65% of sugar consumed is that added to food and beverages by the manufacturers (Fillip 1981).

Sugar intake is a major factor in such degenerative diseases as diabetes and coronary heart disease (Farquhar 1978), as well as contributing to obesity, vitamin deficiencies, psychological disturbances, and dental caries.

Increase complex carbohydrates. Complex carbohydrates contain numerous essential nutrients in addition to calories. Consumption of complex carbohydrates, such as beans, peas, seeds, nuts, and whole grains, results in decreased fat intake and increased dietary fiber, which helps to increase intestinal motility. This helps to reduce elimination problems such as constipation, diverticulosis, and irritable bowel syndrome, and may decrease risk of bowel cancer. Fiber decreases absorption of fat and cholesterol. By binding bile acids, fiber may also reduce their bacterial conversion to secondary bile acids that are potential carcinogens. Fiber may also bind ingested toxins and promote their excretion in the feces. Caliendo suggests, "Cancer-causing agents can be more readily absorbed to the fiber and hence be eliminated more quickly" (1981:290). The water-binding capacity of fiber leads to more frequent and softer stools (Caliendo 1981). Increased fiber is useful for diabetics because the sugar in food moves through the small intestinal wall more slowly in the presence of fiber, decreasing the amount of sugar released into the blood.

Vitamins. In addition to amino acids, fatty acids, and carbohydrates, vitamins are organic compounds that are necessary in small amounts in the diet for normal growth, maintenance of health, and reproduction. The presence or absence of very small amounts of vitamins in the diet makes a difference between normal and abnormal functioning of the body. Good sources of most vitamins include green leafy vegetables, seeds, legumes, and whole grain cereals.

A current controversial issue is whether or not people need vitamin supplements. Many health professionals and nutritionists suggest that individuals who consume a healthy and balanced diet containing foods rich in natural vitamins and minerals have no need for vitamin supplements. Others suggest that there is a wide range of biochemical individuality among people, and everyone would benefit from supplements of some vitamins and minerals. The problem is that there is currently no way of determining each individual's optimum requirements (Ferguson 1981). Some vitamin proponents suggest that an individual take specific vitamin supplements for specific reasons (e.g., vitamin D to aid calcium absorption for older women; B complex for people under stress; vitamin C for upper respiratory infections)(Mindell 1979). The vitamin issue is one to watch as biochemical techniques improve.

OBESITY

Despite national recommendations for the maintenance of ideal weight, approximately one third of the population of the United States is overweight. We focus on obesity rather than other alterations in nutritional health such as anorexia and bulimia because we consider obesity more easily modified through self-care practices.

A person is considered clinically overweight if the weight is 10% more than ideal body weight for height and size of frame. Clinical obesity is defined as weight 20% more than ideal body weight. There is disagreement about how to determine ideal body weight, despite the widespread use of the Metropolitan Life Insurance Table, shown in Table 7-1. Another formula that suggests lower ideal body weight is shown below (Farquhar 1978:144):

Women—height in inches x 3.5 − 108 = IBW (ideal body weight)
Men—height in inches x 4 − 128 = IBW

Obesity, in the majority of cases, is a direct result of calorie intake exceeding calorie expenditure over an extended period. It results either from overeating, which is usually a learned behavior, or from decreased activity—an unbalanced energy equation. Taking into consideration such factors as ethnicity, religious affiliation, socioeconomic status, and heredity, it appears clear that obesity is often a family problem. For example, 60–70% of obese adolescents have one or both obese parents, and 40% of their siblings are also obese (Hammer et al. 1972). Children are often rewarded and/or bribed with food. Because of the behavioral component in overeating, obesity is probably the most preventable and potentially controllable health problem facing us today. However, this is not easy. Knowledge alone is not enough to change behavior!

The problem with obesity is that it leads to metabolic changes such as hyperinsulinemia, impaired glucose tolerance, hyperlipidemia, and hypertension. The Framingham study showed that as the degree of overweight increases, the risks of cardiovascular disease, hypertension, and diabetes increase (Gordon and Kannell 1976). Although controversial, Pritikin (1979) suggests that fat suffocates the tissues by depriving them of oxygen, leading to atherosclerosis and gout, and by impeding carbohydrate metabolism which can foster diabetes. He suggests that physical exercise helps to decrease hyperinsulinemia and serum triglycerides, and improves glucose tolerance tests.

Two clinical types of obesity exist—hyperplasia and hypertrophic obesity. Hyperplasia obesity is characterized by three to five times as many fat cells as normal; in addition, fat cells are enlarged. This type usually begins in infancy or childhood, with fat distributions occurring centrally and peripherally. Permanent weight loss cannot occur easily because there is an increased *number* of fat cells; reducing diets shrink or help to deplete the fat cells of their energy stores. In the second type, called hypertrophic obesity, the size of the fat cell is increased. This type usually begins after puberty, with fat distribution occurring centrally. Although hypertrophic obesity responds to reducing diets, it may also be associated with non-insulin dependent diabetes, hyperlipidemia, and abnormal glucose tolerance tests (Mahan 1979). Exercise can help to decrease fat cell size but not number.

Recently, new ideas about weight loss and obesity have emerged. Among the new theories about weight loss in obesity are the theory of "set point" (Bennett and Gurin 1982) which suggests that the individual has a

TABLE 7-1. 1983 METROPOLITAN HEIGHT AND WEIGHT TABLES

	Men				Women		
Height Feet Inches	Small Frame	Medium Frame	Large Frame	Height Feet Inches	Small Frame	Medium Frame	Large Frame
5 2	128–134	131–141	138–150	4 10	102–111	109–121	118–131
5 3	130–136	133–143	140–153	4 11	103–113	111–123	120–134
5 4	132–138	135–145	142–156	5 0	104–115	113–126	122–137
5 5	134–140	137–148	144–160	5 1	106–118	115–129	125–140
5 6	136–142	139–151	146–164	5 2	108–121	118–132	128–143
5 7	138–145	142–154	149–168	5 3	111–124	121–135	131–147
5 8	140–148	145–157	152–172	5 4	114–127	124–138	134–151
5 9	142–151	148–160	155–176	5 5	117–130	127–141	137–155
5 10	144–154	151–163	158–180	5 6	120–133	130–144	140–159
5 11	146–157	154–166	161–184	5 7	123–136	133–147	143–163
6 0	149–160	157–170	164–188	5 8	126–139	136–150	146–167
6 1	152–164	160–174	168–192	5 9	129–142	139–153	149–170
6 2	155–168	164–178	172–197	5 10	132–145	142–156	152–173
6 3	158–172	167–182	176–202	5 11	135–148	145–159	155–176
6 4	162–176	171–187	181–207	6 0	138–151	148–162	158–179

Weights at ages 25–59 based on lowest mortality. Weight in pounds according to frame (in indoor clothing weighing 5 lbs. for men and 3 lbs. for women; shoes with 1" heels).

From 1979 Build Study, Society of Actuaries and Association of Life Insurance Medical Directors of America, 1980 (used with permission of Metropolitan Life Insurance Co., Health and Safety Education Division, Copyright 1983).

genetically defined control system within him that dictates how much fat is needed. A "thermostat" or "set point" seeks to maintain this amount of fat in an active manner. When dieting and the weight approaches the limit, the individual experiences irritability and anxiety (signs of hypoglycemia) and begins to eat again. It is very difficult to lose weight beyond this set point and, when one does, it is rapidly gained back.

Another theory suggests that fat people eat less than thin people but have internal chemistries that are adapted to low calorie intake (Bailey 1977). Bailey suggests that it is possible to change this internal chemistry (alter metabolism and increased energy expenditure) so that the body has a lessened tendency to make fat out of the food eaten. Overweight people are more proficient than thin people at storing fat and less proficient at burning it off. In addition, the more fat one has, the more one's body chemistry alters to favor the build-up of still more fat. Bailey states that people are *overfat*, not *overweight*, and suggests that the only remedy for obesity is to decrease the proportion of fat on the individual's body through exercise, which converts fat into energy, biochemically (see Chapter 8 on Activity, Rest, and Exercise).

POTENTIALLY HARMFUL SUBSTANCES

Some recommendations on nutrition suggest decreasing consumption of caffeine, alcohol, and food additives such as artificial colors, preservatives, nitrates, and flavor enhancers (e.g., MSG) because of their negative effects on health and potential risks for disease, e.g., cancer. (Farquhar 1978.)

Some individuals find that caffeine precipitates the stress response. Those individuals who drink excessive coffee, tea, or other caffeinated beverages find that they experience shakiness, anxiety, restlessness, heart palpitations, stomach irritation, and diarrhea. As a mild diuretic (Briggs and Calloway 1979), caffeine is thought to decrease or inhibit the absorption of water soluble vitamins (Mason 1980). Animal studies show contradictory results, although one revealed that caffeine-treated female animals had such developmental alterations as cleft palate and digital malformations (Brooten and Jordan 1983). Although no human malformation has been attributed *directly* to caffeine, high daily intake of caffeine (600 mg or above) is associated with human fetal death and birth defects (Brooten and Jordan 1983). The Food and Drug Administration has warned women to avoid or minimize caffeine intake during pregnancy. See Table 7-2 for amounts of caffeine contained in foods and beverages.

In addition to caffeine, other substances have recently been accused of various negative health effects. For example, sulfur dioxide, a preservative found in many foods, can trigger asthma attacks in susceptible individuals. Tommy (see case example) began to wheeze whenever he ate dried sulphured apricots. Dyes, food additives, and salicylates are thought to be related to hyperactivity in children.

TABLE 7-2. CAFFEINE CONTENT IN COMMON BEVERAGES AND DRUGS

Coffee, tea, and cocoa (milligrams per serving—average values)		Over-the-Counter Drugs (milligrams per tablet)	
Coffee, instant	66	Anacin	32mg
Coffee, percolated	110	Aqua-ban	100mg
Coffee, drip	146	Bivarin	200mg
Teabag—5 minute brew	46	Caffedrine	200mg
Teabag—1 minute brew	28	Dristan	16mg
Loose tea—5 minute brew	40	Empirin	32mg
Cocoa	13	Excedrin	64mg
		Midol	32mg
Cola beverages (milligrams per 12-ounce can)		No Doz	100mg
		Pre-mens Forte	100mg
		Vanquish	33mg
Coca Cola	65		
Dr. Pepper	61		
Mountain Dew	55		
Diet Dr. Pepper	54		
TAB	49		
Pepsi-Cola	43		
Diet RC	33		
Diet-Rite	32		

Adapted from Tables 3 and 4 in Bunker M, McWilliams M: Caffeine content of common beverages, Journal of the American Dietetic Association, Vol 74, No 28, pp 28–32, January 1979 (Copyright The American Dietetic Association. Reprinted by permission from Journal of the American Dietetic Association)

Food intolerances and allergies are beginning to receive increased attention in the literature. One of the most common food intolerances is lactose intolerance. The milk-tolerant adult is actually the exception in the world, for lactose tolerance is common only among Northern European Caucasians and their descendents, and two African tribes (Hongladarom and Russell 1976). Allergies are found to be the cause of a number of vague symptoms in many individuals, from headache to stomach pains to difficulty writing and staying awake, and other behavioral changes (Smith 1976, 1979).

Planning for a healthy diet in the presence of food allergies is a challenge for nurses and clients alike. However, there are a number of resources that can be helpful, such as *The Allergy Encyclopedia* (see references). Some people are not aware that an individual food is part of a food family; if an individual is allergic to one member of a food family, there is an increased likelihood of being allergic to another. The first step in diet planning is identifying the problem food(s) through an elimination diet and careful observations, which should be kept in writing. When the foods have been identified, they should be avoided from then on. Clients must learn to read labels carefully and should be encouraged to use creativity in substitutions. For example, a client who is allergic to eggs might substitute yogurt or sour cream for mayonnaise in salad dressings.

There are a number of other topics that are relevant to nutrition and elimination but are beyond the scope of this chapter. With the above recommendations in mind, we turn now to discussing how to help people change their diets to improve their health, the role of diet in elimination, and suggestions for weight reduction. The remainder of the chapter will be presented in the context of the nursing process.

CLINICAL APPLICATION AND THE NURSING PROCESS

Assessing Nutrition

Ethnic and cultural variations influence the value placed on both food and body size. Food habits, nutritional preferences, and values are greatly influenced by the family unit. When assessing and recommending dietary changes, it is important to keep family food preferences and values in mind.

However, before planning any changes, it is very important to have an accurate assessment of what the client is currently eating. Many people plan to limit themselves more severely than is appropriate because they believe that their diets are already limited. Assessment gives the client a good baseline of current food intake. Following an accurate assessment, clients are often surprised to find how little water they drink or how many snacks and/or calories they actually consume.

There are a number of different techniques for assessing nutritional intake. The **food frequency record** is a written tool to list various foods. The client checks the foods he does and does not eat, as well as how often the food is eaten. This can be done in almost any clinical setting, and the nurse can get a general overall idea of the client's dietary patterns and adequacy of nutritional intake.

A second assessment tool is the **food intake diary** which supplements the initial assessment. The food intake diary requires the client to list the time each food or beverage was consumed, comments about how the food was prepared, how much was consumed, and other factors relating to how the client was feeling or the circumstances under which the food was eaten (see Figure 7-1).

24-HOUR FOOD DIARY

Date/Time	What Consumed	Amount	Preparation	Thoughts and Feelings

Figure 7-1. Food intake diary.

Some self-assessment tools such as those in Figures 7-2 (page 141) and 7-3 (page 142) ask questions about food habits, feelings, and thoughts related to food, rather than about specific foods eaten. This kind of tool can be helpful in increasing client awareness about food and its consumption. It may remind the client of questions he wanted to ask, e.g., "What about caffeine?"

Assessing elimination may also be necessary in a complete self-care assessment with a focus on nutrition. Inadequate fluid consumption, lack of roughage, excessive caffeine, inadequate exercise, poor hygienic practice leading to bladder infections, stress, and lack of importance placed on elimination are related to alterations in bowel and bladder functions. Most people do not think about elimination until there is a problem. However, alterations in elimination are common health problems. There are a number of self-care practices that can be taught to clients to prevent and manage such alterations.

Assessment of urinary elimination includes the following questions:

1. How many times the individual voids daily

2. Color, amount, and odor of urine
3. Hygienic practices
4. Urgency, hesitancy, burning, bleeding, and pain.

Assessment of bowel functioning includes the following questions:

1. Frequency of movements
2. Time of day
3. Stool consistency
4. Use of laxatives
5. Pain or bleeding
6. Diarrhea, constipation, or fecal impaction.

Once assessment is complete, long- and short-term goals are set.

NUTRITION SELF-ASSESSMENT

Complete the following self-assessment to help you look at the role of "nutrition" in your life now. On the scale below circle the numbers which best indicate you and your life during the last year:

	Almost Never	Seldom	Often	Almost Always
1. I read the labels for ingredients on foods I consume . . .	1	2	3	4
2. I have two meatless days a week . . .	1	2	3	4
3. I eat food without salting it . . .	1	2	3	4
4. My meals include nonfat or lowfat milk and dairy products . . .	1	2	3	4
5. I limit my meals at fast food restaurants to twice a week . . .	1	2	3	4
6. I limit myself to three alcoholic drinks per week (including wine or beer) . . .	1	2	3	4
7. I limit my caffeine use to three times per week (coffee, tea, cola drinks, etc.) . . .	1	2	3	4
8. I limit sweet desserts to three times per week . . .	1	2	3	4
9. My typical meals include fresh fruits and raw vegetables . . .	1	2	3	4

10. Meal times are pleasant to me . . .   1   2   3   4

Some suggestions for how you might learn from this self-assessment:

1. Connect all the circles down the length of the page. Look at the pattern that your connected line makes. You might also turn your page sideways to get an even more clear visual picture of "nutrition" in your life right now. What does it seem to be saying to you?

2. Now add up your total score: _____

   Circle which range it was in:

   10–19   20–29   30–40

   If your score was in the 10–19 range you might want to make some changes in your nutritional life. Which aspects do you think need the most work? How many "1's" did you mark on this assessment? _____ These might serve as a clue to help you think about making changes in this area of your life.

3. How would you like this self-assessment to look six months from now? Are you interested in planning towards those improvements?

4. Remember to congratulate yourself for the ways in which you are providing good nutrition for yourself. Give yourself a pat on the back; go out and eat something "good" as a way to congratulate yourself.

Figure 7-2. Nutrition self-assessment form (From Baldi S. Costell S, Hill L, Jasmin S, Smith N: For Your Health: A Model for Self-Care. Nurses Model Health, South Laguna, California, 1980, reprinted with permission from Nurses Model Health).

DIET FEELINGS CHECK-OFF

1. Which of the following are descriptive of your eating patterns? Check all those that apply to you:

   ☐ between-meal eating
   ☐ irregular and unpatterned meal and snack times
   ☐ lack of sensitivity to true feelings of hunger
   ☐ thinking about food too much of the time
   ☐ being around food too much of the time
   ☐ eating too many sweets or starch foods
   ☐ lack of knowledge about nutrition
   ☐ eating too quickly

☐ not paying attention to what you are eating
☐ uncontrollable binges
☐ overeating at social events
☐ lack of sensitivity to true feelings of fullness
☐ lack of other satisfactions in life
☐ eating in reaction to tension and depression
☐ eating in reaction to boredom
☐ overeating when you are by yourself
☐ big physical size has a positive effect upon people
☐ unattractive body limits relationships with opposite sex
☐ eating to take your mind off other problems
☐ using eating as a way to control feelings or behavior of others (for example, to make them hungry or to make them do as you wish)
☐ using food as a reward for yourself

2. Which of the following do you use as signals to stop eating?
☐ feeling of fullness
☐ food stops tasting good
☐ feeling of satisfaction
☐ uncomfortable fullness
☐ clean plate
☐ everyone else has stopped eating
☐ you want more, but would feel guilty if you ate more
☐ you want more, but intellectually know that you have had enough

3. Over a three-day period, estimate how many meals _____ and snacks _____ you usually eat.

Figure 7-3. Checklist for Diet Feelings (reprinted with permission of *The American Health Foundation*, 320 East 43rd Street, New York, N.Y. 10017).

Planning and Implementation

Making dietary changes usually involves a number of life-style changes and is a long-term process. The client will be less discouraged and less likely to fail if the process is broken into small, achievable goals. Farquhar (1978) suggests three phases in establishing an alternative food pattern. In phase one, the long-term goal of eliminating sugar begins with the change in the dessert pattern, for example, which is changed by substituting fruit for pies, cakes, or pastry one-third of the time. During the second phase, fruit substitutes for two-thirds of desserts eaten. In phase three, fruit or fruit and nut combinations are the predominant dessert. Phase I of Farquhar's Alternative Food Pattern begins on page 144.

FARQUHAR'S ALTERNATIVE FOOD PATTERN*

Phase I Changes

A. Saturated-Fat and Cholesterol Control

1. Reduce weekly servings of whole milk, cheese (other than low-fat cottage cheese), fatty meats (beef, lamb, bacon, spareribs, sausage, and luncheon meats), and ice cream by one-half (e.g., from the U.S. average of 24 servings a week to about 12 per week). Substitute complex-carbohydrate foods and foods such as fish and poultry in their place. (Do not eat chicken skin.)

2. Change from ice cream to ice milk and from whole milk to nonfat milk. (Infants should preferably be breast-fed. If infants are formula-fed, use the "natural" low-sodium varieties that have recently become available. If they are given cow's milk, use whole milk only up to the age of one year.)

3. Reduce meat fat by trimming and by broiling or roasting instead of frying.

4. Eliminate, except for rare use, intake of organ meats such as liver, sweetbreads, and brains.

5. Change from butter or hard margarine (made with hydrogenated oil) to soft tub margarine (made with unhydrogenated oil).

6. Change from lard to shortening to unhydrogenated vegetable oil, including olive oil if desired. (Although some nutritionists recommend the use of highly polyunsaturated oils, I feel that any type of vegetable oil other than palm or coconut oil [the only saturated fats that are liquid at room temperature] is acceptable. Healthy cultures have used olive oil, a monosaturated oil, successfully for thousands of years.) Avoid use of large amounts of vegetable oils as you want to lower your total fat intake in Phase I from the current U.S. average of 40 percent to about 30 percent of total calories consumed.

7. Reduce consumption of egg yolks to no more than four a week. Use egg whites liberally.

8. Change from creamy peanut butter made with hydrogenated fat to natural peanut butter made without hydrogenated fat.

9. Reduce consumption of fast foods, processed and convenience foods, commercial baked goods, and the like.

*Reprinted from Farquhar JW: The American Way of Life Need Not Be Hazardous to Your Health, 1978 (by permission of W.W. Norton & Company, Inc., copyright 1978, JW Farquhar; originally published as part of The Portable Stanford by the Stanford Alumni Association).

B. Sugar Control
   1. Reduce consumption of soft drinks by half. Limit intake to two or three a week. (U.S. average is five 12-ounce cans or bottles a week.)
   2. Gradually eliminate use of sugar in coffee or tea and on fruit. (Saccharin is discouraged, not only because of its possible role as a carcinogen but also because of the importance of retraining your palate to lowered sweetness levels.)
   3. Switch from heavy to light syrup in canned fruits.
   4. Substitute fruit for pastry, cake, pie, or other sweets in one-third of all desserts.

C. Salt and Caffeine Control

   1. Eliminate, except for rare use, high-salt items such as bacon, ham, sausage, frankfurters, luncheon meats, salted nuts, sauerkraut, pickles, canned soups, canned vegetables, potato chips, and other salted snacks and foods.
   2. Switch from regular table salt to a light salt (one-half sodium chloride, one-half potassium chloride).
   3. Gradually decrease salt use in cooking to about one-third previous levels; simultaneously decrease, and eventually eliminate, salt use at the table.
   4. Explore the use of other flavors in your cooking—spices, herbs, lemon, wine, vinegar, etc.
   5. Limit intake of caffeinated drinks (coffee, tea, cola, etc.) to four cups a day. Try decaffeinated alternatives and herb teas.

D. Complex-Carbohydrate and Fiber Control

   1. Increase intake of complex-carbohydrate foods—including legumes (e.g., beans, peas, lentils), starchy root vegetables such as the potato, as well as other vegetables and fruits—as a partial or full caloric replacement (depending on weight-control needs) for reduced intake of sugar and fatty animal foods.
   2. Gradually introduce lightly milled or whole-grained cereals into your food plan (e.g., whole-wheat bread and flour, bulgur, couscous, cracked wheat, rolled oats, rye, brown rice, etc.).
   3. Increase intake of whole fruits (fruit juices lack much of the fiber contained in whole fruit).
   4. Increase intake of whole vegetables (vegetable juices lack much of the fiber contained in whole vegetables and often contain significant amounts of added salt).

E. High-Caloric-Density Food Control

   1. Reduce intake of HCD foods by one-third (e.g., from average U.S. number of 15 portions per day to about 10 per day). By doing this,

you will also reduce your intake of salt, sugar, and saturated fat.
2. Partially or fully replace such foods with complex carbohydrates (depending on weight-control goals).

F. Alcohol Control

1. Because alcohol may add to weight-control problems and may displace valuable nutrients, limit alcohol consumption so that no more than 10 percent of your total calorie intake is derived from alcohol, e.g., approximately two bottles of beer (24 oz.) or three glasses of wine (9 oz.) or two cocktails (3 oz. liquor) per day.

An understanding of motivation by both the nurse and client is important when changing food patterns. Motivating behavior change is one of the most important but difficult aspects of dietary change. There are a number of techniques that can be used to increase the likelihood that the client will make changes. Use of a behavior contract is one technique (see page 117 in Chapter 6). Accurate record keeping by the client is also helpful. Both work because they encourage the client to actively participate and take responsibility for behavior change. Cost can be a motivating factor in changing dietary patterns (see Figure 7-4 for example).

Other techniques for motivation must also be tried. Mahoney and Caggiula (1978) suggest presenting a clear description of the potential danger or problems associated with maintaining current behaviors. Such discussion can provide cues to health action, as postulated by the Health Belief Model. The nurse's attitude can make a difference. Communicating to the client a firm belief that clients can and will change their eating behavior may improve their health and well-being. The nurse's role also includes modeling healthy eating behavior. Clients are less likely to follow the advice of health professionals who obviously do not follow their own advice.

Techniques used to change dietary consumption are related to theories of learning discussed in Chapter 6. Skinner's pioneering work in operant conditioning is the basis for many diet plans. It has been found that positive consequences are more effective than negative ones in effecting weight reduction (Mahoney 1974; Mahoney, Moura, and Wade 1973). One type of positive reinforcement is shaping. Shaping is reinforcing successively better approximations of a desired behavior. For example, the client may get positive feedback for eliminating red meat once a week. Over time, the client moves toward the long-term goal of reducing meat consumption to twice a week.

Arranging the environment increases the likelihood that a diet will be carried out. This technique can be very difficult and is often neglected. An example of environmental planning is arranging for activities to take the place of snacking, e.g., taking a walk instead of taking a snack. Another

HOW MUCH DO WE PAY FOR EMPTY CALORIES?

Objective: To calculate the portions of the personal and family budget spent on foods with nutritive value, and on empty calorie foods.

Procedure:

1. Have students determine whether the family makes a sound investment in food. (Food is one of the major investments a family or an individual makes.) The student could volunteer to purchase the food for the family or check off the food and prices when the groceries are brought home. (Be sure to add extra items purchased during the week.) COST OR ESTIMATED VALUE OF GROCERIES FOR MY FAMILY FOR ONE WEEK

Vegetables and Juices $ _____
Fruit and Juices   _____
Milk, Cheese, Yogurt   _____
Protein Foods   _____
Bread and Cereal   _____
Other Staple Items   _____
        TOTAL $ _____
Sweets, Cookies, Candy $ _____
Cake, Pastries   _____
Presweetened Cereal   _____
Soft Drinks   _____
Other Empty Calorie Foods   _____ $ _____

2. Processed foods are an expensive addition to the family's food bill. Calculate the portion of your family's food budget spent on relatively unprocessed basics, and the portion on highly processed items (TV dinners, fancy frozen vegetables, casserole kits—such as Tuna Helper®).

3. DISCUSS: What major factors influenced the purchase of good food? What major factors influenced the purchase of poor food?

   How much money is spent on nutritious foods? How much on empty calorie foods?

4. Have students keep track of their own food purchases for a week. Calculate the portion spent on nutritious, wholesome foods and the portion spent on empty calories. Add up class totals.

5. Have students prepare bar graphs of above information.

Figure 7-4. From Katz D, Goodwin M: Where nutrition, politics, and culture meet. Center for Science in the Public Interest, Washington, D.C. (reprinted with permission from the publisher).

helpful change is to preplan meals and snacks for each day and week. By so doing, binges and other means of "cheating" are less likely. Strategies should also be designed for eating away from home, e.g., informing hosts of one's diet, requesting in restaurants that one's food be prepared according to the diet (no added salt, microwaved).

Weight reduction. Recommendations for weight loss include eating small, frequent meals, decreasing calories and alcohol, increasing fiber, increasing energy expenditure with exercise, and enlisting family and social support. Weight loss support/self-help groups such as Overeaters Anonymous and Weight Watchers can be helpful in this regard, providing support and peer group pressure. Remember, knowledge alone is not always sufficient to change behavior, including dieting; the motivational aspects of groups or behavioral changes may be helpful.

The success of any diet depends on how well the diet is followed. A diet will be followed more closely if it fits with client's physical and psychological, familial, and cultural needs. Characteristics of diets leading to long-term weight reduction include the following requirements:

1. Satisfies all nutrient needs
2. Is adapted as closely as possible to the everyday habits of the individual and family
3. Protects the client from hunger as much as possible and leaves him with a sense of well-being
4. Is easy to follow at home and away from home
5. Can be followed over a long period of time
6. Leads to long-term changes in eating habits
7. Satisfies psychological needs and considers feelings.

Some dieters find the following tips useful. Including a 150–200 calorie "treat" daily keeps one from "feeling deprived" and decreases "cheating." One should plan around social or weekend activities by allowing a moderate increase in calories and consuming fewer calories during the work week. It is important to keep foods that are difficult to resist (e.g., ice cream or potato chips) out of the house or at least out of sight or reach. Keeping a food diary on an ongoing basis is a motivating factor, as well as being useful for evaluation. Exercise helps to burn calories, speeds up the metabolism, and reduces frustration or anxiety related to dieting. The client should be encouraged to exercise for at least 20 minutes, three to five times a week. Steady walking is a good beginning (see Chapter 8). Support of family and friends is critical for success in dietary change. These people are in a powerful position to support or sabotage the individual's efforts on a daily basis. For example, the dieter could ask family members to avoid offering "forbidden" foods and help to keep such foods out of the house or to give positive feedback for eating according to the diet.

It is important to acknowledge the possibility of self-defeating behaviors. In the example of weight reduction, the nurse can ask clients what they do to sabotage themselves. This may not be conscious until such a discussion occurs. Common self-defeating behaviors include believing that weight loss is undeserved, or becoming discouraged and going off the diet after reaching a plateau. Another common mistake is rewarding weight loss with food. Some people go off a diet before the goal is reached in response to compliments or finding their clothes larger. Others go off in response to ridicule. Many dieters wait until tomorrow (or Monday) to go back on a diet after "cheating." If overeating occurs at lunch, the client should be instructed to return to the diet plan for dinner and not wait for the next day's meals. One hundred calories above an individual's caloric requirement a day will lead to a one pound weight gain in five weeks. In one year, the weight gain will be 10 pounds, and 100 pounds in 10 years.

Elimination problems. If diarrhea is a problem, it is important to determine and eliminate the cause whenever possible. Management of acute diarrhea involves eliminating all foods for 24 hours (clear liquids only). If the diarrhea slows or stops, low residue, soft lactose-free foods, such as eggs, custards, soups, and toast can be added. Caffeine should be avoided. Add foods one at a time, watching the gastrointestinal tract's response. Management of chronic diarrhea is different. Although caffeine should also be avoided, fiber should be added in the form of fresh fruits, vegetables, and bran.

Constipation is characterized by infrequent bowel movements and may also be associated with dryness of the stool. Self-care techniques to prevent and manage constipation include eating foods high in fiber and natural residues, drinking prune juice and six to eight glasses of water, regular exercise, and stress management. A cup of coffee with breakfast followed by sitting down for one-half hour in a relaxed environment can facilitate a bowel movement.

Urinary tract infections are more common in women because their urethras are shorter. Most are caused by E. Coli from anal and vaginal bacteria, which enter the urethra when the woman wipes back to front. Therefore, bladder infections can often be prevented by wiping front-to-back and keeping the vaginal and anal areas clean. The nurse should suggest the following:

- Drink at least eight glasses of water each day to dilute the urine and provide a less hospitable environment for bacteria
- Urinate every 2–3 hours and after sexual intercourse
- Wear cotton underwear (Ritz and Simmons 1981). Once a urinary tract infection is diagnosed, antibiotics and antispasmotics will often be prescribed. Herbal teas may be helpful in alleviating symptoms (Weiner 1980).

Evaluation

Evaluating diet and elimination changes must be related to the goals that were set and should include three aspects:

1. The extent to which the plans were carried out (e.g., how many glasses of water did the client prone to urinary tract infections actually drink daily?)
2. The extent to which the goals were met (e.g., Did the client lose the desired amount of weight each week?)
3. The nature of the goals and plans (e.g., Was it realistic for the nurse to try to eliminate caffeine on her first rotation to night shift?)

Developing healthy eating habits can lead to an increased sense of well-being, better health, and longevity. However, change in eating habits takes time and effort. Knowledge alone does not ensure behavior changes and food choices satisfy many needs besides hunger. Nurses have a responsibility for assessing nutrition and elimination and recommending diets that are adequate and safe. Nutrition is an area that is critically important and basic to self-care.

SUMMARY

This chapter describes the composition of the North American diet and suggests improvements for better health. We focus on obesity and offer recommendations for self-care. Several tools are provided to encourage nutrition self-care in clients and for nurses themselves.

CASE EXAMPLE

Judith is the mother of three-year-old Tommy, an active and healthy boy with allergies. He has eczema, frequent nasal congestion, and has had to go to the emergency room several times for asthma attacks. Judith sought the help of an allergist, who arranged that Tommy have skin testing. The tests revealed that Tommy was allergic to house dust, animal fur and feathers, molds, grass and weed pollens, and a number of foods. Judith followed suggestions to minimize house dust, get rid of the dog, and keep Tommy indoors on windy days during pollen seasons.

Judith continued to be frustrated and concerned about Tommy's discomfort and decided that she wanted to take a more active approach. She sought to help of her friend Monica, who was interested in self-care. Monica suggested that they do an assessment and devise a self-care plan for Judith to carry out with Tommy. Monica began by asking Judith what she knew about allergies and what she was currently doing. Judith had a good understanding about how allergens trigger symptoms, having read the materials given to her by the allergist. However, she needed practical ways to minimize Tommy's exposure to allergens. Monica and Judith decided that self-care should begin with food and nutrition. They outlined two important goals—avoid foods to which Tommy was allergic and assure that he had a nutritious and balanced diet. Monica suggested a third possibility—that they devise a vitamin supplement* program to help Tommy build up his resistance. Judith and Monica planned to meet on a regular basis to evaluate and plan new strategies. Judith appreciated Monica's interest, advice, and support, because no one else seemed to take Tommy's discomfort so seriously.

Judith's plans for the first two weeks were as follows:

1. Keep a diary of Tommy's daily food intake
2. Begin a modified elimination diet
3. Obtain reference materials for planning
4. Read all labels on food products, and do not buy foods that are not labeled.

Judith obtained an RDA list of nutrients needed for children and taped it to the inside of a kitchen cabinet door. She purchased a nutrition book, *The Allergy Encyclopedia*, and *Earl Mindell's Vitamin Bible for Your Kids* (see references).

Judith began Tommy's elimination diet by limiting him to the foods she was sure he had not had problems with and avoiding those that skin testing had shown to be a problem, such as eggs, potatoes, wheat, citrus, tomatoes, etc. Her trips to the supermarket were enlightening, although time-consuming. She discovered that she had been inadvertently giving Tommy eggs (which caused an acute reaction) contained in the batter of frozen fish sticks and in ice cream. Since he loved ice cream and was complaining about not being able to eat some of his favorite foods, she substituted an inexpensive brand that contained no eggs.

During the first two weeks of implementation, Judith kept a careful diary of Tommy's food intake. Each evening, she spent up to an hour going over his intake and comparing it to the nutrient chart. Judith met with Monica after two weeks to review the self-care plan progress. Tommy's symptoms were improved, particularly his nasal congestion and eczema. Judith had realized that his diet was lacking in B vitamins because she had eliminated all grains except rice. Also, Tommy's nursery school teacher had given him oranges on several occasions during snack time.

Judith and Monica worked out the plan for the next few months. They decided on a vitamin regimen of a multivitamin, extra B-complex, and extra vitamin C. Monica suggested that Judith add vitamin E for Tommy's dry skin, and vitamin A several times a week, although she cautioned her

---

*Authors' note: We acknowledge the controversial nature of vitamin supplements and are in no way prescribing this or any other vitamin regimen for allergic children.

not to overload Tommy with fat-soluble vitamins. Judith decided to meet with the teachers and to prepare a special snack for Tommy to eat on days that he could not eat the class snack.

Over the next six months, Judith continued to read labels, keep a diary, and periodically check the adequacy of Tommy's diet. She added questionable foods, no more than one at a time, with a week in between, and observed Tommy's reactions. She found that he could tolerate some foods, such as citrus, but had definite problems with others, such as walnuts and eggs. Tommy was also learning what foods made him "itchy" and "stuffy" and was beginning to talk about them with his family and the teachers. He loved his snack mix of puffed rice, sunflower seeds, dried apples, apricots, pineapple, and raisins and was content with this substitute for the school snack. His eczema was now limited to his wrists and backs of his legs. Judith attributed some of the improvement to the vitamin E, which had helped his dry skin. The most dramatic improvement was that Tommy's wheezing never became severe enough to necessitate an emergency room visit, which Judith attributed not only to her care around breathable allergens but also to the special vitamin regimen with added pantothenic acid and vitamin B6. Judith now felt that she had the tools she needed for re-evaluating Tommy's allergies and self-care on a continuing basis.

CASE EXAMPLE

Dan is a 28-year-old, white, married public relations director for a municipal bus company. Approximately one year ago he began to have symptoms of mild abdominal cramping, diarrhea, and mild anorexia. He attributed his symptoms initially to a flu virus and later to the stress of his job. The symptoms gradually worsened over the next six months, including a 15 pound weight loss, and increasing sleep requirements to nine to ten hours each night. Finally, he sought medical care when he noticed blood in his stools. The internist in the clinic ordered multiple tests and x-rays, including a sigmoidoscopy, upper gastrointestinal barium series, barium enema, and complete blood count. The laboratory tests revealed a severe microycytic anemia (iron deficiency). The barium enema and sigmoidoscopy were diagnostic of ulcerative colitis involving the entire colon. The physician prescribed iron supplements and sulfathalazine.

Over the next six months, Dan continued to lose weight and have bloody diarrhea up to 20 times daily. The frequency of stools severely impaired his work. He was forced to suddenly leave meetings and was unable to continue visiting clients. His fatigue curtailed his activities and resulted in social isolation. Sexual intercourse was exhausting and frequently stimulated abdominal cramping and diarrhea. At this point, the internist referred Dan to a gastroenterologist.

The gastroenterologist immediately admitted Dan to the hospital for intensive medical treatment and bowel rest with total parenteral nutrition (TPN). Admission to the hospital allowed Dan to relinquish the tight control he had over himself which enabled him to get through each day. Nursing assessment on admission revealed an acutely ill young man—emotionally and physically exhausted. Frequent malodorous daily bowel movements were a great source of embarrassment to him, and a single room afforded him much needed privacy. During the first two weeks of hospitalization, his self-care activities were limited to personal hygiene. The medical treatment consisted of TPN, bowel rest (nothing by mouth, NPO), and intravenous cortcosteroids and antibiotics. His diarrhea subsided to five bowel movements daily, and he gained six pounds.

After two weeks, Dan began to ambulate in the hall and expressed an interest in learning more about his TPN care. Dan's primary nurse recognized this as a sign of the stabilization of disease activity and a readiness to participate in self-care activities. Assessment of his knowledge base revealed that he was an intelligent and independent person but knew very little about managing his illness. He had the mistaken idea that stress was the cause of ulcerative colitis and, therefore, was continually frustrated in his inability to control the illness.

With the information attained through the assessment, Dan's primary nurse realized that his lack of knowledge concerning ulcerative colitis interfered with his ability for self-care. She also realized that the psychosocial component of the disease had never been addressed. A teaching plan was developed to provide him with the knowledge base from which he could develop self-care strategies.

The primary nurse taught Dan the material on the teaching plan with care and consideration. Dan seemed happy with the new knowledge and self-care skills. When Dan had a working knowledge of this material, he was discharged.

Three weeks later, Dan came back to the hospital, pale, weak, and cachectic. He told the nurse that he and his wife were constantly fighting about his diet and disease and stated that he was too overwhelmed "with all these things I have to do for myself to carry out my treatment regimen. All I want is for someone to take care of me."

The nurse, with this new understanding of Dan and his home situation, realized that the teaching plan and self-care skills were unrealistic. New goals would have to be set at a much slower pace, with the assistance of Dan's wife or other close associate to aid in Dan's care.

Note: Not all teaching and self-care plans are successful the first or second time. Plans need to be evaluated and new plans or goals set, if necessary.

SELF-CARE PLAN FOR CASE EXAMPLE

Assessment	Planning	Implementation	Evaluation
Lack of understanding concerning ulcerative colitis.	Increase understanding of pathophysiology and etiology of ulcerative colitis.	Provide the client with patient teaching materials concerning ulcerative colitis and including the following information: • Etiology of ulcerative colitis • Pathophysiological changes in the colon related to symptoms • Increased risk of colon cancer • Potential for a total colectomy	The client verbalizes understanding of pathophysiology and etiology of his disease. The client discusses with family and friends the possible etiologies of ulcerative colitis, correcting their misconceptions.
	Alleviate client's feelings of self-blame.		The client does not blame himself. The client describes disease activity and relationship to symptoms—bloody stools, frequency of stools related to inflammation, and colonic muscle irritability. The client verbalizes an understanding of the risk of colon cancer and takes responsibility for yearly checkups.

Increase client's self-care ability related to diet medication and signs and symptoms of flare

Inadequate self-care activities developed to manage treatment regimes in ulcerative colitis including:
• Diet
• Medications
• Signs and symptoms of impending flare

Describe the trajectory of ulcerative colitis (quiet stage, flare-active stage, recovery stage).

Have client reflect on his illness and identify the initial signs and symptoms of a flare.

Describe to client what is happening at each time and explore with him strategies to cope with symptoms, e.g., initiating a bland, low-residue or clear liquid diet, increasing rest periods, reducing activities, decreasing stress and altering medications.

Give the client medication information pamphlets or cards.

Give client calendars to keep track of daily doses, variations in symptoms, and activities that may affect stress levels and weight changes.

Once stabilized:
• The client manages diet to suit needs.
• Client identifies foods appropriate for clear liquid, bland low residue, high protein, low lactose diets.
• Client adds foods gradually at home and discerns what can and cannot be tolerated.

Client recognizes the onset of a flare and makes changes in his medication regimen, diet, and lifestyle to minimize the debilitation and maximize the treatment effects.

The client describes his medication regimen, potential side effects, and how to handle potential or actual complications such as 1) suppression of the body's ability to fight infection; client describes the early signs of infection and the appropriate steps in prevention, 2) sulfathalazine competition with folate for absorption in the intestine: intake of inadequate folate supplements.

SELF-CARE PLAN FOR CASE EXAMPLE CONTINUED

Assessment	Planning	Implementation	Evaluation
			The client describes the symptoms of flare and verbalizes when and what interventions should be made.
Need for self-care strategies in symptom management.	Increase client's ability to cope with his illness and minimize the interference of symptoms on his life.	Ask the client to list his most disruptive symptoms.	Prior to discharge: • The client identifies the most prevalent symptoms and develops coping strategies to minimize the disruptions or embarrassment.
		Provide examples of social or work situations that may arise. Ask client how he might manage them.	
		Give specific guidelines for symptom management such as arranging schedule to be nearer to the bathroom.	• The client identifies a family member or friend to assist him in developing strategies once he has returned to his usual routines.
		Introduce client to others in the hospital with similar disease or arrange to have a member of the local chapter of the National Foundation for Ileitis and Colitis call or visit.	
		Refer the client to a support group or counseling as needed.	The client seeks out a support group with whom he can share experiences, strategies, and frustrations if needed.

*Case example prepared by Kathleen Fitzgerald, R.N., M.S., Lecturer, Department of Physiological Nursing, University of

Discussion Questions

1. Discuss the role of fats and carbohydrates in weight reduction.
2. Describe the approach you might take when discussing weight reduction with a woman from a culture in which "robustness" is associated with good health.
3. Outline the steps you would take in helping the client to make dietary changes to improve health.
4. How would you assess the adequacy of an adolescent diet? How would you suggest dietary changes?
5. What interventions would you suggest for a client who has chronic constipation alternating with diarrhea?

REFERENCES

American Heart Association, Commission on Nutrition, Diet, and Coronary Heart Disease. Nutrition Today, Vol 9, No 3, p 26, 1974

The Asthma and Allergy Foundation of America: The Allergy Encyclopedia. The C.V. Mosby Company, St. Louis, Missouri, 1981

Bailey C: Fit or Fat? Houghton Mifflin Company, Boston, Massachusetts, 1977

Baldi S, Costell S, Hill L, Jasmin S, Smith N: For Your Health: A Model for Self-Care. Nurses Model Health, South Laguna, California, 1980

Bennett W, Furin J: The Dieter's Dilemma. Basic Books, New York, 1982

Brewster L, Jacobson MF: The Changing American Diet. Center for Science in the Public Interest, Washington, D.C., 1978

Briggs G, Calloway D: Bogert's Nutrition and Physical Fitness, 10th ed. Saunders College Publishing, Philadelphia, Pennsylvania, 1979

Brody J: Jane Brody's Nutrition Book. Bantam, New York, 1982

Brooten D, Jordan C: Caffeine and pregnancy, a research review and recommendations for clinical practice. JOGN Nursing, pp 190–195, May/June 1983

Bunker M, McWilliams M: Caffeine content of common beverages. Journal of the American Dietetic Association, Vol 74, No 1, pp 28–32, 1979

Caliendo M: Nutrition and Preventive Health Care. MacMillan Publishing Co., New York, 1981

Farquhar J: The American Way of Life Need Not Be Hazardous to Your Health. W.W. Norton and Co., New York, 1978

Feingold B: Why Your Child Is Hyperactive. Random House, New York, 1974

Ferguson T, Graedon J: Caffeine. Medical Self-Care, pp 12–19, Fall 1981

Filip J: The sweet thief. Medical Self-Care, pp 8–11, Winter 1981

Foster G, Anderson B: Medical Anthropology. John Wiley & Sons, Inc., New York, 1978

Gordon T, Kannel W: Obesity and cardiovascular disease: The Framingham Study. Clinical Endocrine Metabolism, Vol 5, No 2, pp 267–375, 1976

Hammar L, et al.: An interdisciplinary study of adolescent obesity. Journal of Pediatrics, Vol 80, No 3, pp 373, 1972

Hongladarom G, Russell M: An ethnic difference: Lactose intolerance. Nursing Outlook, Vol 24, No 12, pp 764–765, 1976

Krehl WA: The nutritional epidemiology of CUD. *In* Moss, NH, Mager J (eds): Food and Nutrition in Health and Disease: New York Academy of Science, New York, 1977

Lappe F: Diet for a Small Planet, 2nd ed. Ballantine Books, New York, 1975

Lerner M: The nutrition-juvenile delinquency connection. Medical Self-Care, pp 21–25, Summer 1982

Liebman B, Moyer G: The case against sugar. Nutrition Action, Vol 7, No 12, 1980

Lipson J, Meleis A: Issues in health care of Middle Eastern patients. The Western Journal of Medicine, Vol 139, No 6, pp 854–861, 1983

Mahoney M: Self-reward and self-monitoring techniques for weight control. Behavior Therapy, Vol 5, No 1, pp 48–57, 1974

Mahoney M, Moura N, Wade T: Relative efficacy of self-reward, self-punishment, and self-monitoring techniques for weight loss. Journal of Consulting and Clinical Psychology, Vol 40, No 3, pp 404–407, 1973

Mahoney M, Caggiula A: Applying behavioral methods to nutritional counseling. Journal of the American Dietetic Association, Vol 72, No 4, pp 372–377, 1978

Mahan L: A sensible approach to the obese patient. Nursing Clinics of North America, Vol 14, No 2, pp 229–245, 1979

Mason L: Guide to Stress Reduction. Peace Press Inc., Culver City, California, 1980

Metropolitan Life Insurance Companies: Metropolitan Height and Weight Tables, New York, 1983

Mindell E: Earl Mindell's Vitamin Bible. Warner Books, New York, 1979

Mindell E: Earl Mindell's Vitamin Bible for Your Kids. Rawson Wade Publishers, Inc., New York, 1981

Pariza MW: A perspective on diet, nutrition, and cancer. Journal of the American Medical Association, Vol 251, No 11, pp 1455–1458, 1984

Pritikin N: The Pritikin Program for Diet and Exercise. Grossett and Dunlap, New York, 1979

Ritz S, Simons A: Bladder infections: How to get off the toilet. Medical Self-Care, pp 2–14, Spring 1981

Smith L: Feed Your Kids Right. Dell Publishing Company, New York, 1979

Smith L: Improving Your Child's Behavior Chemistry. Pocket Books, Simon and Schuster, New York, 1976

United States Department of Agriculture: Handbook of Agricultural Charts, No. 524. Washington, D.C., 1977

United States Senate Select Committee on Nutrition and Human Needs: Dietary Goals for the United States, 2nd ed. Government Printing Office, Washington, D.C., 1977

United States Surgeon General's Report: Healthy People. 1979

Wallis C: Salt: A new villain? Time Magazine, Vol 119, No 11, pp 64–71, 1982

Weiner M: Weiner's Herbal: The Guide to Herbal Medicine. Stein and Day Scarborough House, New York, 1980

Williams SR: Essentials of Nutrition and Diet Therapy, 3rd ed. The C.V. Mosby Company, St. Louis, Missouri, 1982

Willett WC, MacMahon B: Diet and cancer—an overview (second of two parts). The New England Journal of Medicine, Vol 310, No 11, pp 697–703, 1984

8

Activity, Rest, and Exercise

"The body is the temple of the soul and to reach harmony of body, mind, and spirit, the body must be physically fit."

Aristotle

There was a time when adequate physical exercise could be achieved by carrying out daily activities and chores. For most people, this just is not so today. We live in a sedentary and mechanized society fostering life-styles with inadequate activity and exercise which, in turn, lead to 'diseases of civilization'. Probably fewer than 30% of American adults meet the American Medical Association's recommendations for at least three periods of exercise each week (Haskell and Blair 1982), although recently many more people have begun exercising. Nurses are in a key position to assess, plan, and help clients implement an exercise program and can provide leadership in the promotion of health through physical exercise (MacNamara 1980).

While evidence on the benefits of adequate physical activity increases, a balance between activity, rest, and exercise is the key. This chapter will discuss the relationship of exercise to health. We will use the nursing process as a means of implementing these concepts in clinical nursing practice.

CURRENT KNOWLEDGE AND RESEARCH

Recently, exercise has become very popular in the United States. One in seven people in the United States jogs regularly and over 13.5 million Americans play tennis. A 1978 Perrier Fitness Study (Harris 1979) determined that the most popular exercise activities were walking, swimming, bowling, bicycling, jogging, and tennis. While the benefits of exercise for the general population have been demonstrated in numerous studies worldwide, more research is needed on the benefits of exercise for individuals with chronic or acute illness.

Questions asked by people who have not exercised in a long time or by those with limitations posed by illness include:

- "How much exercise is appropriate?"
- "What kind of exercise is best?"
- "When is the best time for exercise?"

Nurses can help clients to answer these questions and to help them plan safe and enjoyable exercise activities.

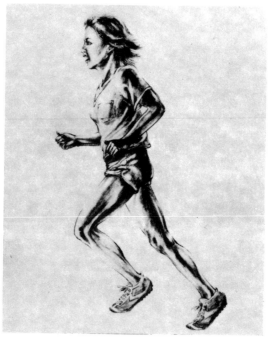

Figure 8-1.

Need for Activity, Rest, and Exercise

Most nurses are acutely aware of the deleterious effects of inadequate activity, especially in hospitalized patients who are on bedrest. This awareness is reflected in the change toward early mobilization of postoperative patients as a standard procedure. But nurses, other health professionals, and the public are less aware of the importance of rest and play periods to relax and disengage from the tensions of daily living. In addition, there is a general lack of awareness of individual differences in the need for sleep and rest.

Need for sleep. Individuals vary in their need for sleep. While some people need as much as ten hours of sleep each night, others feel rested on only five hours of sleep. In the face of increased stress or illness, however, requirements for sleep increase. In fact, an increased need for sleep is often an early sign of stress or illness.

According to Thoresen (1983), the most common type of sleep complaint is insomnia. There are three types of insomnia. In initial insomnia, the individual has difficulty falling asleep. In intermittent insomnia, the individual awakens during the night and has difficulty getting back to sleep. In terminal insomnia, the individual awakens early in the morning and cannot get back to sleep. Insomnia can be caused by stress, depression, drugs and medications, caffeine, and such environmental factors as excessive heat or cold, noise, or light. Approximately one third of American adults complain of insomnia, and an additional 12% consider their sleep chronically disturbed. A regular and sufficient amount of sleep is important for health promotion, disease prevention, and treatment. However, sleep disturbances are common symptoms of tension, anxiety, or depression. Treatment of sleep disturbances will be discussed on page 175 later in this chapter.

Need for play and laughter. Everyone needs some idle time spent without purpose or plans. In a society which values the work ethic, some people feel guilty for spending time in this way. However, play is important to recharge and relax.

Many people confuse exercise and play. If someone says she is "playing golf" and exclaims how well she played a particular hole, you can tell she is playing to win. "Playing to win" has a specific purpose. What we mean by playing are activities that regenerate an individual's body and mind or simply feel good. The individual who plays golf because he enjoys the air, sun, and exercise may not be sure when asked what hole is being played. Thus, exercise may or may not be playful. Running in a race, or for distance or time, is not what we mean by play. But running because you feel like a gazelle, and enjoy the sounds of the ocean or sand under your feet, is play. According to Jasmin and Costell (1980), play is imaginative, creative, equal, supportive, cooperative, self-nurturing, and personal.

Part of play is laughter. Laughter can be effective in reducing anxiety and tension, as well as aiding the body in healing (Moody 1978). Cousins (1977) described his daily use of humor and laughter as an important component of therapy for his life-threatening collagen disease. At present, scientific evidence about the long-term effects of play, laughter, humor, or a positive emotional state are inconclusive. However, we all can appreciate the way in which a good laugh, a funny movie, or a positive attitude can make us feel.

Need for exercise. In the 1981 Surgeon General's Report, Julius Richmond said that exercise does the following:

It improves the efficiency of the heart and increases the amount of oxygen the body can process in a given amount of time. Those who exercise regularly often lose excess weight and improve muscle strength and stamina. Many also develop an improved self-image which can lead to further adoption of positive health behaviors, including that which is related to smoking and nutrition (p. 2).

The benefits of exercise are summarized below.

THE BENEFITS OF EXERCISE

- Increased efficiency of heart and lungs
- Decreased heart rate and blood pressure
- Increased blood flow to all body parts
- Decreased anxiety, tension, depression
- Improved self-image
- Improved appearance

- Increased energy, vitality and well-being
- Increased positive health behaviors
- Increased flexibility
- Increased strength
- Increased coordination
- Increased metabolic rate
- Improved elimination

In addition to the benefits of exercise listed above, regular exercise is useful in the treatment of obesity because it can decrease fat cell size. According to Bailey (1978), the ultimate cure for obesity is exercise. He suggests that an individual burns more calories when physically fit than when unfit, even while asleep.

What is the definition of exercise? What kind of exercise is best? How often should one exercise? Nurses are frequently asked these and many other questions. Exercise is defined as "regular or repeated appropriate use of physical activity for the purpose of training or developing the body and mind for the sake of health" (Halfman and Hojacki 1981). However, according to Pelletier (1981) no single area of research is more clouded with unsubstantiated opinion than the realm of physical exercise and its relationship to health. We will outline some plausible research findings and clinical opinions in the following discussion.

Types of Exercise

Exercise involves the contraction of various muscles. There are three types of muscle contractions:

- Isometric
- Isotonic
- Isokinetic.

Isometric muscle contractions are those in which muscles contract in response to a fixed resistance without movement, such as trying to push a heavy object or pushing one's hands against each other. With isometric exercise there is a minimum of muscle fiber shortening. This type of contraction can lead to increased muscle tone and strength. *Isotonic* muscle contractions enhance physical fitness by a gradual build-up of force, using movement. *Isokinetic* muscle contractions involve resistance that varies at a constant rate using a device with a capacity for variable resistance. This type of exercise is usually used for rehabilitation of knee and elbow injuries. The device allows the muscle to move through a complete range of motion with resistance at every point without stopping the full range of motion.

Activities that use large muscle groups are the most beneficial. Exercise that promotes cardiac conditioning is called *aerobic exercise.* Aerobic exercises are rhythmic, repetitive activities that stimulate the heart and lungs to take up and deliver oxygen to body tissues more efficiently. The most common types are those that use large muscle groups and maintain continuous and rhythmic activity such as jogging, biking, and swimming. For an activity to be considered aerobic, certain criteria must be met; the criteria are frequency, intensity, and time (F.I.T.). *Frequency* refers to the number of times the activity is carried out each week. Authorities range in their recommendations to exercise from three non-consecutive times a week to five and six times a week. Frequency is important in order to maintain the improvements achieved by exercise, and repetition is the only way this can be achieved (Ryan 1978). *Intensity* refers to the maximum heart rate (or exercise heart rate or target pulse rate). The maximum heart rate varies from 60–85% above the resting heart rate, according to different authors, for an exercise to be considered aerobic. This rate is based on age and other health factors, e.g., 60% for people over 65 years old (see Table 8-1 and Table 8-2).

TABLE 8-1. COMPUTING MAXIMUM HEART RATE*

Step 1 ● Take 220 and subtract your age.
220 − (your age) = (A)

Step 2 ● Now subtract your resting pulse rate from the number in A.
(A) − (resting pulse) = (B)

Step 3 ● Multiply B times 65%.
(B) x 65% = (C)
● Also multiply B times 75%.
(B) x 75% = (D)

Step 4 ● Now add your resting pulse rate to the numbers in C and D, separately.
(C) + (your resting pulse) = (low target heart rate range)
(D) + (resting pulse) = (high target heart rate rate)

---

*From Farquhar J: The American Way of Life Need Not Be Hazardous to your Health. W. W. Norton and Co., New York, 1978

TABLE 8-2. TARGET HEART RATE AND HEART-RATE RANGE BY AGE GROUP

Age	Your Maximum Heart Rate* (beats/min)	Your Target Heart Rate (75% of the maximum in beats/min)	Your Target Heart-Rate Range (between 70 and 85% of the maximum in beats/min)
20	200	150	140 to 170
30	190	142	133 to 162
40	180	135	126 to 153
50	170	127	119 to 145
60	160	120	112 to 136
70	150	112	105 to 123

*Maximum heart rate is the greatest number of beats per minute that your heart is capable of. During exercise, your heart rate should be approximately 60 to 85% of this maximum.

Adapted from Kuntzleman CT: The Complete Book of Walking. Simon & Schuster, New York, p 96, 1979

Time of duration refers to how long the heart rate is maintained at the maximum heart rate and how long the acitivity is sustained. Bailey (1978) suggests that 12 minutes of any activity that maintains the target rate is all that is needed for aerobic conditioning. Others think that the exercise activity should be sustained for 20–30 minutes at the target heart rate.

Another type of exercise is *calisthenics*. This systematic, rhythmic bodily exercise usually is carried out without equipment or apparatus. It is a form of isometrics if used only to build strength and endurance. However, calisthenics can also be used to build cardiopulmonary endurance, increase muscle strength and endurance, and increase flexibility. Cooper (1981) states that calisthenics build agility, coordination, and muscular strength, and he recommends sit-ups, toe-touches, and push-ups.

Role of Exercise in Disease Prevention and Health Promotion

Exercise has recently been found to help reduce the risk factors that are associated with chronic diseases such as atherosclerosis, heart disease, and diabetes. Exercise increases vital capacity, increases bone strength, promotes less clotting in the blood, and aids in weight control (Rimer and Glassman 1983). People who exercise regularly have a significant decrease in resting heart rate, systolic blood pressure, and serum cholesterol (Horne 1975). Although exercise cannot stop the aging process, risk of degenerative diseases related to inactivity, such as osteoporosis, is reduced. Thus, the potential benefits of vigorous physical activity outweigh the potential risks of inactivity (Pelletier 1981) and "one cannot escape the conclusion that the long-term effects of exercise are beneficial to health" (Ibraheim 1983:136).

There has been substantial research documenting the benefits of exercise on the cardiovascular system. Routine exercise reduces low-density lipoproteins and increases high-density lipoproteins and triglycerides which have been related to increased risk of cardiovascular disease (Kent 1978; Pollac 1979; and Thomas, 1979). Boyer and Kasch (1970) found that routine exercises led to better control of hypertension, another risk factor for cardiac disease.

Cardiovascular fitness is an observable and predictable benefit of exercise training. It is a state of body efficiency enabling a person to exercise vigorously for a long period of time without fatigue and to respond to sudden physical and emotional demands with an economy of heartbeats and only a moderate rise in blood pressure (Zohman 1974:6). Studies suggest that moderate and vigorous physical activity may have a protective effect against coronary heart disease and also improve the chances for survival from myocardial infarction (Paffenbarger, Laughlin, and Gima 1970; Paffenbarger, Wing, and Hyde 1978).

According to the American Heart Association, "regular exercise and increased cardiovascular functional capacity may decrease myocardial functional oxygen demand for any given level of physical activity" (1980:451A). Paffenbarger and Hale (1975) found that highly active longshoremen appeared to be especially well protected against sudden death syndrome. In addition, the risk of primary cardiac arrest was 55% to 65% lower in persons whose leisure pursuits were high intensity activities (Siscovick, Weiss, Hallstrom, Innui, and Peterson 1982).

Exercise can also increase an individual's ability to handle stress. In contrast, inactivity can lead to depression and frustration, which often perpetuates the inactivity. Increased activity and exercise can lead to feelings of psychological well-being and increased energy (Fair, Rosenaur and Thurston 1979; Farquhar 1978).

Individual perception of the meaning and importance of exercise, as well as how it affects clients, influences when and whether they exercise. In contrast to what nurses might expect and hope for, Laffrey and Isenberg (1983) found in their study of women that the perceived importance of exercise was not consciously associated with the idea of promoting health. They concluded that other intrinsic values associated with exercise must be taken into account. These might include enjoyment, slimness, and attractiveness. In this way, an exercise program can be developed that is personally meaningful to the client (Laffrey and Isenberg 1983). Many people believe that they are too tired to exercise at the end of the day; in fact, exercisers describe feelings of increased energy following an exercise activity, *especially* at the end of the day. Others think that exercise can help one relax when tense and can aid in falling asleep quickly. Some suggest that exercise increases their ability to concentrate and increases work efficiency.

Risks Related to Exercise

What are the risks of exercise? How can the nurse counsel clients most effectively for appropriate self-care in exercise? As we see it, the greatest risk related to exercise is viewing exercise as a chore or work. It is important not only to feel good about the fact that you are exercising but to enjoy the activity in and of itself, spending time in an enjoyable way.

Risks include heart attack and injury. The risk of heart attack or sudden death while exercising is usually highest among individuals with known or documentable cardiovascular disease. There is also potential risk for individuals over 35 who have not exercised in some time, especially if they smoke, are overweight, or have an elevated blood pressure. It is recommended that these individuals get a physical examination before beginning an exercise program (Cooper 1981).

Injuries from exercise are usually classified into two major categories—acute injuries and injuries related to overuse. Nearly 75% involve injury to the lower extremities (Greene 1983), of which two thirds are sprains or strains (Garrick 1977). Acute injuries include:

1. Sprains, which are traumatic twists of joints that result in stretching or tearing stabilizing connective tissue
2. Strains which stretch, tear or cause a rip in the muscle itself
3. Fractures, which are more common in children.

People who sustain injuries related to overuse usually have a long history of excessive amounts of such activities as pitching, swimming, tennis, or running. In adults, most risks related to running increase with increased mileage. Many running injuries, like other injuries related to vigorous exercise, are related to inadequate warm-up and cool-down periods.

Other exercise activities are associated with specific risks of injury, e.g., "tennis elbow" (lateral epicondylitis) caused by throwing, weight lifting, or racquet sports (Greene 1983). Knee injuries, broken bones, and sprains are common in down-hill and cross-country skiing, and in roller-skating. For these reasons, a balance between activity, rest, and exercise is essential, and careful attention to warm-up and avoiding overuse is warranted.

Exercise for special conditions. Pregnancy is a time in which the balance between activity and rest varies. However, regular exercise is important for the woman's well-being and for a healthy delivery (Clark and Affonso 1979; Ketter and Shelton 1984). For the woman who maintained a regular exercise program before pregnancy, continuing the same regimen is usually appropriate as long as she feels well. However, pain or fatigue are signals that should be respected. Women who were inactive before pregnancy should not begin a vigorous exercise program at this time. Such activities as walking and swimming are more appropriate. Pregnant women have increased needs for sleep and rest periods. These needs vary from woman to woman as well as in the same individual over the course of the pregnancy.

For individuals with such chronic diseases as coronary artery disease, renal disease, diabetes, low back injury, and joint injury or arthritis, exercise prescription requires special knowledge and individualized instruction. We used to think that once an individual had an illness or injury, exercise was to be avoided. We now know that exercise benefits most people if prescribed and carried out appropriately. For example, some people with coronary artery diseases became "cardiac cripples" before cardiac rehabilitation programs were established (see case example on page 179). Such programs are carefully monitored by cardiologists and nurses to meet the individual's specific needs. Careful assessment and evaluation includes electrocardiograms, step tests, or treadmill tests; individuals are then prescribed progressive activities from simple deep breathing and range of motion to more vigorous activities. According to Cantu (1980), vigorous programs usually do not begin before six months following a myocardial infarction.

Diabetics who exercise have been shown to require less insulin (Getchell 1979). During exercise, muscles can take glucose from the blood stream without requiring insulin. In addition to lowered insulin requirements, exercise is thought to prevent or delay peripheral vascular complications, if special precautions are taken. These precautions suggested by Getchell (1979) include:

1. Adjustment of the insulin dosage to accommodate exercise (usually under the supervision of a physician)
2. Prevention of hypoglycemia by consuming a controlled amount of carbohydrates before exercise
3. Care of feet, including the use of good shoes and wrinkle-free socks
4. A well-established program under the guidance of a nurse or physician including gradually increased activities balanced with rest to prevent excessive fatigue.

Participation in treatment is generally well-accepted among people who have renal disease. Nurses can use this willingness to encourage exercise self-care. People with end-stage renal disease often have decreased energy because of the disease itself and because of concomitant anemia.

As a result, many individuals with renal disease find themselves enmeshed in the "sick role" and are reluctant to exercise unless specifically encouraged. In renal disease, it is especially important to assess the individual's awareness of the need for a balance between activity and rest and to encourage appropriate exercise. The nurse can encourage exercise by suggesting that several renal clients who have similar exercise tolerances get together to exercise. They can support and help each other assess their needs for activity and rest.

Finally, for people with arthritis or other musculoskeletal problems, regular exercise is important in maintaining flexibility and movement. The balance of rest and exercise is especially important in self-care of these individuals. Too much of the wrong kind of exercise can aggravate rather than relieve joint symptoms. In arthritis, systematic rest helps to control fatigue and joint inflammation. The most important exercises for individuals with arthritis are range of motion and muscle strengthening exercises. Isometric exercises are considered the safest (Simpson and Dickinson 1983). Precautions suggested by Simpson and Dickinson (1983) for exercise for clients with arthritis include:

1. Stop at the point of pain, not discomfort.
2. Exercise in a way that does not cause joint strain.
3. Perform all movements slowly and smoothly.
4. Use swollen, hot, red, painful, or damaged joints as little as possible.
5. Limit the number of repetitions and do not use weights.
6. Change position frequently.
7. Respect your own limitations.

In addition to the need for physical rest, people with arthritis need extra sleep, especially individuals with osteoarthritis, who need 1–2 hours more sleep each night (Simpson and Dickinson 1983). Emotional rest or relaxation is also critically important. Stress reduction exercises can help an individual with arthritis deal more successfully with the stressors of living with chronic pain and physical limitations (see Chapter 9).

CLINICAL APPLICATION: NURSING PROCESS

Barriers to exercise include:

1. Embarassment related to appearance, ability, or physical condition
2. Lack of time
3. Lack of money to buy equipment or clothing required for exercise
5. Weather conditions that prohibit exercise
6. Environmental barriers such as hills, city streets, or street crime
7. Lack of company for exercise.

How can the nurse help clients to overcome such barriers to plan for safe and enjoyable exercise programs? According to Pender, "The nurse should not only instruct, support, and evaluate clients during physical fitness activities, but should serve as a role model of the physically fit adult" (1982:237).

Assessment

When assessing an individual's needs for activity, rest, and exercise, it is important to ask questions about the individual's primary goal for exercise. It is also important to find out if he has participated in other exercise programs, if he is aware of any barriers to exercise, and if there are individuals who have supported or sabotaged his exercise efforts.

According to the American College of Sports Medicine (1975), the purposes of fitness evaluation are:

1. To determine the presence of risk factors for coronary disease
2. To identify the existence of health problems which might modify or preclude exercise prescription
3. To collect information which would permit tailoring the exercise prescription to the individual patient.

The fitness evaluation varies with age, sex, and the individual client's current level of activity. A complete physical examination with blood lipids, a resting blood pressure, an electrocardiogram, and a treadmill test should be obtained for individuals who have a family or personal history of cardiovascular disease, and for individuals over 35 who have not exercised recently.

Having collected an exercise history on the individual and identified any potential risks, the nurse and client assess physical strength. *Physical strength* is defined as the amount of weight that can be moved from one point to another. It can be broken down into total body strength and individual muscle strength. The number of sit-ups an individual can do at one time is sometimes the criteria used for assessing strength.

Another component of exercise or fitness assessment is *flexibility*. Flexibility is the ability to use a muscle through its entire range of motion. It is related to elasticity of muscles and connective tissue. Flexibility decreases with age, illness, or a sedentary life-style. A quick assessment of flexibility is to have clients bend over to see how close to the floor they can touch their hands.

Endurance is another component of the exercise assessment. Endurance is demonstrated by the number of times an activity can be repeated before the muscle fatigues. Strength, flexibility, and endurance all improve with proper training and decrease with disuse.

Another component of the exercise assessment is *cardiovascular function*. Cardiovascular function can be subdivided into:

1. Heart rate, rhythm, and strength
2. Respiratory rate, depth, and rhythm
3. Blood pressure
4. Skin color, temperature, and moistness.

Cardiovascular function improves with regular aerobic exercise. Treadmill stress tests and step tests are used to assess cardiovascular function. The treadmill test is performed in a laboratory with special monitoring equipment by trained personnel. Both tests assess cardiovascular function while the individual performs an activity—walking on the treadmill or stepping 17–18 inches repeatedly (30 steps per minute for men, and 24 steps per minute for women). During the treadmill test, the individual's electrocardiogram is monitored. During the step test, the individual's pulse rate is measured following three minutes of continual stepping; it is checked again at one minute, two minutes, and three minutes following the exercise. Table 8-3 reflects recovery pulse rates.

TABLE 8-3. RECOVERY PULSE RATES FOLLOWING A THREE MINUTE STEP-TEST

	Men	*Women*
Excellent	132 or less	135 or less
Good	150–133	155–136
Average	165–149	170–154
Fair	180–164	190–171
Poor	Above 180	Above 190

*From Getchell B: Physical Fitness, A Way of Life, 2nd ed. John Wiley & Sons, New York, pp 56–57, 1979 *(reprinted with permission from John Wiley & Sons, Inc.)*

Other components in the exercise assessment include speed, agility, coordination, and reaction time. It is important to establish a baseline of the individual's current exercise ability and behavior before implementing a new exercise program. Many individuals think that they are getting more exercise than they actually are; thus, their plans may be unrealistic. The self-assessment tool in Figure 8-2 is provided to help gather that information.

The exercise assessment is complete when all the data required to plan a safe, enjoyable, and realistic exercise program is collected and goals have been set. However, before plans can be made or implemented, it is important that information about the individual's need for sleep and rest is also collected.

EXERCISE SELF-ASSESSMENT

Complete the following self-assessment to help you look at the role of "exercise" in your life now. On the scale below, circle the numbers which best indicate you and your life during the last year:

	Almost Never	Seldom	Often	Almost Always
1. I plan each week to exercise three times . . .	1	2	3	4
2. I end up exercising at least three times for at least 20–30 minutes per week . . .	1	2	3	4
3. I climb stairs rather than riding elevators . . .	1	2	3	4
4. My daily activities include moderate physical activity (rearing young children, working on my feet, etc.) . . .	1	2	3	4
5. I know my "target heart rate" range, and in my regular exercise time I reach it . . .	1	2	3	4
6. I do some form of stretching-limbering exercise for at least 15 minutes twice a week . . .	1	2	3	4
7. I have the necessary items and facilities to engage in my activity properly . . .	1	2	3	4
8. I look forward to my exercise program . . .	1	2	3	4
9. My family/friends encourage me in my exercise program . . .	1	2	3	4
10. I am willing to make the time to exercise 20–30 minutes a day; 3–5 days per week . . .	1	2	3	4

Some suggestions for how you might learn from this self-assessment:

1. Connect all the circles down the length of the page. Look at the

pattern that your connected line makes. You might also turn your page sideways to get an even more clear visual picture of "exercise" in your life right now. What does it seem to be saying to you?

2. Now add up your total score: _____

   Circle which range it was in:

   10–19   20–29   30–40

   If your score was in the 10–19 range you might want to make some changes in your exercise pattern. Which aspects do you think need the most work? How many "1's" did you mark on this assessment? _____ These might serve as a clue to help you think about making changes in this area of your life.

3. How would you like this self-assessment to look in six months from now? Are you interested in planning towards those improvements?

4. Remember to congratulate yourself for the ways in which you are providing good exercise patterns in your life. Give yourself a pat on the back; or go out and "exercise" as a way to congratulate yourself!

Figure 8-2. Self-assessment tool used to gather information on individual's exercise habits. From Baldi S, Costell S, Hill L, Jasmin S, Smith N: For Your Health: A Model for Self-Care. Nurses Model Health, South Laguna, California, 1980 (reprinted with permission from Nurses Model Health)

Sleep and rest. The need for sleep and rest varies from individual to individual as well as for the same individual at different points in time. Each of us has his/her own biorhythms for rest and activity. However, many factors can influence these biorhythms, such as emotional and physical health, and type of work or other physical activity. In addition, changing biorhythms by rotating shifts, for example, can increase an individual's need for sleep.

An individual's assessment of need for sleep and rest is subjective. People who do physical work are usually more in tune with their level of fatigue than are individuals whose work is mostly mental. When assessing sleep patterns and the need for rest, it is important to evaluate the individual's subjective feeling of fatigue or weakness. Many clients cannot explain why they feel tired, yet they know that they are. Others are less aware of their need for rest periods or more sleep. Questions to gather assessment data for sleep and rest are listed on the next page.

Once this information is collected, the nurse and client have a clearer view of the client's sleeping and rest behavior. With this data, the nurse and client can effectively plan and implement a program for exercise and rest.

ASSESSMENT CRITERIA FOR SLEEP AND REST

- How much sleep do you think you need to feel rested and alert?
- How much sleep do you usually get?
- Do you take naps?
- Do you have any routines before going to sleep?
- What time do you go to sleep?
- Does anything help you get to sleep?
- Do you awaken during the night?
- Do you have trouble falling back to sleep?
- What helps you fall back to sleep?
- What time do you get up?
- Do you feel rested when you arise?
- When are you at your "best" (morning, afternoon, evening)?
- How often do you rest during the day?
- What activities do you consider restful? (e.g., music, reading, etc.)

Planning and Implementation

When designing an exercise program, it is important to begin at the client's current level of activity and progress slowly and realistically. Goals that the nurse and client might decide on include:

1. Heighten the body's level of aerobic fitness and endurance through such activities as running, cycling, swimming
2. Enhance the body's level of flexibility through such activities as stretching and yoga
3. Strengthen and vitalize the body and mind through such activities as calisthenics and weight training
4. Improve relaxation and reduce stress through such activities as autogenic training, progressive muscle relaxation, deep breathing, and rest periods (see Chapter 9).

According to Cantu (1980), a good exercise program should be enjoyable, vigorous enough to use 400 calories per hour, increase the heart rate to 70–85% maximum potential for 20–30 minutes (approximately 120–150 beats per minute), rhythmical in movement with contraction followed by relaxation, four to five times each week, and integrated into the individual's life-style. The American College of Sports Medicine (1975) suggests that the *frequency* of training should be three days a week, increasing to five days a week; the *intensity* of the training should be 60–70% of maximum heart rate; the *duration* of training should be 15–60 minutes depending on the intensity (the lower the intensity, the longer the duration); the *type* of activity should be one that utilizes large muscle groups, is continuous, and raises the heart rate to the desired level. According to Bailey (1978), the duration need only be 12 minutes, once the maximum heart rate is achieved. As you can see, there is no consensus among experts on exercise prescriptions. We think that the activity should be enjoyable enough so that the individual will look forward to it at least three times a week for a minimum of 30 minutes. Individual concerns and preferences must be addressed, and we think it is better for an individual to exercise only twice a week for 20 minutes and to really feel good about it, than to exercise more and either wish he/she was doing something else or quit.

When an aerobic exercise program is prescribed, a 10–15 minute warm-up to increase blood flow to the heart and skeletal muscles should be encouraged. Warm-up activities usually consist of stretching, bending, balance, and coordination (MacNamara 1980). These activities improve oxygenation of the tissues and prepare the large muscle groups for the activity to be carried out. Stretching activities are usually followed by heavier exercises (such as sit-ups) to develop strength and endurance. These exercises are usually followed by cardiorespiratory or aerobic exercises such as cross-country skiing, running, jogging, brisk walking, bicycling, swimming, or rowing for the desired length of time. This exercise is followed by a 5–10 minute cool-down to help the body return to normal and can be accomplished by slower and easier movements such as walking and stretching. Cool-down activity prevents pooling of blood in the muscles and promotes the elimination of waste products from muscles. In addition, blood flow is maintained to and from the muscles, and the body temperature and heart rate decrease slowly. All three parts are recommended for safety and effectiveness. Eliminating either the warm-up or cool-down periods can lead to injury, pain, and termination of the exercise program. A sample exercise prescription is shown below.

SAMPLE EXERCISE PRESCRIPTION

Exercise Routine

Warm-up—5–10 minutes of stretching, bending and range of motion exercises, 10 sit-ups.

Conditioning—20–30 minutes, 2–3 times a week for one month of fast walking alternating with jogging. Advance to 25–35 minutes 3–4 times a week of jogging.

Cool-down—5–10 minutes of slow walking, bending and stretching.

---

*Adapted from Fair J, Rosenaur J, Thurston E: Exercise Management. Nurse Practitioner, pp 13–18, May–June 1979

When planning an exercise program, it is important to teach the client when to stop exercising. Exercise activities should be stopped if any of the following symptoms occur: chest, arm, jaw or joint pain; irregular heartbeats; increased shortness of breath; feelings of faintness or light-headedness; nausea or vomiting; unexplained weight loss that may be associated with exercise; or other unexplained changes, such as sudden decrease in exercise tolerance.

In addition to an exercise prescription, increasing daily activity, in and of itself, is helpful. People can increase activity by taking the stairs instead of elevators and escalators, decreasing use of electrical appliances, parking the car further away from their destination or getting off the bus one stop earlier, riding a bicycle or walking instead of driving or taking public transportation. Individuals should consider other possibilities in which they can increase physical activity in their own life-styles.

Sleep and rest. A program for needed rest and sleep should be planned in conjunction with an exercise program. Rest periods should be built into a hectic day or rest will be neglected. Individuals should also plan activities for when they are most rested and alert to be sure they can finish what they need to do. Even if work or other tasks are not finished, the client should leave enough time for sleep each night, to feel rested in the morning.

If the client has a problem with sleep, a number of guidelines are suggested.

- Avoid the use of stimulants, including caffeine.
- Avoid alcohol.
- Increase activity/exercise during the day.
- Establish a regular bedtime.
- Do yoga or other stretching exercises before bed.
- Take a warm bath.
- Take a cup of warm milk, or herb teas, (e.g., chamomile).
- Provide a quiet but not soundproof environment.
- Read something, preferably something boring.
- Listen to soothing music.
- Get a backrub.

Increased activity and adequate rest become regular parts of one's life-style only when they are planned and fit comfortably into it. It is important for increased activity and exercise, balanced with adequate rest and sleep, to become an integral part of self-care and health promotion.

Evaluation

The evaluation of self-care programs in activity and rest is relatively easy because the planning process often involves describing objectives in measurable terms. For example, should clients plan to incorporate two half hour rest periods into their work days, the evaluation process involves noting if rest is incorporated or not; if it is not, then the client and the nurse should discuss whether or not the plan was reasonable, and how it should be modified. Or, for example, if the individual's plan is to undertake an aerobic exercise program with the goal of reducing the resting pulse to 60 beats a minute, taking the pulse will indicate whether or not the goal has been met.

SUMMARY

In this chapter, we have described the positive aspects of activity and exercise and stressed the importance of a balance between activity, rest, and relaxation. We have described the various types of exercise and suggested ways of incorporating these concepts into the nursing process. Nurses as models of health have a role and responsibility to be physically fit adults and advocates of self-care in activity, rest, and exercise.

CASE EXAMPLE

Louise is a 35-year-old, white, married librarian who has a three-year history of rheumatoid arthritis. The disease began in the large knuckle joints of her hands and led to a loss of hand function. For example, she could not open a car door or jars. She was initially treated with aspirin and gold injections, and although she complied with this regimen, she had little effect from either drug. Her joint stiffness has migrated to her neck, jaw, knees, and the balls of her feet.

Louise recently came to the arthritis clinic complaining of right wrist pain and decreased ability to carry on normal activities of daily living. The staff identified the risk of permanent loss of right wrist motion. The treatment plan included the following:

1. Instructing Louise about the disease process so that she would understand the treatment
2. Splinting the wrist
3. Minimal range of motion and strengthening exercises
4. Heat/cold therapies to relieve pain and decrease inflammation
5. Joint protection to minimize pain and deformity
6. Work simplification and energy conservation to reduce fatigue.

Louise's first self-care education session included a simple explanation of the disease process and of the purpose and methods of heat/cold therapy. In addition, she was referred to the occupational therapist for a molded working splint—a splint made to fit the patient allowing considerable hand activity without wrist motion.

Two weeks later, Louise demonstrated decreased right hand inflammation and increased wrist range of motion. Having experienced some relief, she saw the nurse and the regimen as helpful and was ready to take on more and longer range goals. Before proceeding with additional self-care instruction, however, the nurse asked Louise to demonstrate the suggested exercises. The demonstration revealed that Louise was performing her exercises too rapidly and was doing too many repetitions, which would not strengthen muscles and could possibly damage joint structures.

Gradually, over the next few months, Louise learned about joint protection and energy conservation. Her family was encouraged to attend the education sessions and frequently did so. Even though she expressed difficulty in changing old habits and patterns, her family was a major source of support; she learned new and easier ways to do things while protecting her joints, as well as learning the importance of balancing activity and rest. She required assistance in choosing proper lightweight utensils and assistance devices. She was especially pleased with her stationary "V" necked wall jar opener.

After five months of twice-monthly meetings with the nurse, Louise had a basic understanding of self-care management of rheumatoid arthritis. Such management includes information about the disease process, medication, rest (bedrest, joint rest, emotional rest), heat/cold modalities, and exercise. Louise now expressed confidence in coping with her disease, even if remission was not possible. She now has some control over her functioning and no longer feels like a victim. Hopefully, in the next few months, Louise will experience a complete remission. Meanwhile, assessment, reinforcement, and evaluation will continue.

SELF-CARE PLAN FOR CASE EXAMPLE

Assessment	Planning	Implementation	Evaluation
Rheumatoid arthritis of large knuckle joints of hands—decreased hand function	Increase the functions and use of hands	Aspirin and gold injections	Function and ability to use hands
Wrist pain	Decrease pain and increase mobility Increase ability to carry on activities of daily living	Teach about disease process and theory Heat/cold theory Explain purpose	Understanding of disease process and therapy Decrease pain, inflammation, deformity, and immobility
	Hand activity without wrist motion	Refer to occupational therapist for wrist splint	Ability to carry out activities of daily living
		Minimal range of motion and strengthening exercise	Did she carry out the exercises?
Fatigue	Decrease fatigue	Work simplification Energy conservation	Level of fatigue
Week 2			
Decreased hand inflammation Exercising too rapidly	Increase strength without fatigue or damage of joint structure	Repeat exercise regimen Reinforce need for rest	Number of repetitions Joint strength Joint structure

Case contributed by Glenda Dickinson, R.N., M.S., Lecturer, California State University, Hayward

---

CASE EXAMPLE

Daryl is a 42-year-old, plant supervisor who had a myocardial infarction (described in Chapter 5). His cardiologist prescribed a simple exercise program; Daryl is allowed to choose activities that are considered safe for his myocardial function. Following his myocardial infarction, he was only allowed to flex his feet and perform deep breathing exercises to prevent the complications of immobility. Daryl and his wife, Naomi, attach great importance to their role in Daryl's health care. Naomi records the time of each activity and monitors when the next set of deep breathing and foot flexion exercises should be done. She helps Daryl assess and evaluate his need for rest. Daryl is happy to be able to perform any part of his own care and appreciates all the support Naomi offers.

After Daryl is more stable, his activity prescription is reassessed in a patient care conference in which he is involved. It is decided that he should advance to a more active role in his care. The nurse teaches him to take his own pulse and monitor his pulse rate during activity; he is to stop activities when his pulse increases 20 beats/minute over his resting pulse rate. In the beginning, Daryl is frustrated because he fatigues so easily. However, as he gains an understanding of why he becomes so tired and how to balance his activity with rest and sleep periods, his spirits improve.

As the days pass, Daryl participates in more and more activities. His need for rest and sleep, while still vitally important, is reduced substantially. He gains strength daily as he progresses through the cardiac rehabilitation program.

Two days prior to Daryl's discharge, the nurse notes that Daryl is irritable and depressed. He is angry that he will not be able to play basketball or continue weight lifting when he goes home. The nurse explains that weight lifting is an isometric exercise and will strain his heart at this time. Basketball, she continues, involves "arms overhead" movements and bursts of energy. She explains that Daryl will need to recondition his heart before continuing such a strenuous sport. Together, Daryl and the nurse review phase II of the Cardiac Rehabilitation Program. They discuss the benefits of aerobic exercise, such as walking, jogging, cycling, and swimming. Daryl repeats back to the nurse the purpose of warm-up and cooldown exercises and the instructions for monitoring his pulse rate. He is relieved to know he is not a "cardiac cripple."

Daryl is able to describe a safe home exercise program based on his low level treadmill stress test. Daryl is scheduled to begin the aerobic exercise and reconditioning classes six weeks after discharge. When Daryl and Naomi arrive home, they are surprised by their two sons, who wheel a new 10-speed bicycle into the room—a coming home present for the Dad they are so proud of it. Even though Daryl will not be ready for bicycling for several weeks, he feels better knowing it is there.

SELF-CARE PLAN FOR CASE EXAMPLE

Assessment	Planning	Implementation	Evaluation
Limited activities; diminished independence.	Promote cardiac rest. Prevent complications of immobility, especially deep vein thrombosis and atelectesis. Encourage Daryl's participation in his care. Promote Daryl's independence.	Explain need for rest. Provide list of safe activities for myocardial function. Provide paper and pencil for family to record his feeling of well-being. Instruct Daryl on proper deep breathing exercise and foot flexion-extension exercises. Encourage Daryl and family to express feelings about loss of independence, etc. Gradually increase activity level as permitted by cardiologist and Daryl's physiological response to activities. Instruct Daryl and his family on pulse taking, when to stop activity and rest.	Daryl verbalizes rationale for rest and his role in health maintenance. Daryl chooses activities considered safe for his cardiac function. Daryl's family accurately records type, duration, effects of activities Daryl performs. Daryl accurately takes his pulse for 15 seconds. Daryl states parameters for pulse during exercise and when to rest.

Contributed by Cheryl Hubner, R.N., M.S., Vascular Nurse Specialist, Lecturer, Department of Physiological Nursing, School of Nursing, University of California, San Francisco

Discussion Questions

1. What is the role of exercise in weight reduction?
2. Discuss the need for activity and rest of a client in a cardiac rehabilitation program.
3. List the components of an effective exercise program.
4. What exercise would you recommend for a 42-year-old man who was 30 pounds overweight and who hadn't exercised in 20 years?
5. Compare and contrast exercise activities and play activities.

REFERENCES

American College of Sports Medicine: Guidelines for Graded Exercises. Testing and Exercise Prescription. Lea and Felsyer, Philadelphia, Pennsylvania, 1975
American Heart Association Committee Report: Risk factors and coronary disease. Circulation, 62449A-455A, 1980
Bailey C: Fit or Fat? Houghton Mifflin, Boston, Massachusetts, 1977
Baldi S, Costell S, Hill L, Jasmin S, Smith N: For Your Health: A Model for Self-Care: Nurses Model Health, South Laguna, California, 1980
Boyer J, Kasch FW: Exercise therapy in hypertensive men. Journal of the American Medical Association, Vol 211, No 10, pp 1668–1671, 1970
Brown BS: Fitting fitness into your life. Nursing Economics, Vol 93, No 96, 1983
Cantu RC: Toward Fitness: Guided Exercise for Those with Health Problems. Human Science Press, New York, 1980
Clark AL, Affonso DD: Childbearing: A Nursing Perspective, 2nd ed. F.A. Davis Co., Philadelphia, Pennsylvania, 1979
Cooper K: The New Aerobics. Bantam Books, New York, 1981
Cousins N: Anatomy of an Illness as Perceived by a Patient. W.W. Norton and Co., New York, 1979
Department of Health and Human Services, National Institute of Health: Exercise and Your Heart. NIH Publication No. 81-1677, 1981
Fair J, Rosenaur J, Thurston E: Exercise management. Nurse Practitioner, Vol 4, No 3, pp 13–18, 1979
Farquhar J: The American Way of Life Need Not Be Hazardous to Your Health. W.W. Norton and Company, New York, 1978
Garrick J: Sports medicine. Pediatric Clinics of North America, Vol 24, No 4, pp 737–46, 1977
Getchell B: Physical Fitness: A Way of Life, 2nd ed. John Wiley & Sons, Inc., New York, 1979
Greene JC: Prevention and treatment of sports injuries. Nurse Practitioner, Vol 8, No 10, pp 39–40, 44, 1983
Halfman MA, Hojnacki LH: Exercise and the maintenance of health. Topics in Clinical Nursing, Vol 3, No 2, pp 1–10, 1981
Harris L & Associates: The Perrier Study: Fitness in America. Study No. 52813, New York, 1979
Haskell W, Blair S: The physical activity component of health promotion in the occupational setting. In Parkinson R (ed): Managing Health Promotion in the Workplace. Mayfield Publishing Co., Belmont, California, 1982

Horne W: Effects of a physical activity program on middle-aged sedentary corpora-
    tion executives. American Industrial Hygiene Association Journal, Vol 36, pp
    241–245, 1975
Ibraheim M: In support of jogging. American Journal of Public Health, Vol 73, No 2,
    pp 136–37, 1983
Jasmin S, Costell S; Play. *In* Baldi S, Costell S, Hill L, Jasmin S, Smith N: To Your
    Health: A Model for Self-Care. Nurses Self-Care Model, South Laguna, Califor-
    nia, 1980
Kent S: Does exercise prevent heart attacks? Geriatrics, Vol 33, No 11, pp
    95–104, 1978
Ketter DE, Shelton BJ: Pregnant and physically fit, too. MCN, Vol 9, No 2, pp
    120–122, 1984
Kuntzleman CT: The Complete Book of Walking. Simon & Schuster, New York, 1979
Laffrey SC, Isenberg M: Participation in physical activity during leisure. Interna-
    tional Journal of Nursing Studies, Vol 20, no 3, pp 187–196, 1983
MacNamara EL: Fitting nursing into fitness. The Canadian Nurse, Vol 176, No 4, pp
    33–35, 1980
Moody RA: Laugh after Laugh. Headwaters Press, Jacksonville, Florida, 1978
Paffenbarger R, Laughlin M, Gima A: Work activity of longshoremen as related to
    death from coronary heart disease and stroke. New England Journal of Medicine,
    Vol 282, No 20, pp 1109–1114, 1970
Paffenbarger R, Hale W: Work activity and coronary heart mortality. New England
    Journal of Medicine, Vol 292, No 11, pp 545–550, 1975
Paffenbarger R, Wing A, Hyde R: Physical activity as an index of heart attack risk in
    college alumni. American Journal of Epidemiology, Vol 3, pp 161–175, 1978
Pelletier K: Longevity: Fulfilling our Biological Potential. Delacorte Press, New
    York, 1981.
Pender N: Health Promotion in Nursing Practice. Appleton-Century-Crofts, Nor-
    walk, Connecticut, 1982
Peters RK, Cady LD, Bischoff DP, Bernstein L, Pike MC: Physical fitness and
    subsequent myocardial infarction in healthy workers. Journal of the American
    Medical Association, Vol 249, No 22, pp 3052–3056, 1983
Pollack ML: Exercise—a preventative prescription. Journal of School Health, Vol
    49, No 4, pp 215–219, 1979
Price JH, Luther SL: Physical fitness: Its role in health for the elderly. Journal of
    Gerontological Nursing, Vol 6, No 9, pp 517–523, 1980
Rimer B, Glassman B: The fitness revolution: Will nurses sit this one out? Nursing
    Economics, Vol 1, No 2, pp 84–89, 144, 1983
Ryan AJ: Sports medicine today. Science, 200919-924, 1978
Simpson CF, Dickinson GR: Exercise: Adult arthritis. American Journal of Nursing,
    Vol 83, No 2, 1983
Siscovick D, Weiss N, Hallstrom A, Innui T, Peterson D: Physical activity and primary
    cardiac arrest. Journal of the American Medical Association, Vol 248, No 22, pp
    3113–3117, 1982
Thomas GS: Physical activity and health: Epidemiologic and clinical evidence and
    policy implications. Preventive Medicine, Vol 8, No 1, pp 89–103, 1979
Thoresen CE: Disturbed sleep: Taming the gentle tyrant. Healthline, Vol 2, No 4, pp
    1–3, 1983
United States Surgeon General's Report, 1981
Zohman L: Beyond diet . . . exercise your way to fitness. CPC International, 1974

9

Stress Management

Stress and stress management are topics of current interest among professionals and lay individuals. There are debates among experts about what stress is, whether stress is positive or negative, how much is beneficial or harmful, and, indeed, whether it is the cause or effect of various conditions. Some stress is inherent in every kind of daily life. Although research is inconclusive, inadequately managed stress is now viewed as a major contributor, directly or indirectly, to six of the leading causes of death in the United States—cardiac disease, cancer, respiratory disease, accidental injuries, cirrhosis, and suicide. This chapter discusses current knowledge and controversy about stress, incorporating relevant research. A discussion of the clinical application of stress management using the nursing process will be followed by a description of stress management techniques available for self-care.

CHARACTERISTICS OF STRESS: ISSUES AND RESEARCH

The word "stress" is used by many to refer to both a cause (stimulus) and an effect (e.g., "This stress is making me sick" or "I feel stressed"). For the purpose of this chapter, we differentiate *stressor* from the *stress response*. A stressor is a stimulus and can be defined as any condition, event, or situation that demands change on the part of an individual or family. The stress response is "the nonspecific response of the body to any demand made on it" (Selye 1976).

Responses to Stressors

Hans Selye, a pioneer in stress research, described the body's response

to stress as the General Adaptation Syndrome (GAS). This response consists of three stages:
1. Alarm reaction
2. Resistance
3. Exhaustion.

During the alarm phase, one experiences predictable physiological changes activated by the sympathetic nervous system that allow the individual to meet the demand of the situation. This has been called the "flight or fight response" (see below). During the resistance phase, the sympathetic nervous system acts to attempt to return the body to normal. The stage of exhaustion follows the body's repeated attempts to return physiological processes to the normal, pre-alarm conditions.

PHYSIOLOGICAL RESPONSES TO STRESS

- Increased heart rate
- Increased blood pressure
- Increased respiratory rate
- Increased muscle tension
- Increased gastric motility

- Increased blood glucose
- Pupil dilation
- Peripheral vascular constriction
- Adrenalin release

These physiological responses to perceived threats are protective mechanisms without which humans and animals would be unable to protect themselves. However, many events in daily life trigger a state of excitement or readiness unnecessarily—alarm clocks, constant telephone ringing, driving in traffic. High stress occupations, such as police work, many areas of nursing, or accounting (especially during tax season) lead to greater than usual daily pressures, and the individual may experience chronic stress. With chronic stress, one's body and mind are fatigued, often exhausted, and physical and emotional symptoms become apparent. (See list below of emotional responses to stress.)

EMOTIONAL RESPONSES TO STRESS

- High-pitched, nervous laughter
- Stuttering
- Impulsive behavior
- Insomnia
- Irritability
- Depression
- Anxiety

- Inability to concentrate
- Emotional instability
- Overpowering urge to cry or run and hide
- Nightmares
- Accident proneness
- Loss of appetite or overeating

An example of a common stress-related disorder is headache (Carini and Owens 1978). In general medical practice, headaches are the major complaint of approximately one-third of the patient population. The majority are tension or muscle contraction headaches (Philips 1977). A tension headache is pain that is usually described as bilateral, dull, bandlike, and persistent for hours.

Chronic stress also weakens the body's immune system, increasing the individual's susceptibility to infection and disease. According to Pelletier (1979), there is scientific evidence that stress has an adverse effect on the immunological system, including suppression of T-lymphocytes and macrophages, the body's own cancer-fighting cells. Thus, stress can be the major causal factor in a variety of physical disorders. Common, stress-related conditions can be grouped by system (see Table 9-1).

TABLE 9-1. CONDITIONS THAT MAY BE RELATED TO CHRONIC STRESS

Gastrointestinal

- Ulcerative colitis, duodenal ulcers
- Regional enteritis, heartburn
- Nausea and vomiting
- Diarrhea, constipation

Integumentary

- Hives, acne
- Psoriasis, eczema

Cardiovascular

- Migraine headaches
- Hypertension, premature atrial tachycardia
- Raynaud's Syndrome

Musculoskeletal

- Neck and backache
- Arthritis
- Chronic pain

Respiratory

- Asthma

Types of Stressors

Stressful events range in intensity from mild everyday annoyances to overwhelming life events. Over time, such events may be brief and time-limited, may occur intermittently, or may be repeated chronically. Stressful events may be classified as situational stressors (external conditions) and developmental stressors (maturational changes). (See Table 9-2 for examples.)

Researchers disagree about how stressful various kinds of events actually are to individuals and families. Holmes and Rahe (1967) ranked life events from the most to the least stressful and suggested that the greater the number of large life changes an individual experienced in a period of time, the higher the risk of illness. Their Social Readjustment Rating Scale (SRRS) (Table 9-3) has been used to study connections between life

TABLE 9-2. EXAMPLES OF TYPES OF STRESSORS

Situational	Developmental
Normal daily demands—e.g., commuting in traffic, work pressure	Maturational—e.g., adolescence, childbirth, menopause
Abnormal daily stressors—e.g., rapid pace of social change, threat of war, economic collapse, or nuclear holocaust.	Social—e.g., kindergarten entry, leaving home for college, marriage or divorce, "empty nest"
Stressful events—e.g., illness, immigration, loss of job	

changes and subsequent illness. By itself the SRRS is not predictive of illness, and more recent work indicates that individuals differ in their abilities to cope with major life changes and one mediating factor is the quality of the individual's social support.

The SRRS contains some outdated items and some not appropriate for the elderly or for women. Norbeck (1984) modified a life events questionnaire for relevance to women of childbearing age. She reworded some items to reduce bias from sexist assumptions about marital status and socioeconomic factors, and added such new items as change in childcare arrangements, becoming a single parent, custody battles, and conflicts with partner about parenting. However, illness, in and of itself, may precipitate more life changes such as those marked by asterisks in Table 9-3.

In contrast to Holmes and Rahe's focus on important life events, Lazarus (1981) takes the position that the everyday hassles and annoyances—the mundane details of life—contribute more to stress, illness, and depression than do major life event changes. Examples include commuting in traffic, home or office equipment breaking down, minor disagreements with co-workers, and constant interruptions. Links between kinds of stressors, numbers of stressors, and illness is an area in which there has been much recent research; however, definitive findings are yet to be published.

Although it is not clear whether daily events or major life changes are more taxing to individuals, an individual's *perception* of an event as more or less stressful is known to be a factor in determining the amount of stress he experienced. The subjective experience of a stressor contributes to the magnitude of the physical and emotional response to it. The same event might be regarded as devastating by one person and as a minor

TABLE 9-3. SOCIAL READJUSTMENT RATING SCALE

Event	Value
Death of spouse	100
Divorce	73*
Marital Separation or End of Relationship	65*
Jail Term	63
Death of Close Family Member	63
Personal Injury, Illness, Abortion, or Miscarriage	53*
Marriage	50
Fired from Work	47
Marital or Relationship Reconciliation	45
Retirement	45
Change in Family Member's Health	44
Pregnancy	40
Sexual Problems	39*
Addition of New Family Member	39
Business Readjustment	39
Change in Financial Status	38*
Death of Close Friend	37
Change to Different Line of Work	36*
Change in Number of Marital Arguments	35*
Mortgage or Loan over $10,000	31
Foreclosure of Mortgage or Loan	30
Change in Work Responsibilities	29*
Son or Daughter Leaving Home	29
Trouble with In-Laws	29
Outstanding Personal Achievement	28
Spouse Begins or Stops Work	26*
Starting or Finishing School	26
Change in Living Conditions	25*
Revision of Personal Habits	24*
Trouble with Boss	23
Change in Work Hours or Conditions	20*
Change in Residence	20*
Change in Schools	20
Change in Recreation	19
Change in Church Activities	19
Change in Social Activities	18*
Mortgage or Loan under $10,000	17
Change in Sleeping Habits	16*
Change in Number of Family Gatherings	15*
Change in Eating Habits	15*
Vacation	13
Christmas	12
Minor Violation of the Law	11

From Holmes TH, Rake RH: The social readjustment scale. The Journal of Psychosomatic Research, Vol 11, No 2, p 216, 1967 *(reprinted with permission of Pergamon Press, Ltd.)*

interruption by another. Current research efforts are devoted to exploring what other factors modify the individual's response to a perceived stressful event (Kobasa, Hiker, and Maddi 1979).

Equally important as type of stressor and the individual's perception of it is the *coping style* of the individual. Again, some individuals seem to get through seemingly traumatic experiences nearly unscathed, while others are immobilized by what seem to be minor circumstances. Personal factors that have been linked with successful adaptation to stress include having a sense of control of one's life, being flexible and optimistic, and having a good social support system (Antonovsky 1980).

The issue of the individual's perceived sense of control is interesting. During the 1970s, scientists proposed a link between personality type, stress, and incidence of illness. The Type A personality (the stereotypical busy executive, with much responsibility who is impatient, angry, and hurried) was thought to have a higher stress level than more relaxed individuals, which led to higher rates of heart disease (Friedman and Rosenman 1974). However, recent studies (Kobasa et al., 1979; Pines 1980) have suggested that pressure or amount of responsibility may not be as hazardous as one's sense of control over one's life. Individuals who have less responsibility or pressure (e.g., assembly workers, garment stitchers, cooks, middle managers) but who also have little control over their work have been found to have more symptoms of stress and higher rates of heart disease than their bosses. Thus, control over one's own situation seems to be related to improved health status. A desirable goal would be to promote a sense of control in the area of health and stress management. Self-care is a logical place to promote this.

A number of self-care techniques have been shown to be effective in stress management. As early as 1939, Jacobsen advocated progressive muscle relaxation to treat anxiety. Other relaxation techniques, such as meditation, yoga, autogenic training, visualization, biofeedback, and hypnosis have been shown to produce a physiological response that is the opposite of the stress response. Further, recent studies have documented the effectiveness of relaxation techniques for reducing blood pressure (Patel and North 1975) and for controlling pain (Mooney 1983; Zahourek 1982). These techniques will be described beginning on page 194 of this chapter.

The negative effects of stress can also be seen in the acute care setting. Research suggests that anxiety increases both discomfort and physical complaints (Parker 1981). Illness itself is a stressor, not only because of obvious physical stresses, but because it requires temporary or long-term life changes. However, stress management techniques are underutilized in the acute care setting. An important part of the nurse's role is to work with clients to help them cope with stressors affecting their health. With this thought, we turn to clinical application of stress management techniques, using the nursing process.

CLINICAL APPLICATION

Nurses can help their clients to manage stress. However, nurses themselves would also benefit from using stress management to cope with stressors inherent in nursing practice. Stress management can be organized into four categories:

1. Avoiding or eliminating the stressor
2. Reducing the stressor
3. Altering the individual's perception of the stressor
4. Altering the individual's response to the stressor.

Consider the example of a daily commute in heavy traffic as a stressor. Avoiding the stressor would entail taking public transportation. Reducing the stressor might entail car pooling to work, thereby reducing the number of days per week the individual was exposed to the stressor. Altering the perception of the stressor might entail self-talk (talking to oneself) about what options are and are not possible although, in this case, an individual's self-talk may actually be more destructive than the stressor itself. Altering response to the stressor might entail using stress reduction techniques.

For the hospitalized patient who requires a painful dressing change, T.I.D., eliminating or reducing the stressor is inadvisable. However, the patient's perception can be altered by having an understanding of how the procedure contributes to healing rather than perceiving that it is simply a painful assault. The patient's perception and response could also be modified by premedication or use of relaxation techniques. Before considering how to proceed with stress management, the first step must be for the nurse and client to determine what stressors exist for the individual and how the individual responds physically and emotionally to those stressors.

Assessment

The major goal of the assessment process is for the individual to become a more sensitive observer of what events or situations in daily life lead to feelings of being "stressed." During this process, it is also useful for the individual to identify the physical and emotional sensations experienced when stressed. One way of gathering this information is through a detailed nursing history. A better way is through a systematic self-assessment, done daily over a period of at least one week. The outline on page 190 gives an example of a written tool that can be used by clients or nurses.

Another approach focuses on assessment of adequate relaxation rather than identification of stressors; Figure 9-1 could be used alone or in conjunction with the first tool.

Since clients may be unaware of physical parameters of stress, it is important for the nurse to collect data on physical symptoms. Such assessment can also be used to teach clients to be more aware of physical manifestations of stress. See Table 9-4 for guidelines.

STRESS SELF-ASSESSMENT TOOL

Date	Time	Stressor	Physical Response	Emotional Response

Planning and Implementation

Of major importance in planning a stress management program is tailoring the program to the individual's needs, personality, life-style, and culture. Specific techniques may be helpful to one client but not to another. Some individuals may have to try more than one technique to find one with which they are comfortable. For example, for a Middle Eastern woman, practicing assertive communication as a stress management technique may have repercussions in her marriage, while deep breathing or meditation may fit much better with her life-style. In addition, it is often better to teach clients stress reduction or relaxation techniques before introducing other techniques, such as assertive communication, which in and of themselves may be stressful initially.

The nurse should also assess the individual's motivation for reducing stress. Consider busy executives who say that they know that they need to implement a stress management program, but somehow cannot find the time during the day to do so; in this case, stress management techniques seem to have a lower priority than work. Another approach, in which individuals engage in stress management in the same manner that they approach everything else—as a job—may result in the stress reduction plan becoming one more stressor. In this case, individuals need to be encouraged to make time in the day for play or for something that they consider to be relaxing or fun. The nurse and client should explore these activities in the interest of choosing the ones that are most effective for the individual. Some people enjoy massage, while others get a lift from activities that pamper them in some way, (e.g., facial, manicure, haircut). Some people find saunas or jacuzzis relaxing, while others prefer casual visiting with friends or taking a walk when feeling stressed. For instance,

RELAXATION SELF-ASSESSMENT

Complete the following self-assessment to help you look at the role of "relaxation" in your life now. On the scale below circle the numbers which best indicate you and your life during the last year:

	Almost Never	Seldom	Often	Almost Always
1. It is easy for me to find a place to be alone in my house . . .	1	2	3	4
2. My feet are warm when I go to bed at night . . .	1	2	3	4
3. My neck and shoulders are relaxed . . .	1	2	3	4
4. I fall asleep within ten minutes of going to bed . . .	1	2	3	4
5. When I shake hands with people my palms are dry . . .	1	2	3	4
6. I practice deep breathing when I am tense . . .	1	2	3	4
7. When I put my hands to my face they are warm . . .	1	2	3	4
8. I am able to function in an emergency situation . . .	1	2	3	4
9. When I notice that I am tense I am able to calm down . . .	1	2	3	4
10. It's easy for me to focus my attention and block out distracting noises . . .	1	2	3	4

1. Connect all the circles down the length of the page. Look at the pattern that your connected line makes. You might also turn your page sideways to get an even more clear visual picture of "relaxation" in your life right now. What does it seem to be saying to you?

2. Now add up your total score: _____

   Circle which range it was in:

   10–19   20–29   30–40

192 Self-Care Nursing: Theory & Practice

If your score was in the 10–19 range you might want to make some changes in how and when you play. Which aspects do you think need the most work? How many "1's" did you mark on this assessment? _____ These might serve as a clue to help you think about making changes in this area of your life.

3. How would you like this self-assessment to look in six months from now? Are you interested in planning towards those improvements?

4. Remember to congratulate yourself for your efforts to learn to relax.

Figure 9-1. Relaxation self-assessement tool (From Baldi S, Costell S, Hill L, Jasmin S, Smith N: For Your Health: A Model for Self-Care. Nurses Model Health, South Laguna, California, 1980, reprinted with permission from Nurses Model Health).

TABLE 9-4. PHYSICAL PARAMETERS FOR ASSESSING STRESS

Head and Neck
- Dilated pupils
- Complaints of headaches
- Tightness of face and jaw
- Bruxism
- Dry mouth
- Pale lips

Respiratory
- Increased rate of breathing
- Decreased depth of breathing
- Breath holding
- Use of accessory muscles
- Frequent upper respiratory complaints
- Wheezing or asthma symptoms

Cardiac
- Increased blood pressure
- Increased heart rate
- Abnormal rhythm
- Bounding pulse
- Palpitations
- Pale nailbeds
- Cool skin
- Ashen color
- Clammy palms
- Cold hands and feet
- Increased temperature

Gastrointestinal
- Increased or decreased appetite
- Loss or gain of weight
- Diarrhea
- Constipation
- Indigestion
- Nausea
- Vomiting
- Flatus
- Distension

Musculoskeletal
- Pain or tightness in neck and back

Psychological
- Impulsive behavior
- Instability
- Weakness
- Dizziness
- Fatigue
- Insomnia
- Hyperexcitation
- Irritability
- Depression
- Anxiety
- Frequent accidents
- Increased or decreased response to pain

one of us advised a graduate student preparing for an oral examination to choose the activities she found most enjoyable and relaxing and to engage in them the day before the examination. Her stress reduction assignment for that day was to take a walk by the ocean, to spend most of the day clothes shopping, and to avoid studying.

The most important points to remember in planning a stress management program are:

1. Does the plan meet the individual's need?
2. Can it be incorporated into a daily or weekly pattern?

If implemented regularly, the program will achieve its maximum benefit. A thorough discussion of likes and dislikes and the issues of making time for such activities may be all that is needed for individuals to feel that they have a "right" or "permission" to take some time for themselves each day.

Attention to nutrition and exercise are also important points of stress management. Balanced nutrition is influential in determining the individual's response to stress. Poor food choices can contribute directly to increased stress in an individual. Consider caffeine and sugar, which precipitate the stress response. We are all aware of the "lift" obtained following ingestion of a cup of coffee or a candy bar, just as we are aware of the "letdown" when our systems return to normal following this artificial stimulation. Another example is alcohol, which can stress the body by depleting it of magnesium and other water soluble vitamins (Mason 1980). Some people use the so-called "stress vitamins" as nutritional supplements during stressful periods. These vitamins include C and B complex and minerals such as calcium, potassium, and zinc. However, scientific data to support these ideas are missing, and their use remains controversial.

Effective coping can improve a stressful situation by initiating effective action. Coping promotes health if used effectively. However, some intrapsychic methods of coping, such as denial or avoidance, can be used either effectively or maladaptively. Denial can decrease feelings of threat and stress to manageable levels so that the individual can carry out normal daily functions. Such denial or avoidance can be helpful for the short run but, over time, becomes maladaptive if it interferes with more positive adaptive behaviors that require action or medical intervention. Applebaum (1981:200) classifies coping mechanisms into four categories:

1. Coping via information search, in which individuals under stress seek information as to the nature of the situation and what can be done to alleviate the pressure
2. Coping via direct action, in which individuals under stress attempt to change the situation by altering the fit between themselves and the environment
3. Coping via the inhibition of action, in which individuals under

stress do not attempt any direct action but maintain a psychological distance from the situation by waiting until the initial tension and ensuing reactions are at a lower level

4. Coping via intrapsychic modes, in which individuals under stress use such defense mechanisms as denial or sublimation.

Despite the fact that many people turn to such coping methods as overeating, excessive use of alcohol, or drugs when feeling stressed, these methods are not recommended as effective for long-term stress management.

Physical activity may be a more effective stress reduction strategy, since it helps to keep muscles in tone and free of tension. Some exercise, whether gentle or strenuous, can prevent or reduce the symptoms of stress. Hospitalized patients can do bed exercises, and most other people can at least incorporate walking into their everyday lives. Gentle exercises include slow movements, such as yoga, which directs awareness to sites of tension. Gentle stretching is useful in preventing or reducing headaches or neckaches. Active or aerobic exercise helps the cardiovascular system, clears the lungs, burns calories, and decreases skeletal tension. Moderate to active exercise such as walking, hiking, jogging, swimming, or bicycling are very effective techniques for stress management.

RELAXATION TECHNIQUES

Relaxation techniques are designed to produce a physiological reaction that is the opposite of the stress response—"The Relaxation Response" (Benson 1976). This parasympathetic response can be produced by a number of techniques and consists of the following:

- Decreased respiratory rate
- Increased depth of respiration
- Decreased heart rate
- Decreased blood pressure
- Increased blood flow to the extremities
- Skeletal muscle relaxation
- Decreased metabolic rate.

Benson (1976) suggests that it does not matter if a person practices a formal relaxation technique, as long as four basic components are included:

- A quiet environment
- An object on which to concentrate
- Passive attitude
- A comfortable position.

One can achieve the relaxation response without special training or by incorporating the four basic components in one's own way, as long as regular practice is maintained. Table 9-5 gives examples of the relaxation response produced by different relaxation techniques.

Breathing

Deep breathing is an integral part of many different relaxation techniques, such as yoga, hypnosis, visualization, meditation, autogenic training, and progressive muscle relaxation. However, deep breathing is in and of itself a powerful stress-reducing technique, one that often is utilized inadequately in clinical nursing practice.

Effective breathing increases oxygenation and helps to relax muscles. However, as tension increases, many people hold their breath or breathe in a shallow and rapid manner. It is helpful to instruct clients to breathe deeply and slowly and attempt to fill the lungs. A review of anatomy may help clients to visualize their lungs. In addition, visualization can be used in conjunction with deep breathing to enhance the effects. The nurse can suggest that the client visualize the inhaled air nourishing the body and relaxing tired muscles. On exhalation, the client can be instructed to visualize blowing away the tension.

Breathing techniques can be used anywhere and are especially useful during stressful situations or when symptoms appear. The advantage of deep breathing is that a special time, place, or arrangement is not required, and it can be incorporated into a busy schedule. Mason (1980) suggests taking at least 40 deep breaths a day, inhaling and holding the breath for ten seconds, then exhaling through the mouth with a sigh. It is useful to incorporate reminders to deep breathe throughout the day, such as each time the telephone rings or at each stop sign or traffic light while driving a car.

Autogenic Training

Autogenics, a powerful relaxation technique described by the German neurologist Schultz (1932), produces a state similar to that produced by hypnosis. Autogenic training is a systematic way of teaching the body and mind to respond to verbal suggestions that produce relaxation. Schultz found that a relaxed state could be achieved by thinking of heaviness (which promotes deep muscle relaxation) and warmth (which promotes peripheral vasodilation) in the extremities. Key phrases of autogenic training are listed below.

Individuals beginning autogenic training are instructed to assume a comfortable reclining position and to loosen tight clothing and remove eyeglasses or jewelry. They are asked to repeat each of the key phrases three times. It is not important whether or not they actually feel heaviness or warmth in the beginning; with practice, individuals will achieve the

TABLE 9-5. DIFFERENT TECHNIQUES ELICITING THE PHYSIOLOGIC CHANGES OF THE RELAXATION RESPONSE

Technique	Oxygen Consumption	Respiratory Rate	Heart Rate	Alpha Waves	Blood Pressure	Muscle Tension
Meditation	Decreases	Decreases	Decreases	Increases	Decreases*	Not Measured
Zen and Yoga	Decreases	Decreases	Decreases	Increases	Decreases*	Not Measured
Autogenic	Not Measured	Decreases	Decreases	Increases	Inconclusive	Decreases
Progressive Relaxation	Not Measured	Not Measured	Not Measured	Not Measured	Inconclusive Results	Decreases
Hypnosis with Suggested Deep Relaxation	Decreases	Decreases	Decreases	Not Measured	Inconclusive Results	Decreases

*In patients with elevated blood pressure.
From Benson H: The Relaxation Response. William Morrow and Company, Inc., New York, pp 70–71, 1975 (reprinted with permission of the publisher)

AUTOGENIC TRAINING: KEY PHRASES

- My arms and legs are heavy.
- My arms and legs are warm.
- My heartbeat is calm and regular.

- My breathing is calm and regular.
- My solar plexus is warm.
- My forehead is cool.

desired state of relaxation. It is recommended that the exercise be practiced at least daily. Following the exercise, individuals should sit quietly and gradually return to a normal state of alertness.

Autogenic training is particularly helpful for hyperventilation and asthma, gastrointestinal disturbances, hypertension, cold hands and feet, and headaches. It can also help reduce anxiety, irritability, and fatigue. In addition, autogenics can help moderate pain (Zahourek 1982) and increase resistance to the harmful effects of stress. Therefore, autogenic techniques can also be quite useful for hospitalized patients.

Visualization

The purpose of visualization is to use a mental picture to create a response from the body, using visual imagery to change a mental or physical state. Visualization is the use of positive, conscious suggestions to affect unconscious processes. For example, patients who have an infection might be asked to picture their own antibodies moving to the site of the infection to battle the bacteria. Simonton, Simonton, and Creighton (1978) suggest that their cancer patients use such vivid images to aid their fight against cancer. Visualization is useful in labor and delivery, e.g., visualizing contractions opening the cervix, deep inhalations nourishing the body, and exhalations blowing away tensions.

Visualization can be used in conjunction with other relaxation techniques, such as autogenics. Mason (1980) suggests that the individual practicing autogenics visualize thoughts that occur as bubbles in a glass of carbonated water, which float to the top of the glass and burst. Visualization can also be used to anticipate and rehearse a worrisome upcoming situation to reduce stress associated with the situation.

Progressive Muscle Relaxation

Developed by the physiologist Jacobsen in 1939, this relaxation technique focuses on specific muscles and muscle groups. A comfortable position is helpful, and deep breathing is essential. This technique increases awareness of both tension and relaxation through systematic muscle contraction alternated with subsequent relaxation. For example, hands and forearms are contracted by making a fist. The client is instructed to hold the fist tighter and tighter, becoming increasingly aware of the tension. The client is then instructed to release the fist, becoming aware of the sense of relaxation. The same instructions are given for other muscles throughout the body (see below).

PROGRESSIVE MUSCLE RELAXATION

Instructions by Muscle Groups

- Make a fist—hands, forearm
- Flex upper arm, pull elbow to side—upper arms, shoulder
- Bring toes toward head—calves, feet
- Push feet against floor—thighs
- Curl toes—toes, feet

- Wrinkle forehead, squint eyes, clench jaws—face
- Raise shoulders and tighten muscles—shoulders and neck
- Tighten abdominal muscles— abdominal muscles
- Tighten buttocks—buttocks

Progressive muscle relaxation is effective for a number of stress-related conditions, especially those that are related to specific muscle groups. It helps to control nausea and vomiting in patients receiving chemotherapy (Cotanch 1983). It is easy to practice in almost any setting, but it is also important that it is practiced regularly.

Biofeedback

Although this technique is newer than others, it has also been used successfully in many stress-related disorders. Biofeedback is defined as the process by which an individual learns to influence physiological responses that are not ordinarily under voluntary control (Blanchard 1978). For example, it is now used as a treatment tool for urinary incontinence (Sugar 1983). Biofeedback requires a monitoring device that provides a measure of autonomic function, such as a line on a graph, a blinking light, or a buzzer. Through trial and error, individuals learn to achieve and maintain a desired level of bodily function as measured by the instrument.

The biofeedback instrument monitors such functions as heart rate, skeletal muscle tension, and other autonomic functions, such as those outlined on page 199.

For example, an electromyelograph (EMG) measures the nerve impulses to a muscle and translates skeletal muscle tension into an audible or visible signal. By noting whether the signal increases or decreases, the individual can learn to tighten or relax any muscle.

Smooth muscle relaxation is also possible with biofeedback, although it is entirely different from skeletal muscle control. Biofeedback measures skin temperature as one index of vascular constriction or dilation. Learn-

AUTONOMIC PROCESSES CONTROLLED BY BIOFEEDBACK

- Heart rate and rhythm
- Blood pressure
- Skin surface temperature
- Muscle tension
- Alpha wave, EEG

- Electrodermic response
- Sexual response
- Stomach acid levels
- Sphincter control

ing to raise skin temperature in the hands and feet is especially effective for tension and migraine headaches. When an individual is relaxed, the arteries can dilate enough so that the skin reaches 90 to 95°F.

Skin moisture can be used in biofeedback to assess tension and relaxation. When an individual becomes tense or frightened, perspiration increases. Conversely, when relaxed or resting, the skin is drier. Thus, the Galvanic Skin Response (GSR) or electrodermal response (EDR), which measure electrical conductivity of the skin, can be useful in assessing tension and also help an individual learn to reduce the body's physiological response to a stressor. Uses of biofeedback are outlined below.

FOUR BASIC OPERATIONS OF BIOFEEDBACK

- Detection and amplification of bioelectrical potential
- Conversion of bioelectrical signals to easy-to-process information

- Feedback of information to the client
- Voluntary control of target response through learning based on the feedback

Other Stress Reduction Techniques

The techniques described previously are helpful in modifying an individual's physical and mental response to stress. However, avoiding or reducing stressors should be considered to be as important, if not more important, than altering the response to stress. We will discuss two types of activities here that are particularly applicable to nurses—assertive communication and time management.

Being in a situation in which one is unable or not allowed to express one's thoughts or feelings is a major cause of stress for many people. However, because communication styles differ across ethnic or cultural groups, we will not suggest that *assertive communication* should be a general goal for everyone in every situation. Rather, we will confine the discussion to nursing, in which assertive communication can improve some of the difficulties that nurses often experience.

TABLE 9-6. COMPARISON OF ALTERNATIVE BEHAVIOR STYLES

	Passive	Assertive	Aggressive
Characteristics	Allow others to choose for you. Emotionally dishonest. Indirect. In win-lose situations, you lose. If you do get your own way, it is indirect.	Choose for self. Appropriately honest. Direct. Self-respecting, self-expressing, straightforward. Convert win-lose to win-win.	Choose for others. Inappropriately honest, tactless. Direct, self-enhancing. Self-expressive, derogatory. Win-lose situation which you win.
Your Own Feelings on the Exchange	Anxious, ignored, helpless, manipulated. Angry at yourself and/or others.	Confident, self-respecting, goal oriented, valued. Later: accomplished.	Righteous, superior, depreciatory, controlling. Later: possibly guilty.
Others' Feelings on the Exchange	Guilty or superior. Frustrated with you.	Valued, respected.	Humiliated, defensive, resentful, hurt.
Others' View of the Exchange	Lack of respect. Distrust. Can be considered a pushover. Do not know where you stand.	Respect, trust, know where you stand.	Vengeful, angry, distrustful, fearful.
Outcome	Others achieve their goals at your expense. Your rights are violated.	Outcome determined by above-board negotiations. Your and others' rights respected.	You achieve your goal at others' expense. Your rights upheld; others violated.
Underlying Belief System	I should never make anyone uncomfortable or displeased	I have a responsibility to protect my own rights; I respect others but not necessarily their behavior.	I have to put others down to protect myself.

From Steinmetz J et al.: Managing Stress. Bull Publishing Co., Palo Alto, California, 1982 (reprinted with permission from the publisher)

Assertive communication is the appropriate expression of one's thoughts and feelings about a situation without being indirect or putting others down. Assertive communication is helpful in situations that threaten self-respect and self-esteem and is an important part of self-care. See Table 9-6 for examples of three communication styles. Many nurses are unassertive. If we improve our ability to express ourselves in a straightforward manner, we will gain self-respect as well as the respect of the other members of the health care team and our clients. By demonstrating assertive communication, we become better teachers and models for our clients as well. There are a number of books and classes currently available for improving one's abilities to communicate clearly and in a straightforward manner (Steinmetz, Blankenship, Brown, Hall, and Miller 1982).

Another area that leads to stress is an *inability to manage time*. In nursing, effective time management can decrease some occupational stressors and improve the quality and quantity of nursing care. Daily pressures mount and countless people complain about having too much to do in too little time. In our fast-paced world, a few suggestions are offered. The first guideline is to keep an appointment calendar. Making plans on a yearly, monthly, weekly, and daily basis is a helpful way of keeping track of activities. Making lists (see Figure 9-1) further helps to choose priorities for tasks on a daily basis and to remember all the details that need to be done. In setting priorities, it is helpful to ask yourself the question, "Will this matter next week or next year?" As you accomplish each task on your list, check it off and reward yourself for a job well done. Once a list is made, major tasks or problems can be broken down into smaller, more manageable parts. At this time, tasks can be delegated and assistance requested. However, when you have acted on all these suggestions and you still feel overwhelmed, it is important to practice assertive communication and learn to say no.

SUMMARY

In this chapter, we have defined the concepts of stress, stressor, and the stress response. We have reviewed patterns of physical and emotional stress responses as well as the conditions that may be related to chronic stress. Techniques of stress management were presented with tools and strategies for assessment and intervention designed to modify stress. We hope that readers can find ways to apply this information in their personal and professional lives.

CASE EXAMPLE

Sam is a 40-year-old, married, Jewish executive in a large manufacturing company. During his yearly physical, he was informed that his blood pressure was 180/120. The employee health nurse referred Sam to his physician who immediately prescribed diuretics. Sam's diet was restricted to 2 grams sodium a day.

Following one month of treatment, Sam's blood pressure had dropped to 140/90. The employee health nurse then referred Sam to a stress management class as an adjunct to medical management, because she realized the nature of his work entailed considerable pressure. Because Sam's wife, Susan, who was a writer, was also under considerable pressure to meet deadlines, the employee health nurse suggested that both Sam and Susan attend the classes.

During the first class, the nurse described the difference between stressors and the stress response and explained the role of the individual in enhancing health. She advocated such self-care practices as healthy diet, adequate exercise, and self-expression. She stated that these practices were important before illness occurred and should also be done as part of long-term management of illness. The participants were asked to keep a record of the stressors they faced on a daily and weekly basis as well as their physical and psychological responses to each stressor. The class was also encouraged to practice deep breathing on a regular basis as a stress management technique.

After the class, Susan asked the nurse why it was necessary to prepare restrictive diets and practice stress management, rather than to just take the pills the doctor prescribes. The nurse asked Sue to describe the medications and the difficulty she was having in preparing food without sodium. Then, the nurse explained that sodium-restricted diets and relaxation aided in the treatment of hypertension, which was the reason Sam was at the class. She also reiterated the importance of active participation in improving health, explained that a sodium-restricted diet could be prepared without too much inconvenience, and offered to talk to Susan in more depth. They set up an appointment for the following week.

At their next meeting, Sue explained that Sam was on a 2 MG. sodium diet. The nurse questioned whether it was 2 MG. or 2 GM., and Sue was not sure. She was quite clear about how difficult it was to locate low-sodium milk. The nurse asked Sue to clarify the diet order and also discussed the use of a vegetable steamer to prepare fresh vegetables instead of using canned vegetables which are high in sodium. She also gave Sue a list of herbs and spices that could be substituted for salt.

In the subsequent classes, the nurse taught several relaxation techniques including progressive relaxation and autogenic training. Sue and

Sam practiced regularly. Sue preferred progressive muscle relaxation for specific muscles (her hands and arms from typing, her neck and lower back from sitting), while Sam preferred autogenics for more generalized relaxation. They completed most of the homework assigned.

Sue verified, with great relief, that the dietary restriction was 2 GM sodium. She now felt she could begin to conquer the diet. In addition, after three weeks in class Sam's blood pressure was 130/80 and his medication was reduced by the physician.

During the next meeting, the nurse suggested that students read Farquhar's book, *The American Way Of Life Need Not Be Hazardous To Your Health* (1978). She elaborated on other cooking techniques, but by this time Sue was feeling she had mastered the task and was anticipating writing an article on how to prepare a tasty low sodium diet in no time at all.

At the end of the class, Sue and Sam told the nurse how much they both had learned. Sue had lost five pounds, and Sam had started a running program as another component of his stress management program.

The employee health nurse continued to follow Sam's blood pressure. Two months after his participation in the stress management series and one month after he began running, his blood pressure was 120/76 with no medication. He practiced his autogenic exercises regularly and ran three times a week, and he and Sue both felt it was far better than "depending on pills!"

NOTE: Although this is a true case, not all cases of stress-related hypertension can be managed this quickly and easily.

CASE EXAMPLE

Ralph is an 18-year-old, male gas station attendant who was admitted to the emergency room following an automobile accident. He sustained a severe fracture of his left femur which required pinning to reduce. He also required an exploratory laparotomy for abdominal bleeding and a temporary colostomy. Ralph was admitted to the intensive care unit postoperatively, where he required high doses of narcotic analgesics every two hours to control his pain.

Ralph's behavior was demanding. He frequently shouted such statements as, "Someone come over here right now and help me!" "Doesn't anyone hear me?" or "Doesn't anyone care about me?" The nurses reassured Ralph that they did hear him and cared about him and that he was receiving as much medication as ordered by the physician. He continued to demand attention frequently, despite the nurses' efforts.

When his condition was stable, Ralph was transferred to the medical-surgical unit. His demands continued, and the nurses requested consultation by the Clinical Nurse Specialist (CNS). They stated that Ralph was abusive to the nurses, and he kept a record of time of administration of his pain injections; exactly three hours after receiving one, he "was on the bell for another shot." The nurses questioned Ralph's need for this much medication on his third postoperative day.

The CNS reviewed Ralph's chart and then did an assessment of his pain. The following problems were revealed:

1. Pain secondary to fracture and abdominal surgery
2. Inadequate pain management
3. Altered body image secondary to traction and colostomy
4. Loss of control of self secondary to pain and immobility, leading to
5. Decreased sensory input.

The CNS talked with Ralph about his own role in pain assessment and management. She asked him to rate his pain at the present time on a scale of one to ten. He said it was nine. She gave him a pain assessment flow sheet and asked him to keep a record of his pain, assessing it before receiving pain medication and one hour after receiving it, to see how well the medication was working. At this time, the medication regimen was changed from Demerol 100 mg PRN to Demerol 75 mg q 4 hours, and a nonsteroidal anti-inflammatory agent was added.

In addition, the CNS explained to Ralph that there were self-regulation techniques that he could use to reduce the pain while waiting for his medication; these techniques would supplement the narcotics. She also explained that medication alone would not get rid of all the pain. She asked if he were interested in learning techniques to help control the pain instead of having the pain control him. Ralph really responded to the idea of regaining some control and complained that one of the worst parts of "being tied to a pole" was that he could not *do* anything.

The CNS began by teaching deep breathing techniques. She asked Ralph to visualize the air he breathed in nourishing his body and relaxing each muscle; she instructed him to visualize blowing away the pain each time he exhaled. Ralph was encouraged to visualize his favorite place and to visualize himself there when his eyes were closed. Following the teaching session, Ralph stated that he was feeling more relaxed and that the pain seemed lessened. He liked these exercises and would do them when the pain worsened.

Later that day, the CNS brought Ralph a tape recorder and a relaxation tape and instructed him on how to use the tape. She called the switchboard and asked that outside calls be held and placed a sign on the door that said "no visitors for 30 minutes." Ralph listened to the tape. The CNS returned when it was over, and Ralph seemed very relaxed and in good spirits. He said, "The pain is gone. Maybe I don't need any medication any more." The CNS explained that he might still have some pain, but because he was controlling it, it would be less and less. She suggested that his Demerol dose could be decreased and that he should use the tape and the medication when necessary.

SELF-CARE PLAN FOR CASE EXAMPLE

Assessment	Planning	Implementation	Evaluation
Pain secondary to fracture and abdominal surgery	Increase client's participation in pain assessment and management.	Teach client to assess pain q 2–3h, before receipt of narcotics, after receipt.	Client assesses pain q 2–3h before receipt of pain medication and 1h after.
		Teach client self-regulation techniques such as deep breathing, visualization, and deep relaxation techniques.	Client verbalizes knowledge of self-regulation techniques and gives the nurse a return demonstration.
		Provide client with tape and tape recorder. Have client listen to tape prn at least once a day and before sleep.	Client listens to tape at least BID.
Increased need for narcotics	Taper intramuscular medication with MD orders and titrate p.o.	Explain rationale of tapering narcotics and increase deep breathing to prevent pneumonia.	Client verbalizes understanding of need to employ deep breathing and decrease narcotics.
Altered body image	Client verbalizes concerns and anxiety about body image.	Explain postoperative course and that colostomy is temporary.	Client verbalizes understanding of postoperative course, questions, and anxiety.
		Encourage verbalization of questions and fears.	
		Call ostomy support group to aid client.	Talks with ostomy group member.
		Encourage verbalization about fractured femur and need for traction.	Verbalizes fears, concerns, and questions about femur.

Discussion Questions

1. Explain the difference between a stressor and the stress response.
2. List five physiological stress responses.
3. List five emotional stress responses.
4. Discuss the differences in everyday hassles and annoyances and major life event changes.
5. What factors modify an individual's response to a stressor?
6. Name the four components required to produce the relaxation response.

REFERENCES

Alle JE: Biofeedback: A mind-over-body matter. Medical Self-Care, pp 32–35, Fall 1982

Antonovsky A: Stress and Coping. Jossey-Bass Publications, San Francisco, California, 1980

Appelbaum S: Stress Management for Health Care Professionals. Aspen Systems, Rockville, Maryland, 1981

Baldi S, Costell S, Hill L, Jasmin S, Smith N: For Your Health: A Model for Self-Care. Nurses Model Health, South Laguna, California, 1980

Benson H: The Relaxation Response, William Morrow & Company, Inc., New York, 1976

Blanchard E, Epstein L: A Biofeedback Primer. Addison-Wesley, New York, 1978

Claus KE, Bailey JT: Living with Stress and Promoting Well-Being. The C.V. Mosby Company, St. Louis, Missouri, 1978`

Corini ___, Owens ___: Neurological and Neurosurgical Nursing, 7th ed. The C.V. Mosby Company, St. Louis, Missouri, 1980

Contanch PH: Relaxation training for control of nausea and vomiting in patients receiving chemotherapy. Cancer Nursing, Vol 6, No 4, pp 277–283, 1983

Conway-Rutkowski B: Getting to the cause of headaches. American Journal of Nursing, Vol 81, No 10, pp 1846–49, 1981

Davis M, Eshelman E, McKay M: The Relaxation and Stress Reduction Workbook. New Harbinger Publishing, Richmond, California, 1980

Duldt BW: Anger: An occupational hazard for nurses. Nursing Outlook, Vol 29, No 9, pp 510–18, 1981

Farquhar JW: The American Way of Life Need Not Be Hazardous to Your Health. The Portable Stanford, Stanford, California, 1978

Ferguson T: Getting organized to deal with stress. Medical Self-Care, pp 22–24, Spring 1981

Friedman M, Rosenman RH: Type A Behavior and Your Heart. Alfred A. Knopf, New York, 1974

Goldway E: Inner Balance: The Power of Holistic Healing. Prentice-Hall Inc., Englewood Cliffs, New Jersey, 1979

Grant JW: Stress and the nurse: A selected bibliography. Journal of Nursing Education, Vol 19, No 6, pp 58–63, 1980

Hastings AC, Fodimer J, Gordon S: Health for the Whole Person. Westview Press, Boulder, Colorado, 1980

Holmes TH, Rahe RH: The social readjustment rating scale. The Journal of Psychosomatic Research, Vol 11, No 2, p 216, 1967

Jacobsen E: Variations of blood pressure with skeletal muscle tension and relaxation. Annals of Internal Medicine, Vol 12, pp 1194–1212, 1939

Kahn A: Assertiveness training. Medical Self-Care, pp 28–29, Spring 1982

Kenzer NS: Stress and the American Woman. Ballantine Books, New York, 1978

Kobasa SC, Hiker R, Maddi S: Who stays healthy under stress? Journal of Occupational Medicine, Vol 21, No 9, p 595, 1979

Lazarus R: Little hassles can be harmful to your health. Psychology Today, pp 58–62, July 1981

Mason LF: Guide to Stress Reduction. Peace Press, Culver City, California, 1980

Mooney NE: Coping with chronic pain in rheumatoid arthritis: Patient behaviors and nursing interventions. Rehabilitation Nursing, pp 20–25, March/April 1983

Mulray R: Tension Management and Relaxation. The C.V. Mosby Company, St. Louis, Missouri, 1981

Nath C, Rinehart J: Effects of individual and group relaxation therory on blood pressure in essential hypertensives. Research in Nursing and Health, Vol 2, No 3, pp 119–126, 1979

Norbeck JS: Modifications of Life Events questionnaires for use with female respondents. Research in Nursing and Health, Vol 7, No 1, pp 61–71, 1984

Numerof R: Managing Stress. Aspen Systems, Rockville, Maryland, 1983

Parker K: Anxiety and complications in patients on hemodialysis. Nursing Research, Vol 30, No. 6, pp 334–336, 1981

Patel C: 12 month followup of yoga and biofeedback in the management of hypertension. The Lancet, Vol 1, No 7898, pp 62–64, 1975

Pelletier KR: Holistic Medicine. Delacorte Press, New York, 1979

Peper E, Ancoli S, Quinn M: Mind/Body Integration: Essential Leadership in Biofeedback. Plenum Press, New York, 1979

Philips C: Headaches in general practice. Headache, Vol 16, No 6, pp 322–29, 1977

Pines M: Psychological hardiness. Psychology Today, p 34, December 1980

Reinhardt A, Quinn M: Coping with life stressors: A life-style approach. Family and Community Health: The Journal of Health Promotion and Maintenance, Vol 2, No 4, pp ix–xix, 1980

Selye H: The Stress of Life. McGraw-Hill, New York, 1956, 1976

Simonton OC, Matthews-Simonton S, Creighton J: Getting Well Again. J.P. Tarcher, Inc., Los Angeles, California, 1978

Sparacino J: Blood pressure, stress and mental health. Nursing Research, Vol 31, No 2, pp 89–93, 1982

Steinmetz J, Blankenship J, Brown L, Hall D, Miller G: Managing Stress. Bull Publishing Company, Palo Alto, California, 1982

Sugar E: Bladder control through biofeedback. American Journal of Nursing, Vol 83, No 8, pp 1152–54, 1983

Veninga RL: Work, stress and health: Four major conclusions. Occupational Health Nursing, Vol 30, No 6, pp 22–44, 1982

Wallis C: Stress. Time Magazine, pp 48–55, June 6, 1983

Zahourek RP: Hypnosis in nursing practice—Emphasis on the problem patient who has pain—Part 1. Journal of Psychiatric Nursing and Mental Health Services, Vol 20, No 3, pp 13–17, 1982

10

Psychological and Spiritual Well-Being

The concepts of psychological and spiritual well-being are abstract and have no generally agreed-upon definitions. These areas are highly subject to individual and cultural interpretation. While essential to good health, psychological well-being and spirituality are often neglected in nursing care in favor of more observable and "acute" needs of clients who show significant physical or psychiatric pathology. Recent criticism of the disease-oriented medical model is based on increasing realization that emotional and spiritual needs of clients are intimately related to their health status and, thus, must be considered in relation to professional care and to self-care.

This chapter focuses on the broad categories of psychological well-being and spirituality in the context of health and self-care and will *not* address psychopathology or theology. We define and describe these areas and suggest that there are broad variations in practices that promote health and growth. We also address research and issues relevant to health and healing for clients and nurses and provide suggestions for clinical application using the nursing process.

CURRENT KNOWLEDGE AND ISSUES

The first assumption on which the subsequent discussion is based is illustrated by the following poem, by William Carlyon, which suggests that one cannot be totally healthy through correct health practices alone.

The Healthiest Couple*

By William Carlyon

They brush and they floss
with care every day,
But not before breakfast
of both curds and whey.

He jogs for his heart,
she bikes for her nerves;
They assert themselves daily
with appropriate verve.

He is loving and tender
and caring and kind,
Not one chauvinist thought
is allowed in his mind.

They are slim and attractive
well-dressed and just fun.
They are strong and well-
    immunized
against everything under the sun.

They are sparkling and lively
and having a ball.
Their diet? High fiber
and low cholesterol.

Cocktails are avoided
in favor of juice;
Cigarettes are shunned
as one would the noose.

They drive their car safely
with belts well in place;
at home not one hazard
ever will they face.

1.2 children they raise,
both sharing the job.
One is named Betty,
.2 is named Bob.

And when at the age of
two hundred and three
they jog from this life
to one still more free,

They'll pass through those portals
to claim their reward
and St. Peter will stop them
"just for a word."

"What Ho" he will say,
"You cannot go in,
This place is reserved
for those without sin."

"But we've followed the rules"
she'll say with a fright.
"We're healthy"—"Near perfect"—
"And incredibly bright."

"But that's it" will say Peter
drawing himself tall.
"You've missed the point of living
By thinking so small."

"Life is more than health habits,
Though useful they be,
It is purpose and meaning,
the grand mystery."

"You've discovered a part
of what makes humans whole
and mistaken that part
for the shape of the soul."

"You are fitter than fiddles
and sound as a bell,
Self-righteous, intolerant
and boring as hell."

The second assumption underlying our discussion is the belief that body, mind, and spirit are intimately connected and that any influence in one area influences the other two areas and the person as a whole (see Figure 10–1).

---

*Reprinted with permission of William Carlyon

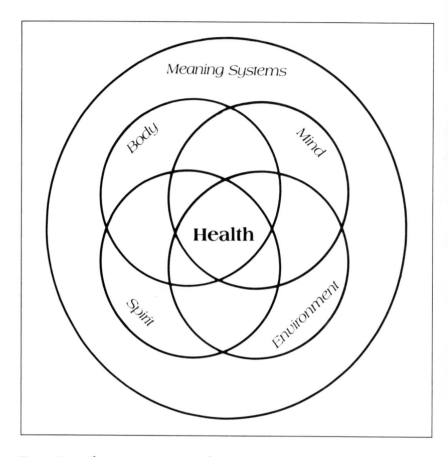

Figure 10–1. The Integrative Approach in Nursing

Jaffee illustrates the interdependence of body, mind, and spirit with the suggestion, "Once you recognize that disease is not simply a physical struggle but may also involve psychological, spiritual, and social dimensions, then it becomes clear that the appearance of any physical symptom—especially a serious or chronic one—ought to evoke a deep personal inquiry into your life" (1980:18). The holistic health movement is based on the assumption that mind, body, and spirit are inextricably linked and all of these must be considered in health and illness.

Although connections between stress and such disorders as ulcers and headaches have been known for decades, research has only recently begun to uncover neurological connections between psyche and soma. Examples include the brain's limbic system, which contains pleasure and punishment centers, biochemical and genetic contributors to psychiatric disorders (Kety 1979), and increased levels of the amino acids tyrosine and tryptophan, which are precursors of neurotransmitters and, in effect, act like drugs (Wurtman 1982).

Similarly, beliefs about the connections between health and illness and religious faith are as old as human society. Beliefs are part of explanatory models (Kleinman et al. 1978) and influence individual and cultural perceptions of health and illness. However, more recently research and clinical investigation is beginning to uncover the mechanisms by which beliefs and attitudes affect the body's capacity to heal. A recent example is the finding that laughter (Moody 1978; Cousins 1979) has a role in increasing the brain's output of beta-endorphins, which may decrease pain (Guillemin 1978).

The third assumption underlying our discussion is that the client's "world view" must be considered when discussing psychological well-being or spirituality. World view refers to an outlook on life, the whole meaningful universe as seen by the people of a particular culture, and it influences perception of everyday events. Because human beings live in a meaningful universe, not simply a world of physical objects and events, meaning is derived from the belief system of the cultural group (Hallowell 1942). Redfield (1960) defined world view as individuals' particular view of the world, the way the world looks to them, in particular, the way they see themselves in relation to all else. Most importantly, human beings see their world as having some order and including elements that in English are connoted by the words, "man," "nature," and "god."

Of particular importance to our discussion is that world views differ radically between different cultural groups. Nurses cannot understand the clients' perceptions of health, psychological well-being, or spirituality unless they have some understanding of their world view.

Definitions and Distinctions

We confine ourselves to a few definitions rather than distinguishing between such concepts as psychological well-being, emotional well-being, positive well-being, and mental health. Despite somewhat differing definitions, there are many areas of overlap. Dupuy (1972) views mental health as ". . . a relatively enduring positive state wherein the person is well-adjusted, has a zest for living, has developed his capability, and is attaining self-realization" (1972:509). Assessing these variables involves determining whether or not, for example, an individual has significant health concerns (and are they realistic?) or to what degree the individual experiences tension or anxiety.

Jourard (1968) describes the healthy personality as the people who take alert and responsive care of themselves, and who find life meaningful with some satisfactions and some accepted suffering. They love and are loved, they can fulfill reasonable social demands, and they know who they are and do not apologize. Healthy people find meaningful values and challenges in life, have an element of focus and direction, live in and with their body, and are not afraid of solitude.

The family is the context in which psychological well-being develops and is played out. Sedgwick states, "As an emotional environment, the family is embued with the responsibility of creating an atmosphere conducive not only to group living and cooperation, but to individual development as well" (1981:4). Jaffee (1980) views the family as a protective envelope, forming a first line defense and protection against the environment; the home is like a social skin and the people within that skin are like the organs of the body, functioning as a harmonious whole or as conflicting elements. Individual psychological or spiritual distress or physical ill-health can either precede or result from family disharmony.

Spirituality also has numerous definitions, from narrow to broad. Maloney states that ". . . the term spirituality refers to the particular way in which one conceives and realizes the ideal of his or her religious existence" (1983:2). Broader perspectives define spirituality as "the lived expression of world view," "an organization of the purpose and meaning of human life" or "a search for meaning" (Smith 1983).

In the strict classical sense, spirituality always includes the transcendent. Transcendence, used in theology, means that which exists apart from the material universe. In philosophy, transcendence means moving beyond the limits of human experience and knowledge. However, a broader and more recent usage of spirituality includes the humanistic perspective, which may not include ideas of transcendence (Duncombe 1984). The humanist perspective suggests that the main purpose of human life is to work for human well-being and freedom on this earth and that human beings have the potential they need within them to solve the problems of the human race, without depending on a superhuman being or force (Wilson and Kneisl 1983).

Religion is a social institution in which a group of people participate, rather than an individual search for meaning. Spiro (1966) defines religion as an institution of culturally patterned interactions with culturally postulated superhuman beings. Geertz suggests that a religion provides a comprehensive order of meaning that affirms, or at least recognizes, "the inescapability of ignorance, pain and injustice on the human plane while simultaneously denying that these irrationalities are characteristic of the world as a whole" (1966:24).

Some writers suggest that spirituality is basic to psychological well-being. Maslow (1969), for example, suggested that individuals who have never had a "core religious experience" might be said to be in a "lower-lesser state" in which they are not fully functioning. Jourard (1968) suggests that the healthy personality has free access to the unconscious and seeks transcendental or mystical experiences for the purpose of personal fulfillment beyond rationalism.

Both psychological well-being and spirituality are important in health, yet most individuals emphasize one aspect more heavily than the other. Some persons think that it is possible to have well-developed spirituality without psychological well-being, such as the mystic who cannot deal with people or whose experience is very painful, or the psychotic who has a mystical experience. In these examples, we must consider the perspective of the evaluators—the same individual might be considered to be simply crazy in one culture and a saint to whom the truth has been revealed in another. However, we consider spirituality, defined broadly as a sense of meaning, as part of psychological well-being and recognize that people experience spirituality in a variety of ways—through religious rituals, meditation, prayer, walking in a beautiful place, working toward a cause in which one deeply believes, or creating music or art.

Practices that allow individuals to have inspiring experiences beyond their everyday concerns and usual boundaries, to feel connections with the larger scheme of things, are important to psychological well-being. Individuals need to maintain, at least at times, a sense of meaning and purpose to their lives. Psychological and spiritual self-care allow individuals to get in touch with their feelings and this broader scheme and to arrange their lives so that they have the time to meet their emotional and spiritual needs on a regular basis.

Health and Healing: Issues and Research

Evidence of strong interrelationships between psychological, spiritual, and physical elements in health and healing often come from examples that are not clearly understood in Western medicine. The strict separation of medical and religious systems in the United States is not the rule around the world. In many cultures, illness-related ideas and practices are inseparable from religious beliefs and practices. Illness is thought to be caused by such supernatural beings as gods, ghosts, angry ancestors, demons, or spirits. In some cultures, illness is seen to be caused by human beings who are able to mobilize unusual powers, such as witches, sorcerers, or shamans. In the United States, faith is the basis of healing in many religious and ethnic groups. In some groups, such as among fundamentalist Christians or Christian Scientists, faith is seen as the major route to healing. It appears, suggests Glick (1967), that we must think about how and where "medicine" fits into "religion," rather than thinking of them as separate systems.

A central question in both religion and medicine is who or what has the *power* to make one sick and to heal? If individuals believe that sickness is caused by a human or superhuman agent, such as a god, a demon, or a witch, then they literally are victims, and nothing will convince them that self-care measures are likely to heal—unless, of course, self-care measures are based on faith and prayer or carrying out specific rituals prescribed by a healer. On the other hand, if individuals believe that illness is due to natural forces, such as weather, bacteria, an imbalance in the elements of the body, or decreased resistance due to stress, they are more likely to take some personal responsibility for instituting self-care measures. The locus of control construct is interesting in this regard. Locus of control studies distinguish between "internals" (people who perceive events to be the result of their own actions) and "externals" (people who perceive events as beyond their control, due to luck, fate, or chance, or due to control by powerful others). Health locus of control studies measure expectation of control over health and illness, attempting to predict health behavior (Wallston and Wallston 1978). With some exceptions, studies have found "internals" more likely to engage in health promotion behaviors. Most studies used middle-class people as subjects and focused on prevention. However, Coreil and Marshall (1982) studied Appalachians and Haitians, who are described as having a fatalistic world view, e.g. "health problems are due to the 'will of God' and there is little we can do about it." They found that people in both groups perceive a greater degree of control over treatment of illness than prevention and found considerable heterogeneity within groups.

Thus, personal beliefs based on a world view powerfully influence interpretations of illness and what actions the individuals are willing to take on their own behalf. Nurses must assess such beliefs before they assist in planning self-care. *Nursing Update* (1975) surveyed 32 religious denominations in the United States for customs associated with birth, death, health crisis, diet, and health and illness beliefs. In reference to birth, some examples are the necessity of infant baptism (Episcopalian, Eastern Orthodox, Greek Orthodox, Russian Orthodox, and Moravian). In reference to death, last rites are practiced among Armenians, Buddhists, Eastern Orthodox, Episcopalians, Greek Orthodox, and Roman Catholics. Special handling of the body (e.g, washing, shrouding, chanting, handling only by certain people) is required among Buddhists, Muslims, Mormons, Hindus, and Jews. Muslims, Mormons, Jews, and Russian Orthodox do not believe in cremation. Muslims do not believe in autopsies or embalming. Examples of dietary practices include prohibition of coffee and tea (Adventists, some Baptists, Christian Scientists, Mormons), alcohol (Adventists, Baha'i, Christian Scientists, Mormons, Pentacostals), and pork (Black Muslims, Muslims, Jews). However, these data were collected in the early 1970s, and theological concepts and religious practices change over time. The best rule is to ask clients about their religious beliefs and practices.

An extreme example of the power of beliefs can be seen in accounts of voodoo death in many parts of the world. Death follows an incident in which individuals believe that they have been the target of witchcraft or have been marked out for death by a sorcerer because of some transgression against the society. The death occurs more quickly than expected of someone who gives up hope and stops eating, and demonstrates that the psychic pain of extreme distress can result in massive somatic damage. Lex's (1974) review of research suggests that death results from the combination of a sorcerer's suggestion and the victim's strong belief in witchcraft; this combination affects the tuning of the nervous system, resulting in overactivity in both the sympathetic and parasympathetic systems which begin to fire simultaneously. Engel (1968) has described the "giving up/given up complex" as an emotional frame of mind that facilitates disease; it often follows a stressful event with which the individual "feels unable to cope."

Beliefs and expectations also have the power to heal. In contrast to individuals who sicken or die because of their perception of events in their lives are those with terminal illnesses who experience spontaneous remissions or "miracle cures." Jaffee (1980) suggests that one possible explanation of "miracle" healings is that some patients rediscover a transcendental or spiritual purpose in life or experience love and feelings of connection with a spiritual power or community. In a study of heart attack victims, White and Liddon (1972) described five out of ten recovered heart-attack victims who experienced what they called a "transcendental redirection"—a spiritual experience of rebirth and transformation which they felt benefited their healing.

Some individuals have reported spiritual or "out-of-body" experiences when near death, e.g., being greeted by dead relatives, watching the health team resuscitating their own bodies, or seeing a light at the end of a tunnel (Kubler-Ross 1981). By informing themselves about the process of dying and experiences associated with it, nurses can appreciate that such experiences occur. Such knowledge can encourage more openness and sensitivity to dying individuals' needs.

These examples illustrate some relationships between beliefs, attitudes, and health. An especially important attitude is hope. Lange (1978) suggests that loss of hope has a deleterious effect on the human being, resulting in giving-up behavior which may lead to physical and emotional disequilibrium. She states, "In many clinical situations, the nurse plays a crucial role in recognizing, maintaining, and restoring hope" (1978:172). She compares hope and despair behaviors in Table 10–1.

The power of expectation and hope in altering physical responses can also be seen in studies of the placebo effect. The only active ingredient in a placebo is the power of the belief, of positive expectations that the treatment indeed does help. Countless studies show that a significant percentage of people given placebos do experience objective improvement in the symptoms. The nurse's view of the therapy can influence the client's view. If the nurse is negative about the treatment or the physician, the client can be adversely affected. Conversely, a positive attitude can lead to a different outcome. This does not suggest false reassurance or saying what you do not believe; it does mean that you do not take hope from the client.

The Simontons' work with terminal cancer victims whose cases are considered hopeless demonstrates the power of the individual's beliefs,

TABLE 10-1. COMPARISON OF HOPE AND DESPAIR BEHAVIORS

Hope	Despair
Activation	*Hypoactivation*
Feeling vitality, vibrancy	Feeling all excitement, vitality
Having energy and drive	gone
Feeling inner buoyancy	Feeling empty, drained, heavy
Seeming to be more alert and wide	Being understimulated
awake	Feelings seeming to be dulled
Experiencing everything fully	Feeling tired, sleepy
Feeling interest and involvement	Feeling dead inside
Feeling like singing	Feeling mentally dull
Comfort	*Discomfort*
Having a sense of well-being	Having a lump in one's throat
Feeling harmony and peace within	Sensing loss, deprivation
Feeling free of conflict	Heart seeming to ache
Feeling loose, relaxed	Not being able to smile or laugh
Feeling general release, lessening	Having whole body tense, wound up
of tension	inside
Feeling safe and secure	Having feeling of being trapped,
Feeling life is worth living	boxed in
Feeling optimistic about the future	Being easily irritated, hypersensitive
	Feeling under a heavy burden
Moving toward People	*Moving away from People*
Having an intense positive relationship with another	Having a sense of unrelatedness
Reaching out	Wanting to withdraw, be alone
Having a sense of being wanted	Lacking involvement
and needed	Not caring about anyone
Feeling much respect and interdependence	Feeling a certain distance
Wanting to touch, hold, be close	Wanting to crawl into oneself
Sensing emphathetic harmony with	
another	
Competence	*Incompetence*
Feeling strong inside	Feeling that nothing one does is
Having a sense of sureness	right
Feeling taller, stronger, bigger	Sensing regret
Being more confident in oneself	Feeling vulnerable and totally helpless
Having a sense of accomplishment,	less
fulfillment	Feeling caught up and overwhelmed
Really functioning as a unit	whelmed

Being motivated

Having no sense of control over
situation
Longing to have things as they
were
Feeling unmotivated and afraid to
try

From Lange SP: Comparison of hope and despair behaviors. *In* Carlson CE, Black-well B (eds.): Behavioral Concepts and Nursing Intervention, 2nd ed. J. B. Lippin-cott Co., Philadelphia, Pennsylvania, p 175, 1978 *(reprinted with permission of J. B. Lippincott Co.)*

attitudes, and self-care practices in contributing to healing and remis-sion. The Simonton program uses a multifaceted approach including visualization, positive mental images, journal keeping, exercises, pain management techniques, and use of the family support system, with remarkable results for a number of their clients (Simonton, Simonton, and Creighton 1978).

In the opinion of some healers, clinicians, and researchers, people use only a miniscule proportion of their abilities to harness healing powers, citing examples of yogis who so discipline their minds and bodies that they are able to walk on fire without being burned. Krieger (1979) suggests that we have untapped power to heal others as well and has taught the art of therapeutic touch to many nurses. Nurses use this therapeutic tool to decrease symptoms and often see significant improvement in their cli-ents, family, and friends.

Psychological well-being in the nurse. An integral part of self-care application is the psychological well-being of nurses. We think that nurses in general are not fully effective in working with their clients unless they are aware of their own emotional and spiritual well-being. Nurses who do not take care of themselves sufficiently often burn out or do not have energy to give clients what is needed. Burnout is a state of emotional exhaustion, which occurs as a consequence of work-related stress over a period of time. Nurses who burn out have "a sense of being consumed, of losing a crucial aspect of identity or satisfaction, or of having a part of themselves changed, submerged, or emptied" (Patrick 1981:114).

Burnout can be prevented or interrupted once the nurse becomes aware of her psychological state. The following assumptions are similar to those that we advocate for all areas of self care:

● Self-assessment and sensitivity to the amount and character of one's emotional exhaustion
● Taking responsibility for an active role in achieving and maintaining optimal levels of self-care
● Shifting from a medical model to a holistic model of health care with

a personal commitment to wellness (Patrick 1981).

Unfortunately nurses are not always good role models for psychological well-being. They often ignore principles of good physical, psychological, and spiritual health that they encourage for their clients. It is vitally important for nurses to care for themselves at least to the extent that they care for their clients, not only for their own sakes, but for their clients' sakes as well. Nurses who have a well-developed spirituality and/or who seem to radiate good psychological well-being often seem to have a very positive effect on their clients and their co-workers. Somehow, people feel more positive in their presence.

Nurses' psychological and spiritual well-being become considerably strained by some aspects of nursing care, especially in the face of such ethical issues as termination of life support or abortion. Death of a client is a particularly difficult experience for most nurses, especially if the client "breaks the rules" by dying. The person who is "not supposed to die" often raises such spiritual questions in nurses as:

- "Why did God let him die?"
- "What was the meaning of his life?"
- "Why does a beautful innocent child die and a killer live?"
- "I feel so vulnerable, it could happen to me."

Such incidents push nurses to face their values, beliefs, and feelings with an intensity unusual in everyday life. Despite the painful nature of these experiences, these are rich opportunities to examine one's philosophy of life and values and to become more aware of the status of one's emotional and spiritual well-being. To take advantage of such moments of insight helps one to care for oneself emotionally and spiritually. The nurse's awareness can allow her to support clients who face death. The clearer she is about her own spirituality, the more comfortable she is likely to be in talking about life and death with clients.

In addition to facing your values and feelings during such critical times, it is important to develop your own awareness of these areas on a daily basis. There are ample opportunities in all areas of nursing for examining your values and your sources of emotional and spiritual strength. Each experience with a client that moves you in some way can help you to learn more about who you are and how you fit into the world. In addition, you can systematically assess your view of life, your coping style, and your emotional, spiritual, and interpersonal resources with an eye toward devising a self-care plan. For example, Kleinman et al.'s (1978) scheme for uncovering a client's explanatory model of illness (see Chapter 3) is equally useful for the nurse's recognition of what elements are part of her world view. With these thoughts in mind, we shift to how the nurse uses the nursing process to encourage self-care (of clients and self) in the areas of emotional well-being and spirituality.

CLINICAL APPLICATION: THE NURSING PROCESS

Although psychological well-being is often given at least lip service in care of clients, spiritual well-being is usually neglected. With the emphasis on the medical model found particularly in acute care settings, nurses often do not recognize that a client's spiritual "dis-ease" may be as important, if not more so, than the physical illness. We stress this point as an important part of nursing care and self-care, because so little attention is given to it in nursing education and clinical nursing practice.

Before describing assessment, we raise an issue that troubles many nurses. To what extent, if any, should nurses intervene when clients' problems appear to be spiritual? In their own searching, clients often reach out to nurses, asking such questions as "Do you think there is a heaven?" or "Do you believe in God?" Nurses face such questions with reactions that range from anxiety and no response to eager participation in a theological discussion. Clients may have difficulty broaching spiritual concerns when nurses respond at either extreme—from the nurse who refuses to discuss spiritual issues of any kind to the intensely religious nurse whose beliefs spill over into the care of all patients. We take a middle position which suggests that assessment of spiritual concerns is an important part of health assessment, and nurses should intervene only to the extent to which they feel comfortable, keeping the following guideline in mind—nurses should make every effort to support the client's and family's own spiritual beliefs, rather than attempting to impose their own.

Assessment

The first part of assessment of both psychological and spiritual well-being is the attempt to get an idea of the client's world view. Only in this context can the nurse understand a client's psychological or spiritual status. Eliciting the client's explanatory model of illness provides insight into his world view, at the same time being more acceptable to the client than such general questions as "Do you believe in _____?" A cultural assessment is also helpful in this regard, at least including some questions about family national background, religion, and cultural traditions that the individual considers important.

It is often difficult to distinguish psychological and spiritual concerns. The nurse should consider both the content of the concern and the context in which it is expressed. For example, clients who want to talk about difficulties with their spouses and who seem uninterested in discussing the meaning of life in general are most likely concerned mainly with the psychological realm. However, if a client feels quite guilty for having "sinned" through adultery, it is likely that both psychological and spiritual realms are involved. The guidelines for assessment, listed below, although based on Christian concepts, offer examples of some spiritual dimensions of experience.

GUIDELINES IN PASTORAL DIAGNOSIS

---

1. Awareness of the holy. What, if anything, is sacred to the person? Has he ever experienced a feeling of awe or bliss?
2. Providence. Does the person ask such questions as "Why me?" or "What have I done to deserve this?"
3. Faith. Does the person have an affirming or negative stance toward life? Does he embrace life and experience or is he cautious and tends to shy away from them?
4. Grace or gratefulness. Does the person seem "too thankful" in the face of excruciating problems or feel unworthy of forgiveness?
5. Repentence, repenting. Does the person initiate changes that will take him from less to greater well-being or from sinfulness to saintliness?
6. Communion. Does the person reach out to care about, and feel cared about by others? Does he align himself with the "company of the faithful?" Or is he alienated or estranged from others?
7. Sense of vocation. Does the individual put his talents to work as a participant in the process that moves the universe toward increasing integrity? Does he have a sense of purpose and investment in his work?

Adapted from Pruyser PW: Guidelines for pastoral diagnosis. *In* The Minister as Diagnostician: Personal Problems in Pastoral Perspective. The Westminister Press, 1976

Readers will recognize that these same kinds of variables can be also addressed by such terms as being in touch with the unconscious, guilt, optimism, rigidity, growth orientation, and interpersonal relationships. Indeed, psychological and spiritual concerns overlap in many ways, and self-care approaches may be similar. However, we do not see the nurse's major task as diagnosis or intervention in either realm. Rather, the point of assessment is to encourage clients to describe their concerns and to work with them within the frame of reference that they choose to devise a self-care plan that addresses their concerns. Having some sense of whether a problem is mainly psychological or spiritual is most helpful if the client needs the help of another professional. For example, a hospital chaplain can be helpful in the diagnostic realm.

Baldi and Paquette (1985) suggests that assessment of spirituality has a twofold purpose:

1. Learning about how well the spiritual part of the person's life is going and whether and to what extent his spirituality is a strength to him at the current time
2. Learning if there is an identifiable problem related to spirituality that needs addressing. An important aspect of assessment is

learning to what extent the client is aware of this component of life and to facilitate the client making a decision whether to do something about it or not.

Clients' concerns about psychological or spiritual well-being can be assessed indirectly or directly. Indirect assessment may occur through conversation about other topics, as the nurse becomes aware that something is not right in the client's life. Questions that raise the issue will indicate whether or not spiritual or psychological well-being are indeed problem areas and whether or not the client is willing to talk about these areas with the nurse.

Another approach is more structured and direct and includes specific questions as part of the nursing history, or use of separate tools, such as those below. The outline below contains selected questions from Dupuy's General Well-Being Schedule (1977), which is a research tool. The Spiritual Assessment list below is useful in assessing people from various ethnic groups.

SELECTED QUESTIONS FROM
THE GENERAL WELL-BEING SCHEDULE

During the past month:

- Have you been bothered by nervousness or your "nerves?"
- Have you felt so sad, discouraged, hopeless, or had so many problems that you wondered if anything was worthwhile?
- Did you feel relaxed and at ease or high strung and keyed up?
- How much energy, pep, or vitality did you have or feel?
- Have you felt tired, worn out, used up, or exhausted?
- Have you been waking up fresh and rested?

Adapted from Dupuy H: General well being schedule. In Fazio AJ (ed): Concurrent Validation Study of the NCHS General Well Being Schedule. (DHEW Pub No (HRA) 78-1347, Series 2, No 73), Hyattsville, Maryland, National Study for Health Statistics, 1977

SPIRITUAL ASSESSMENT

1. Does the way people live have anything to do with health/illness? In what ways?
2. Have you ever felt that you were ill spiritually? Explain.
3. Do you feel that health and illness are divinely sent?
4. Does illness increase or decrease your spiritual contacts or beliefs?
5. Do your religious beliefs serve as a comfort to you?
6. Do your religious beliefs cause conflicts within you?
7. Are there religious ceremonies that are important in the prevention, treatment, and/or cure of illnesses?
8. Who are the important persons for ministering to your spiritual needs?

9. Have you ever had to go against your beliefs and values in order to get medical care?
10. Will you let us know if we suggest something to you that goes against your beliefs and/or religious practices?

From Paxton R, Ramirez M, Martinez C, Walloch E: Nursing assessment and intervention. In Branch MF, Paxton PP (eds.): Providing Safe Nursing Care for Ethnic People of Color. Appleton-Century-Crofts, New York, pp 169, 1976 *(reprinted with permission of Appleton-Century-Crofts)*

The most important part of the assessment process is not simply learning that clients have a concern or problem in the psychological or spiritual sphere but learning what the concern means to them in the context of their world view. Physical symptoms should receive similar attention. Pain, for example, may be interpreted by the nurse as something that clients simply want to get rid of. However, pain may have a different meaning to clients. Is pain a sign of weakness and should they avoid showing their "weakness" to others? Is pain and suffering seen as ennobling? Is pain something to be avoided at all costs, even at risk of suppressing one's involvement with life? Is pain welcomed as absolving an individual from wrongdoing if he believes he has been sinful? Is pain a way of getting attention? Assessment of the client's spiritual and psychological well-being allows the client and nurse to talk about perceived concerns and problems, to put them in the client's philosophical context, and to suggest areas on which to focus the self-care plan that will be congruent with the client's beliefs, world view, and life-style.

Planning and Implementation

At the juncture of the assessment process and planning process is goal-setting. However, with some clients, the assessment process alone may serve as the intervention. Once clients realize just what their concerns are, they may only need "permission" to do what they already know they need to do. Talking about the problems in the open may be the catalyst for change. For example, a woman who is juggling career and family may recognize that she just wants to have some time for herself each day. Following assessment and her own and the nurse's "permission," she may begin to include such time.

However, it may be more effective for the client and nurse to write out goals for a self-care program based on their assessment. The clients' goals can be quite varied, such as increased awareness of their feelings or their powers of introspection, being able to include more quiet time in everyday life, or having the time to spend some focused attention on spiritual matters. A goal may be to learn to lift oneself out of mild depression, or to intervene in the early stages, or to be able to give onself "permission" to address emotional and spiritual needs on a regular basis. The nurse's goal is to facilitate and support clients in improving their own psychological and spiritual well-being.

An important part of the planning process is encouraging clients to assign priorities to their goals so that they can address the most important needs. Setting priorities means making choices. Such choices involve thinking about what is most and what is least important to the clients and to the significant people in their lives. For example, ask the client about what is most important today and if it will be important in the long run. Would it be more helpful to accomplish just one more task at work at the end of the day? Or should clients put it aside for tomorrow so they can come home in a more relaxed frame of mind and have the emotional energy to spend time with the children? This kind of discussion with the nurse will help the client to decide what is most important in developing a self-care plan.

When planning self-care for psychological and spiritual well-being, it is also useful to specify measurable behavioral objectives. For example, objectives like I will feel "better," or "more peaceful," or "more aware" are not measurable; on the other hand, objectives like, "I will set aside 20 minutes daily for prayer or meditation," or "I will write in my journal every day" are measurable. The individual either does or does not accomplish the objective and, thus, can evaluate whether or not the plan is effective. (See Chapter 6 for a review on how to write objectives.)

The client should also be encouraged to make time for pleasurable or spiritual activities on a regular basis. "Once in awhile" activities are enjoyable and enrich life, but to be most effective for health promotion, regular attention to psychological and spiritual needs is best. Weekly church services meet such needs for some people, while a solitary walk twice weekly in a beautiful place does it for others. Some individuals will want to schedule an hour a day to do whatever appeals to them most at the time, as long as the activity meets the criteria of, for example, making them feel happy or peaceful, or leading to introspection. Such activities might include reading poetry or an inspirational book, meditating, or writing letters to good friends.

Another part of the planning process is determining what clients can accomplish through self-care and when professional care should be sought. For example, a mild depression might resolve with self-care behaviors, but if the depression interferes with the individuals' functioning at work or home, or with eating or sleeping, professional help should be sought. Similarly, individuals who are experiencing a spiritual crisis, who have lost a sense of meaning in their life, who feel they cannot go on in this way, should seek the help of a clergyman or other spiritual advisor. Nurses need to be acutely aware of their own limits and the limitations of self-care.

Another responsibility of the nurse in self-care planning is providing the client with ideas for community resources that address psychological and spiritual arenas. For example, many self-help groups that focus on specific problems also address members' emotional needs (see Chapter 12). Cesarean support groups, for example, provide self-care information but also help women to resolve negative feelings associated with a previous cesarean birth. Other self-help groups specifically focus on psychological needs, such as Emotions Anonymous, Recovery Incorporated, and grief support groups. The nurse should be aware of classes and other community resources that can be suggested to clients.

Referral to community resources might include suggesting some of the alternative therapies that have developed in the United States during the past two decades. Some of these therapies specifically address body-mind awareness and consciousness development. Such therapies as transcendental meditation, encounter groups, and assertiveness training reflect a shift from the treatment of symptoms toward the general improvement of mental health, achieved through techniques for enriching experience and facilitating human relationships (Sayre 1983). Although some of these therapies necessitate working with a trained therapist, others are oriented to self-care and can be learned with practice (see Table 10–2 for other examples).

There are many useful techniques for psychological and spiritual self-care, some of which have been mentioned throughout this chapter. However, we focus here on one tool that is excellent for developing one's skills for introspection and awareness of inner processes and can facilitate growth both spiritually and psychologically. For people who enjoy writing, journal keeping can be invaluable for working through difficult situations, coping with stress, or increasing personal awareness of emotional and spiritual directions.

Individuals can keep a variety of types of journals, but there are a few general principles to guide the journal keeper. The first is that the individual should "shut off the censor" and try to write as freely and unself-consciously as possible. Keeping the journal in a private place for one's eyes only is helpful in writing freely. Concerns with spelling, grammar, or making perfect written sense can interfere with the purposes of the journal, which are self-expression and exploration. Secondly, a journal is more effective if it is kept in a bound book or a looseleaf notebook so that notes are made in chronological order and loose pieces of paper are not lost. Dated journal entries give writers perspective; they can look back to get a sense of where they have been and can become more aware of patterns in their life.

Different kinds of journals include dream journals, in which dreams written down provide insight into the person's unconscious, and food intake and emotions logs for dieters. One woman began a journal when her first child was born and chronicled her feelings and the child's development regularly over time. She plans to share her observations of him when he is older, if he is interested.

Psychological or spiritual self-care can also be implemented through an "intensive journal" (Progoff 1975). An intensive journal is a tool to help one deal with difficult times in one's life. It can also be called a crisis journal, in which the individual uses writing to work through and find direction during a difficult event. For example, a mother of a sick premature baby in an intensive care nursery found that writing in a journal helped her to realize that some of her distress was due to her ambivalence toward her sick baby and her guilt about feeling unable to bond with him. These insights occurred in the middle of the night, and the journal provided a therapeutic companion; after writing out her thoughts, she could return to bed, feeling relieved. The "intensive journal" is based on the premise that each person possesses self-directing, self-healing capacities that are not always accessible on a daily basis or conscious level. Progoff suggests that an intensive journal helps one to gain entry to the inherent wisdom and direction in one's life and leads to the kinds of growth and self-awareness that might otherwise be available only through psychotherapy or counseling.

For people who cannot or never express themselves in writing, setting aside some regular time for solitary reflection serves some of the same purposes as using a journal. Individuals might spend 15 minutes in the morning thinking about what they want out of the day and visualizing how they would like to handle the tasks ahead, including planning some time for enjoyment. Along with a morning reflection time, some individuals enjoy reflecting on the day's events at its end and affirming what went well. The point is to include time for self-reflection on a regular basis to be sure that one's emotional and spiritual needs are not being neglected.

Journal keeping and self-reflection are only two of a variety of self-care techniques which focus on psychological and spiritual well-being. Others, such as meditation or prayer, use of play, humor, and creative activities have been mentioned throughout the chapter. Whatever the client chooses, however, evaluation of the self-care plan and implementation is important.

Evaluation

Since the focus of psychological and spiritual self-care is growth and achieving feelings of peace and comfort in the inner sphere, self-care practices heavily emphasize self-awareness and staying in touch with one's feelings. Evaluation should be encouraged on a regular basis, such as by the daily inquiry, "How am I doing today? Have I spent some time addressing this area of my life?" It is important to evaluate on a continuing basis and to remain in the present, rather than focusing on the future or the past. Evaluation should also include a periodic look at the self-care plan and its implementation, with a view to changing it when goals are met, or improving it so that self-care goals can be reached.

TABLE 10-2. ALTERNATIVE HEALING THERAPIES

Therapy	Name of Originator	Therapeutic Goals	Central Techniques
Body discipline and body-mind awareness therapies			
Primal scream	Arthur Janov	To release primal pain caused by early frustration of need to be loved	Producing emotional flooding by breaking down personality defenses
Rolfing or structural integration	Ida Rolf	To realign body with gravitational forces, opening up chronic muscle blocks, which prevent free functioning	Massage and manipulation of deep connective tissues; encouraging expression of feelings about body and related experiences
Bioenergetics	Alexander Lowen	To reintegrate body and mind	Stressor and releasor exercises; emotional catharsis
Gestalt	Frederick Perls	To resolve significant emotional experiences and increase ability to choose experience	Fantasy; role playing; emotional catharsis; group work; discussing dreams and body language
Therapeutic touch	Dolores Krieger	To rebalance body energies	Deliberate transfer of energy from healer to healee through touch
Orthomolecular nutrition	Linus Pauling	To provide for ingestion of optimal levels of nutrients	Diet counseling; megadoses of vitamins
Biofeedback	Originated from work of Neal E. Miller	To gain conscious control over some autonomic functions such as heart rate and blood pressure	Mechanical feedback while client attempts to control autonomic function

Psychological growth therapies

Therapy	Originator(s)	Goal	Technique
Transactional analysis	Eric Berne	To improve social interaction; to increase self-esteem and ability for intimacy	Analyzing components of interaction to recognize and eliminate destructive forms
Encounter marathon	Fred Stoller, George Bach, William Schutz, Elizabeth Mintz	To increase ability for intense and honest communication	Nonverbal techniques; structured interpersonal exercises to break down personality defenses
Esalen encounter ("open encounter")	William Schutz	To break through self-deception in order to know and like the self	Nonverbal techniques and structured interpersonal exercises
Morita therapy	Masatake Morita	To relieve depression, obsessive fears, and acute anxiety	Period of stimulus deprivation followed by specific instructions to behave in a non-neurotic way
Reality therapy	William Glasser	To satisfy needs for self-esteem and love in a responsible way	Involvement with the therapist leads to ability to care for others, increased awareness of effectiveness and social acceptability of personal current behavior
Psychosynthesis	Roberto Assagioli	To arouse and develop the will	Exercises to sublimate sexual and aggressive energies into creative activities
Rational-emotive therapy	Albert Ellis	To eliminate irrational beliefs; to change specific behavior	Explaining irrational beliefs; positive reinforcement of effective behavior; group marathon encounters

Continued

TABLE 10-2 CONTINUED

Therapy	Name of Originator	Therapeutic Goals	Central Techniques
Assertiveness training	Robert Alberti, Michael Emmons, Sherwin Cotler, etc.	To decrease anxiety in social settings; to develop effective social skills	Role playing in group settings; teaching basic human rights and social skills
Sex therapy	William Masters, Virginia Johnson	To remove inhibitions that produce sexual problems such as impotence, premature ejaculation, and orgasmic dysfunction	Process of reconditioning during which couple engage in gradual and nonthreatening sexual encounters
Synanon: addiction group therapy	Charles Dederich	To eliminate destructive aspects of identity to enable client to stop using drugs	Direct attack on defensive behavior in peer group setting
Direct decision therapy	Harold Greenwald	To make a specific decision to change a behavior	Exploring life choices and alternatives for action
Psycho-imagination therapy	Joseph Shorr	To find true identity	Role playing in imaginative situation; exploring subjective reactions
Confrontation problem-solving therapy	Harry Garner	To reconstruct past and current erroneous perceptions; to increase social responsiveness	Confronting problems; fostering reality testing

Consciousness development therapies

Arica	Oscar Ichazo	To recover the true self lost through socialization	Eclectic blend of meditation and body awareness techniques
Living Love	Kenneth Keyes	To develop higher consciousness; to rid the self of desires	Instruction about levels of consciousness; reprogramming by mental exercises
Erhard Seminar Training (est)	Werner Erhard	To liberate the self from the fallacies of logical thinking; to accept total responsibility for life	Lecture; mental exercises; testimonials
Transcendental Meditation	Maharishi Mahesh Yogi	To make contact with the creative intelligence underlying existence; to relieve specific problems	Lecture; instruction in use of mantra and meditation techniques
Silva Mind Control	José Silva	To achieve alpha consciousness, which makes possible harmony with inner processes and gives ability to diagnose illness and solve emotional problems	Relaxation training; hypnosis; techniques of sensory projection
Eriksonian hypnosis	Milton Erikson	To maximize behavioral potential and treat organic and psychological problems	Autohypnosis
Neurolinquistic Programming	Richard Bandler and John Grinder	To enable client to learn new patterns of behavior	Imitative learning; reframing; dissociation from problem situations

From Sayre J: Alternative healing therapies. In Wilson HW, Kneisl CR: Psychiatric Nursing, 2nd ed. Addison-Wesley, Menlo Park, California, 1983 (reprinted with permission of publisher)

SUMMARY

This chapter discussed an important but often neglected area of health in which self-care can be very beneficial. The nurse's role in psychological and spiritual well-being is that of catalyst to find the best path by which to help clients achieve well-being. Nurses also need to pay attention to their own well-being, because nurses who neglect themselves are less effective with their clients. We hope that readers will use this chapter for their own growth and awareness, for their own sakes and for the sake of being good role models for their clients.

Psychological and spiritual well-being are concepts that are heavily influenced by world-view and more strongly subject to cultural and individual variation than such subjects as exercise, nutrition, or safety. Thus, *subjective* cues to well-being can be more important than objective cues. Individuals need to select criteria by which they decide if they do or do not experience psychological and spiritual well-being, and based on that assessment plan, how best to institute self-care in the context of their own personalities, cultures, and religions.

CASE EXAMPLE

Wendy G. is a 30-year-old, single, Italian-American nurse who works on a busy psychiatric unit of a large county hospital. She lives alone and is somewhat isolated because she works the evening shift, her boyfriend travels a lot in his work, and her family is in another city. The unit has been completely full with a larger-than-usual number of severely ill patients for the past six months, following government funding cuts to the chronically mentally ill. All the staff have been overstressed and overworked, but Wendy has been finding it especially hard to come to work each day. For the past month, she has taken several sick days because she just felt "too tired" to face the emotional needs of too many sick patients. She has also been awakening during the night and finding it difficult to get back to sleep and feeling particularly tired and bothered by headaches the next day.

Wendy visited her nurse practitioner and stated that she had felt mildly sick for a few weeks. The nurse found no physical problems but told Wendy that she seemed depressed. Wendy was relieved: "Of course! That's exactly what's wrong with me, but I've been too busy at work and too dragged out at home to pay attention." She felt no need to consult a psychotherapist but did think that she should do something, because this depression did not seem to be lifting by itself. She decided to talk with a fellow staff nurse, John, who was a "holistic health nut" and convinced of the importance of self-care.

Wendy and John went to dinner together, and she told him how she had been feeling and asked if he knew of any self-care techniques for depression. John said that he was flattered that she sought him out and suggested getting together the next day before work to set up a self-care plan.

Wendy and John started the assessment process by describing the details of Wendy's feelings and activities during the last months. She realized during their discussion that she had had difficulty accomplishing anything more than getting to work, getting through her shift, and going home to sleep. She had not engaged in her usual outdoor daytime activities with the excuse that it had been raining. But she had not even been doing her favorite indoor activities, like weaving, because as she stated, "I just don't feel like it." She blamed her lack of energy on disturbed sleep, resulting from the high pressure situation at work recently. When John asked Wendy what she had done for fun lately, she started to cry.

John said, "O.K., that's where you can start. But first, why don't you take a baseline for a week to get a good sense of your feelings and how you are treating yourself before we talk about changes?" John suggested keeping a journal with daily entries on energy level (several times during the day) physical exercise, sleep pattern, any dreams that she remembered, moods, and, in particular, writing down any thoughts that got her into a negative frame of mind.

During the week, Wendy dutifully recorded data on the subjects John had suggested in a small notebook that she kept in her purse. As the week went on, she realized that she was not paying attention to her own emotional well-being, and was quite surprised. She prided herself on her self-awareness in her work with psychiatric patients but seemed to have forgotten herself the rest of the time. As she began to put herself down for being "so unaware for a psychiatric nurse," and failing to apply to herself what she knew about mental health, she caught herself and remembered to note these "negative thoughts" in her journal. By catching herself in the act of subverting her outlook, she was able to turn her thoughts to more positive ones and congratulate herself for having taken responsibility to begin to turn the depressive process around.

Wendy had not seen John at work because he had been off. He arrived at the coffee shop where they were to meet before work the following week with a stack of books—some humorous novels that he had enjoyed, *Control Your Depression* (Lewisohn, Munoz, Youngren, and Zeiss 1978) and an article by Franklin (1982) on depression self-care. Wendy was enthusiastic about her self-awareness assignment and shared the following realizations:

- She put herself down all the time for what she was not accomplishing.
- These negative thoughts became a vicious cycle and produced more lethargy.
- She was not getting any physical exercise.

John explained that exercise has recently been shown to work as an antidepressant and mood elevator, by increasing beta-endorphins in the brain.

Wendy and John outlined the following self-care plan:

1. Get some vigorous exercise daily—use the mini-trampoline when it was raining, jog when it was dry.
2. Structure time at home—make a list of small tasks and accomplish at least one each day.
3. Engage in some activity that is fun or pleasurable one hour daily, at least three times a week.
4. Continue to write in the journal, but use it to express herself and maintain awareness of her moods and thoughts.
5. Expose herself to humor at least three times a week—a movie, a book, records.

During the week, Wendy implemented the self-care suggestions and reported to John the following week that she was in considerably better spirits. She was convinced that exercising had been a major factor, giving her more energy and improving her sleep. She was enjoying her work at the hospital more and had spent time at home cleaning out her closets and drawers. She said that "getting rid of a bunch of clothes and other things I don't use feels like a new start for me." And though she does not like the rain, she was not letting it stop her from getting out of the house during the day. She thanked John for his help and for letting her "unload" on him. As she handed back some of his books, she said, "Thank goodness I'm not in as bad shape as some of the depressed people in that self-care book. However, I did buy my own copy because the suggestions are useful for anyone."

CASE EXAMPLE

Mr. Mahmoud Said is a 66-year-old, Palestinian immigrant who entered the hospital because of progressive left-sided weakness. Exploratory surgery revealed an inoperable brain tumor which could not be treated by other means. Although he had an uneventful recovery from surgery, the nursing staff considered him "a difficult patient" with an even more difficult family. Mahmoud was accompanied by his wife, son, two daughters, and his sister-in-law. His wife slept on a cot in his room, and other family members were in constant attendance most of each day. His wife made constant demands on the nursing staff and at times interfered with his care. Because the nurses complained of feeling "burned out" after caring for Mahmoud after one day, the clinical specialist was asked to work with him and his family.

After talking with the family several times, the clinical specialist realized that the problems in giving care were not related to the family but to cultural differences. She consulted an Arab-American nurse from another hospital, who explained that the Said family was behaving normally—indulgence of a hospitalized relative, never leaving him alone, and making many demands on staff to show their caring for him. She also warned the clinical specialist that the Saids were not likely to be terribly cooperative until they got to know and trust the staff and that changing nurses daily only made them more anxious and more demanding. The clinical specialist also expressed her concern about Mahmoud's flat refusal to talk about the results of the surgery. The Arab-American nurse explained that Middle Eastern patients do not communicate openly about grave illness or impending death, believing that only God knows what an individual's prognosis is; in their culture, to anticipate death would indicate giving up hope and, thus, forfeiting God's help. She suggested that the best way to handle communication about the prognosis would be for the doctor to communicate with the oldest son.

The clinical specialist arranged a staff conference to discuss Mahmoud's care and to communicate what she had learned from the Arab-American nurse. Over the next three days, she and another nurse shared caring for Mahmoud and noticed a dramatic difference in their behavior. Mrs. Said's demands decreased markedly, and the family became extremely warm, not only to the two nurses, but to other staff. The doctor talked with the son who said that he would communicate the medical information to the family when the time was right. When Mahmoud was discharged, they gave candy and other small gifts to the staff as a measure of their appreciation; many staff members stated that they would miss this family.

Four months later, Mahmoud was readmitted as terminal. Nursing care was not a problem because the family trusted the staff and was eager to participate in his care. Family members competently took over more of his care as his condition grew worse. The clinical specialist was mainly concerned about whether Mahmoud knew he was going to die in order for him to prepare himself. She talked with the son, who grew angry and stated that under no condition should Mrs. Said or the family be told that he would die. She asked him if a religious official should visit him, and the son said no, that was only for when someone was dying, and God would take care of his father.

Although the staff was disturbed by such strong "denial," they respected the Saids' wishes, never contradicting them when they talked about Mahmoud's recovery. The family maintained a cheerful vigil in the room. Out of the room, the daughters appeared concerned but stated only "He will get better, God willing, God will take care of him." When Mahmoud died, two weeks later, he was surrounded by his family, strong until the end. When he was pronounced dead, the family began loudly crying and wailing and were taken to a private room in which they could mourn in the customary manner. The Imam was called, and arranged for an official to wash and wrap the body according to Moslem customs.

The clinical specialist arranged another brief case conference to allow the staff members to discuss their feelings about Mahmoud's death. Several staff members felt very close to the Saids and had felt that it was ethically wrong not to tell Mahmoud that he was dying and to "support the family lie." The Arab-American nurse, who attended the meeting, helped the staff understand how Moslems' strong faith in God, continued hope, and apparent "denial" is a cultural style of coping with bad news or disaster; in this case, to interfere with their style would have been unethical. She said that despite the staff's discomfort, they had given culturally sensitive care.

Discussion Questions

1. How do you describe emotional well-being in yourself? How do you know that you enjoy it or not?
2. What is the relationship between religion, spirituality, and psychological well-being?
3. How would you assess a client's needs in the area of psychological well-being?
4. State four questions that are useful in eliciting a client's explanatory model of illness.

REFERENCES

Baldi S, Paquette M: Spirituality. In Hill L, Smith M: Self-Care Nursing: Promotion of Health. Prentice-Hall, Inc., Englewood Cliffs, New Jersey, 1985

Coreil J, Marshall PA: Locus of illness control: A cross-cultural study. Human Organization, Vol 41, No 2, pp 131–138, 1982

Cousins N: Anatomy of an Illness as Perceived by the Patient. Norton, New York, 1979

Duncombe D: Personal communication, 1984

Dupuy H: The Psychological Section of the Current Health and Nutrition Examination Study. Proceedings of the Public Health Conferences on Records and Statistics and National Conference on Mental Health Statistics, 14th National Meeting, Rockville, Maryland, U.S. DHEW, PHS HRA, June 1972

Engel G: A life setting conducive to illness: The giving-up/given up complex. Annals of Internal Medicine, Vol 69, No 2, pp 292–300, 1968

Franklin N: Dealing with the blues and depression. Medical Self-Care, pp 10–16, Spring 1982

Geertz C: Religion as a cultural system. In Banton M (ed): Anthropological Approaches to the Study of Religion. ASA Monograph No. 3, Tavistock Publications, New York, pp 1–46, 1966

Glick LB: Medicine as an ethnographic category: The Gimi of the New Guinea Highlands. Ethnology, Vol 6, pp 31–56, 1967

Guillemin R: Peptides in the brain: Endocrinology of the neuron. Science, Vol 202, No 27, pp 390–402, 1978

Hallowell AI: Culture and Experience. University of Pennsylvania Press, Philadelphia, Pennsylvania, 1955

Jaffee DT: Healing from Within. Bantam Books, Toronto, Ontario, Canada, 1980

Jourard SM: Disclosing Man to Himself. D. Van Nostrand, Princeton, New Jersey, 1968

Kety S: Disorders of the human brain. Scientific American, Vol 241, No 3, pp 202–218, 1979

Kleinman A, Eisenberg L, Good B: Culture, illness and care: Clinical lessons from anthropologic and cross-cultural research. Annals of Internal Medicine, Vol 88, No 2, pp 251–258, 1978

Krieger D: The Therapeutic Touch. Prentice-Hall Inc., Englewood Cliffs, New Jersey, 1979

Kubler-Ross E: Living with Death and Dying. Macmillan, New York, 1981

Lange SP: Comparison of hope and despair behaviors. In Carlson CE, Blackwell B (eds): Behavioral Concepts and Nursing Intervention, 2nd ed. J.B. Lippincott Company, Philadelphia, Pennsylvania, 1978

Lewisohn PM, Munoz RF, Youngren MA, Zeiss AM: Control Your Depression, Prentice-Hall, Inc., Englewood Cliffs, New Jersey, 1978

Lex BW: Voodoo death: New thoughts on an old phenomenon. American Anthropologist, Vol 76, pp 818–823, 1974

Maloney GA: Pilgrimage of the heart. Harper and Row, New York, 1983

Maslow A: Religion, Values and Peak Experience. Ohio State University Press, Columbus, Ohio, 1969

Moody R: Laugh after Laugh. Headwater Press, Jacksonville, Florida, 1978

Nursing Update: Beliefs that can affect therapy. Vol 6, No 7, pp 6–9, 1975. Reprinted in Pediatric Nursing, pp 40–43, May/June, 1979

Patrick PKS: Burnout: Antecedents, manifestations and self-care strategies for the nurse. In Marino LB (ed): Cancer Nursing. The C.V. Mosby Company, St. Louis, Missouri, 1981

Paxton R, Ramirez M, Martinez C, Walloch E: Nursing assessment and intervention. In Branch MF, Paxton PP (eds): Providing Safe Nursing Care for Ethnic People of Color. Appleton-Century-Crofts, New York, 1976

Progoff I: At a Journal Workshop: The Basic Text and Guide for Using the Intensive Journal. Dialogue House Library, New York, 1975

Pruyser PW: Guidelines for pastoral diagnosis. In The Minister as Diagnostician: Personal Problems in Pastoral Perspective. The Westminster Press, Philadelphia, Pennsylvania, 1976

Redfield R: The Little Community. The University of Chicago Press, Chicago, Illinois, 1960

Sayre J: Alternative healing therapies. In Wilson HW, Kneisl CR: Psychiatric Nursing, 2nd ed. Addison-Wesley, Menlo Park, California, 1983

Sedgwick R: Family Mental Health: Theory and Practice. The C.V. Mosby Company, St. Louis, Missouri, 1981

Simonton OC, Matthews-Simonton S, Creighton J: Getting Well Again. J.P. Tarcher Inc., Los Angeles, California, 1978

Smith SJ: Personal communication, 1983

Spiro M: Religion: Problems of definition and explanation. In Banton M (ed): Anthropological Approaches to the Study of Religion, ASA Monograph No. 3, Tavistock Publications, New York, 1966

Wallston BS, Wallston KA: Locus of control and health: A review of literature. Health Education Monographs, Vol 6, No 2, pp 107–117, 1978

White RL, Liddon SC: Ten survivors of cardiac arrest. Psychiatry in Medicine, Vol 3, No 3, pp 219–225, 1972

Wilson HS, Kneisl CR: Psychiatric Nursing, 2nd ed. Addison-Wesley, Menlo Park, California, 1983

Wurtman RJ: Nutrients that modify brain function. Scientific American, Vol 245, No 50, pp 56–60,

Sexuality

11

by
Toni Ayres, R.N., Ed.D.

Sexuality is a pervasive aspect of each person's life; it shapes personal identity and expression regardless of whether that person chooses to engage in sexual activity. A person's sexuality includes identity as feminine or masculine, presentation of self to others, interactions with others, and sense of self as attractive, worthwhile, grown-up, self-reliant, sophisticated, respected, and loved. People's feelings about their sexual selves, either positive or negative, influence how they operate on a daily basis, including choosing such things as what to wear, what postures to adopt, what to eat, how much to exercise, whether to relate intimately to another person, and how such an interaction will occur. Thus, people's sense of their own sexuality will influence, and are influenced by, a multitude of factors including self-esteem, body image, current physical state of health, psychological well-being, and past experiences.

This chapter discusses the emergence of the concept of sexual health, barriers or hurdles that must be overcome in the promotion of sexual health, and the clinical application of sexual health principles, using the nursing process.

CURRENT KNOWLEDGE AND ISSUES

We have come a long way since the Victorian Era (1837–1901) when sexual desire and intercourse were considered a threat to health. Because the Victorians believed that all references to sex should be censored from literature and conversation, sex became a dark, frightening, and dangerous force that had to be constantly kept under control (Haeberle 1978). Sigmund Freud (1856–1939) moved Western thinking past this obsession with sexual censorship to a time when psychoanalysts believed that all

236

sexual material in a person's mind must be released from repression. Freud's theories spread rapidly to reshape the foundations of knowledge about human sexuality. Such ideas included developmental fixations, complexes, immaturity of masturbation, vaginal versus clitoral orgasms, and female passivity. However, Freud studied very few actual patients (approximately 50) and based his theories on patients who were considered "neurotic." Victorian and Freudian thinking suffered from prejudices and was unable to transcend the limitations of the sexual perspective prevailing in that time and place (Brecher 1969).

Havelock Ellis (1859–1939), who wrote at the same time as Freud, based his information on his knowledge of the experience of sex for normal men and women and their problems in ordinary life. Ellis was the first researcher to begin with the assumption that not everyone is alike. He studied sexual behavior and how people felt about it rather than basing his ideas on what the prevailing mores dictated people should do. Ellis challenged the viewpoint that sex was frightening and mysterious; he did so by studying sexual customs in many other cultures and providing insight into a variety of sexual experiences as a natural expression of human existence.

Although for centuries scientific inquiry in other areas utilized quantitative methods, there were no such studies in sexuality. Alfred Kinsey (1894–1956) was the first sex researcher to use quantitative statistical methods. Kinsey's two famous studies were published in 1948 and 1953. They reported detailed sexual behavior patterns of more than 12,000 Americans of both sexes, all ages, various religions, all economic and educational levels, many varied life-styles, and from every state including urban and rural settings. One of the reasons for Kinsey's success in collecting such detailed data was his ability to put the subject at ease with his honesty and non-judgmental attitude. He assured his respondents of confidentiality and his interviewing was so sincere and skillful that respondents felt an almost compulsive need to be completely honest with him. It is these traits of sincerity, honesty, and objectivity which are important today for health professionals in the incorporation of sexual health into the total picture of health care.

Thus, in approximately 100 years there has been a complete change in the view of human sexuality as a threat to health to its establishment as an important "health entity" (Fulton 1965). Today, the study of sexuality has been broadened to a field of investigation called sexology. Sexology is a multidisciplinary study of sex in all of its aspects—anatomical, physiological, psychological, medical, sociological, anthropological, historical, legal, religious, literary, and artistic perspectives.

Sexual Health

While there had already been some attempts to promote sexual health in American society by the Sex Information and Education Council of the United States (SIECUS), it was not until 1975 that the World Health Organization (WHO) made the first attempt to concretely define sexual health:

Sexual health is the integration of the somatic, emotional, intellectual, and social aspects of sexual being in ways that are positively enriching and that enhance personality, communication, and love. Every person has a right to receive sexual information and to consider accepting relationships for pleasure as well as for procreation. (WHO, 1975)

This definition begins to provide a way for health care providers to recognize and evaluate their efforts to promote sexual health.

Maddock (1975) further developed the concept of sexual health by offering a definition of a sexually healthy person and a description of the components of sexual health care. According to him, "Sexually healthy individuals have, first, a certain amount of cognitive knowledge about sexual phenomena; second, a degree of self-awareness about their own attitudes toward sex; third, a well-developed usable value system that provides input into sexual decisions; and finally, some degree of emotional comfort and stability in relation to sexual activities in which they and others engage." These criteria are not automatically bestowed on people at a certain time in their lives. Sex is a natural function, but good sex does not always happen naturally. Positive sexual functioning is learned.

The basis of promoting sexual health and sexually healthy individuals is based on positive attitudes, e.g., the belief that sex is a good thing, capable of enhancing personal health and enriching relationships. Health professionals need to begin by exploring their attitudes regarding the promotion of sexual health. "How do I feel about providing sexual information, counseling, and support in order that my clients can have a better sexual future?" If health providers are not comfortable with sexuality, they need to refer clients to others who are sexual health resources.

Consumers are currently seeking sex-related health services in greater numbers than they ever have in the past. Consumer demands have gone beyond the more "legitimate" areas of concern, such as reproduction, family planning, and child development. A growing number of health consumers, regardless of their own current level of wellness or illness, now want information on erections, orgasms, types of lovemaking activities, sexually transmitted diseases, jealousy, sexual anxieties, and relationship complications. People want to understand their own sexual feelings and behavior. Maddock (1975) lists the following components that should be included in a system that delivers sexual health care:

1. *Awareness.* The recognition that sexual function and satisfaction are a legitimate concern of health care professionals. This basic

component gives the direction for all other services and practices.
2. *Information.* The facts that can be made available to clients. Increasing emphasis on preventative medicine has shown that patient education is effective and a majority of clients with sexual concerns simply need appropriate information.
3. *Enrichment.* Community programs that provide opportunities to discuss sexual concerns and problems in a supportive group atmosphere. Family planning clinics, social service agencies, and organizations specifically focusing on sexuality are the most sophisticated providers, often using a multidisciplinary approach.
4. *Counseling.* The resources that offer therapy at the level of primary care. Such health providers may be doctors, nurses, or other professionals who have sufficient awareness, training, and commitment to help clients deal with their sexual anxieties and simple relationship problems, and facilitate sexual decision making.
5. *Therapy.* High quality programs of therapy for individuals or couples experiencing severe sexual dysfunction or incompatibility. Severe sexual problems contribute to other individual and relationship problems such as alcoholism, drug dependency, psychosomatic illness, and low work productivity; thus, a sex therapist should be available in major medical centers.
6. *Clinical Services.* Those services related to the healthy functioning of sexual organs for sexual purposes. Specialties such as urology, gynecology, and andrology (the study of diseases of males, especially male sex organs) should be able to separate the sexual and reproductive aspects of a client's life.
7. *Community Support.* The social and community support systems that make possible the delivery of high-quality sexual health care. Financial and institutional support must permit the dissemination of sexual information to the public and the performance of sex research.

Problems in the Delivery of Sexual Health Care

The primary obstacle to the delivery of sexual health care is the low value placed on sexual health by many medical and nursing personnel. Sexuality is seen as a "luxury" budget item that will only get attention when everything else has been taken care of. This accounts for the lack of funding for both sex research and sex education and for the little time spent with patients really listening to their sexual concerns.

Other obstacles include problems in research, lack of professional training, personal beliefs such as fear of offending clients, and effects of illness on sex. Without adequate sex research, the information on human sexuality that we would like to see available simply is not available. In an age of rapidly expanding research, information on human sexuality has

many large gaps. For example, most research on the effects of medications, surgery, or illness on sexual function has been done on men. It is
very difficult to find more than a few studies on the sexual consequences
of myocardial infarction in women; those studies that are available are
biased toward a disease model rather than a health maintenance model.
Men, in fact, are much easier to study because their erections are both
observable and quantifiable. In order to measure the same phenomenon
(the arousal stage) in women, one would have to measure the amount of
lubrication that the woman produces. Vaginal lubrication is much harder
to quantify, and subjective reports from research subjects create problems
of validity and reliability. However, it *is* time that subjective reports from
women about their psychosocial and physical experience of sex were
taken more seriously. In American culture, there is a widespread view that
women do not know what they are feeling during sex because they basically do not know or are not supposed to know anything about sex. This bias
has permeated the medical profession in particular and is closely associated with the myth that clients do not know anything about how their
bodies work and should not be told because they would not understand it
anyway.

   An additional problem with past research is that many researchers had
very little background in human sexuality; because of this, the studies
were concerned almost exclusively with intercourse between heterosexual
married couples. In these studies, adequate sexual functioning for women
is often measured by the ability to have orgasm during intercourse. Since
anywhere from 50% to 60% of women *do not* have orgasm simply from the
stimulation of intercourse, this criterion is an inadequate measure of
sexual achievement (Hite 1976; Kinsey et al. 1953). Men, too, are denied
the fullest expression of their sexuality by this constant focus on intercourse, as if that were the only socially approved outlet. Sex research,
therefore, should begin to include criteria for evaluation that reflects real-
life practices, experiences, and life-styles. Only then will we see data that
addresses single people, gays and lesbians, and such practices as oral
sex, uses of vibrators, and masturbation. Although there are numerous sex
books, academic and popular, that focus on these topics, the traditional
medical model has not incorporated these topics into their studies or
publications.

   A final problem with current research is that it may not reflect the
improved prognosis for sexual functioning that occurs with sexual counseling. For example, medical literature estimates that the rate of erection
problems for the male diabetic is at least 50% by 50 years of age. This fact
has been known for quite some time. What the research fails to address,
however, is the percentage of individuals experiencing sexual dysfunction
whose situations improve when competent sex therapy is provided. For
example, one sex therapist worked in sex therapy groups with 34 diabetic
males who had been told that they were impotent or considered them-

selves impotent. By the end of the group's sessions, 83% were able to regularly get erections firm enough for intromission (Bohannon, Zilbergeld, Bullard, and Stocklosa 1982). There have been other studies with patients who have had radical pelvic exteneration surgery and patients with spinal cord injuries demonstrating the increased self-esteem which accompanies successful sexual adaptation and which leads to increased productivity, return to work, and positive quality of life (Anderson and Cole 1975; Capone, Good, Westie, and Jacobson 1980). These are a few of many examples of the positive potential of sex counseling and therapy.

The third major barrier to the delivery of sexual health care is the lack of knowledge on the part of health care professionals. In the past, nurses have simply referred clients to physicians if a sexual concern became apparent. Realistically, however, physicians have little training in human sexuality, and it is unreasonable to assume that they have any particular expertise about sex simply by virtue of their medical education. During the 1970s, nearly all medical schools instituted at least some training in human sexuality, even though in some cases it may have been quite limited. There are very few nursing schools which provide courses in human sexuality. Sexuality is usually integrated into maternity content, with nothing specific on sexuality and adolescence, aging, or men. This situation represents a gap in nursing curricula since nurses are in an excellent position to provide information, counseling, or support. There are currently many books for nurses concerning the promotion of sexual health (Kolodny, Masters, Johnson, and Biggs 1979; Mims and Swenson 1980; Woods 1984). Although these texts provide much of the necessary didactic material, awareness of attitudes and behaviors that facilitate or inhibit nurse-client interactions regarding sexuality are often best learned in a group setting that includes discussion and role playing. We must not assume that all nurses will be interested in doing patient teaching or counseling regarding sexual matters. However, those who are interested need further training beyond their own life experiences.

Personal beliefs are another barrier to the delivery of sexual health care. These beliefs can block communication about sex, particularly when there are differences in life-style or values. As in any other nursing interaction, the nurse's personal beliefs and feelings need to be acknowledged but not communicated to the client in such a way that the client feels chastised. An example might be a nurse's feelings about taking care of a homosexual client when the nurse disapproves of homosexuality. That client deserves the same quality of care as any other person and should not be made to feel judged by the health care system where help has been sought. The result of feeling such disapproval could be that the client will be reluctant to seek help.

The fifth barrier is the fear of offending the client by introducing the subject of sex. Many health professionals believe that if the client has a concern about sexual functioning, the client will be comfortable enough to bring up the concern in a forthright manner. Studies that have asked clients about their comfort with bringing up the subject of sex have reported that 60% to 80% of clients would prefer the health care professional to introduce the subject. This is particularly true in settings in which the possibility of future sexual functioning is in question, such as a trauma ward, rehabilitation ward, cardiac unit, orthopedic unit, diabetic clinic, or radical surgery unit. Clients are often very relieved that someone in authority, and who is supposed to know about sex, brought up the subject.

Clients will often drop hints that they have sexual concerns by making a joke about sex, hinting that they are "no good anymore," or are "unattractive now"; other clients will ask questions "for a friend." There are many different ways that these clues surface. Health providers usually take such hints or questions at face value and do not realize that there is a sexual question underneath. Sometimes patients who are in the hospital will grab or pinch a nurse, constantly make sexual references in conversation, expose themselves, or do something else that has sexual overtones. Some psychiatric clients act out their problems in a sexual manner. The usual result of this behavior is that the patient gets labeled by the staff as being "a weirdo" or a "problem patient." Staff subsequently try to avoid this patient as much as possible. Often the patient is assigned to a new nurse every day, which prevents any rapport from being established. Sometimes the patient's behavior is reported to the doctor who may then say things like, "Mr. Blue, you stop giving the nurses a bad time!" In this way the sexual issues or concerns that may have motivated the original behavior are not addressed. One staff person who can address this patient's concerns and provide information and feedback about inappropriate behavior can prevent the patient from losing his dignity any further and can unify the staff rather than using up all the staff energy avoiding the problem.

Related to this is the belief that someone else on the health team (e.g., the physical therapist, the enterostomal therapist, the discharge planner, the social worker, the doctor) will surely be the appropriate one to talk about possible sexual concerns with the client. This problem could be easily solved by members of the health team by including sexuality as part of case conferences so that team members may know who was the best prepared or had enough rapport with the client to discuss sexual health.

The final barrier to delivery of sexual health care is the belief that illness or age ends the capacity for sex. This belief is perpetuated by the client's family and the health profession. The result is that everyone keeps the subject of sex in the closet and presumes an asexual attitude on the part of the client. If in fact there is no further interest in sex or no physical capacity for sex, it does not mean that the client has no desire to discuss sex. Some clients may need to grieve over the loss of sexual function or loss of sexual partner. Their recovery from their sadness will be facilitated by encouraging the grieving process, allowing expression of tears, frustrations, and other feelings. In addition, people who have wanted to stop having sex may find a surgery or illness a useful excuse. They may have partners who will want to talk to someone about this change in sexual behavior. Certainly there should be no pressure put on any clients to feel they should be interested in sex when in fact they are not.

CLINICAL APPLICATION AND THE NURSING PROCESS

Assessing sexual health is often difficult for nurses and clients. Discussing sexuality openly may be embarrassing for one party or the other. Cultural constraints also impede discussion of sexuality. In many cultural and ethnic groups, sex is only to be discussed between husband and wife; sex may not even be mentioned between marital partners, just practiced. Because of difficulties associated with open discussion of sexuality, some individuals may not realize that they have a sexual problem, and others may not mention a problem until it becomes a major one.

In light of difficulties surrounding discussion of sexuality, the following framework will be useful. The P-LI-SS-IT model, formulated by Annon (1974) is useful for guiding interventions for promotion of sexual health.

THE P-LI-SS-IT MODEL

P	Permission
LI	Limited Information
SS	Specific Suggestions
IT	Intensive Therapy

At the first level, the nurse brings up the subject of sex and, thus, gives permission to talk about sexual feelings and to legitimize the existence of sexual feelings, thoughts, and desires, indicating that clients are not alone in their concerns. The next level of intervention is giving limited information which is pertinent to the client's concerns. This information may be all that is necessary for a client to solve the problem. The third level, giving specific suggestions, necessitates that the nurse take a Sexual Problem History. Finally, intensive therapy is provided by a sex therapist or sex counselor when the client needs more in-depth interventions.

In sexual health promotion, the nurse's role is that of a facilitator who encourages clients to use their own resources and abilities to care for themselves and their own sexual relationships. Most nurses are not prepared to intervene beyond the level of giving limited information unless they have had special training. However, assessment of sexual problems from minor to more serious ones is often appropriate for the nurse or for self-assessment by the client.

If the health history questions or the self-evaluation tool indicate a need for the specific suggestion level of intervention, more in-depth assessment is necessary. The outline below provides guidelines for a Sexual Problem History adapted by Annon (1974).

SEXUAL PROBLEM HISTORY

I. Description of the current problem (what the client sees as the problem).
  A. Ask about the effect on the patient:
   • "How does this affect you?"
   • "How do you feel about it?"
  B. Explore the effects on the partner:
   • "How does this concern affect your partner?"
   • "How has your partner dealt with the problem?"
  C. Explore the severity:
   • "How often do you have this difficulty?"

II. Onset and Course of the Problem
  A. Onset (gradual or sudden, precipitating events, consequences):
   • "When did this start occurring?"
   • "What was the situation the first time this occurred?"
  B. Course (changes over time; increase, decrease, or fluctuation in severity, frequency, or intensity; relationship of problem to other variables).

III. Client's Concept of the Cause and Maintenance of the Problem
  (Explore psychological, biological, sociological, and environmental influences that client thinks may be contributory factors.)

IV. Past Help With the Problem and Outcome
  A. Medical Evaluation (specialty, date, form of treatment, results, currently on any medication for any reason).
  B. Other professional or paraprofessional help. (Specialty, date, form of treatment, results. Include questioning that covers alternative treatments such as biofeedback, special diets, polarity, movement, etc.)
  C. Self-help (what, when, results)
   • "How have you tried to solve the problem up until now?"
  D. Partner Communication
   • "Have you discussed this with your partner?"
   • "What were the results?"
  E. Current Expectations and Goals (specific vs. general)
   Explore how the client would like things changed.
   • "How would you like the situation to be different?"

The client should be encouraged to give specific details of the problem and to describe a typical situation in which the problem occurs. It is common for clients to use euphemisms and vague statements that make it hard to get an accurate picture of the problem. The nurse must continue to clarify or ask the client to clarify each statement that could be misinterpreted. The taboo in the culture that says it is not o.k. to talk about sex makes it difficult to remember to keep asking the client to be specific.

Assessment

"Giving permission" is the first step in assessing sexual health. The subject of sexuality may be brought up in various ways. The nurse needs to be alert to the client's concerns by observing such nonverbal clues as facial expressions, dramatic sighs, or questions dealing with how much physical activity is possible, jokes about sexual performance, or questions that show concern over body image. One way to bring up the subject is to use such open-ended questions as "People with your _____ (disease, surgery, etc.) sometimes experience problems in the area of sex. How has this affected your life?" If the client does not have a particular health problem, the question might be more general, such as "Some people want to ask me sexual questions they may have. What questions do you have?" If the client has no difficulties, the nurse should go on to another area of health assessment. However, the door has been opened, and clients will know that they can come back to the topic at a later time.

In contrast to the open-ended approach of broaching the subject, a more formal approach involves including questions about sexuality in the health history. This approach also gives permission for sexual concerns to be discussed. This line of questioning is suggested by Kolodny (1979) and is provided below.

HEALTH HISTORY QUESTIONS

---

1. Are you currently active sexually? If yes, what is the approximate frequency of sexual activity?
2. Are you satisfied with your sex life? If not, why not?
3. (For Men) Do you have any difficulty obtaining or maintaining an erection? Do you have any difficulty with the control of ejaculation?
4. (For Women) Do you have any difficulty becoming sexually aroused? Do you feel you have enough lubrication? Do you ever experience pain during intercourse? Do you have difficulty being orgasmic?
5. Do you have any questions or problems related to sex that you might like to discuss?

Nurses must keep in mind the importance of eye contact and body language while asking these questions. Not looking at the client while addressing these questions may convey the message that the nurse is not sincerely interested in his answers or is too embarrassed to really hear them. It is also helpful to take the most abbreviated notes possible. Too much note-taking can make the client feel ill-at-ease.

A different approach to assessment is the self-evaluation format, in which the client takes responsibility rather than the nurse. The tool below (Inventory for Self-Evaluation) can be used privately by the client and/or facilitated by the nurse. This inventory serves the dual purpose of assessment and intervention, as it has the capacity to increase self-awareness and growth and suggest techniques.

INVENTORY FOR SELF-EVALUATION

---

1. Are you at the level of physical fitness that feels good to you?
2. Are you aware of your emotions, feelings, and moods?
3. Do you take drugs or medications or have an illness that can hinder your optimum sexual functioning?
4. Have you made peace with your own body? Can you stand in front of the mirror and touch every touchable part of you while saying out loud what is delightful, charming, or nice about that part?
5. How do you feel about touching your own body? Can you enjoy self-pleasuring without feeling guilty or self-indulgent?
6. Could you write out or relate one of your favorite erotic fantasies? Or would you be "too embarrassed?" Do you give yourself permission to be flooded with sensual images and imagine what, for you, are arousing, erotic behaviors?
7. What do you deeply believe and value about your sexuality? Do you have a system of sexual values with which you are comfortable? Are your sexual values consistent with your desires and your actual behaviors?
8. How do you rate your gender preference? How do you feel about your gender preference now? Where would you like your gender preference to be five years from now?
9. What do you expect in a "typical" sexual encounter? Are your expectations reality oriented? Or do you expect "too much" too quickly?
10. If you and your partner do not choose pregnancy, can you plan ahead for your sexmaking and use your chosen contraceptive method effectively? If you are a woman relying on a diaphragm-spermicide method, will you be assertive about taking the time to put it in? If you are a man relying on the condom-foam combined method, are you relaxed and confident enough about your masculinity not to panic if you lose your erection while putting on the condom?
11. Are you knowledgeable about the symptoms of sexually transmitted diseases (STD's)? Can you recognize them in yourself? In a partner? Are you willing to take the responsibility for talking about the possibility of STD's—yours or your partner's—before sexmaking with a new partner? Can you openly suggest and use measures to minimize risks if you and your partner decide to go ahead with sexmaking?
12. If you have an ongoing relationship, how satisfied are you with its overall quality? Do you like your partner? Do you accept or receive pleasure as well as give it (not necessarily during the same episode of pleasuring)? Are either of you spectators of your own performances? In other words, do you view your sexual behavior as an audience might view a sporting event, or are you so involved you do not have time to be a spectator of your own sexmaking?
13. What sex language turns you on? Turns you off? Is there anything about your sexual self that you fear to reveal? Can you tell what about your sexual identity (masculinity and/or femininity) that you most enjoy? Least enjoy?

From Nass G, Libby R, Fisher MP: Sexual Choices: An Introduction to Human Sexualty. Wadsworth, Inc., 1981 (*reprinted by* permission of Wadsworth Health Sciences, Monterey, California)

Finally, in cases in which a client has a chronic illness or trauma, had surgery, or takes medications that may interfere with sexual functioning, the assessment format provided in Figure 11-1 can be used.

CAUSES OF SEXUAL DYSFUNCTION

	Psychological Factors	Biological Factors	Sociological Factors
Before the event (illness, surgery, RX, etc.)			
During the event			
After the event or as a result of the event			

Figure 11-1. Format to assess causes of sexual dysfunction.

For example, problems with ejaculation and erectile potency are often associated with antipsychotic, antidepressant, and antihypertensive medications (Segraves 1977).

Most people simply assume that a disease itself caused a sexual dysfunction. Often the disease is not the cause of the problem but the individual's reaction to the diagnosis or disease itself, e.g., depression or anxiety contributes to sexual dysfunction. Filling in all the categories in the grid is useful in allowing the nurse and client to visualize different influences and separate new problems from those that are antecedent to the event or illness.

Planning and Implementation

Once the nurse and client have a clear idea of the client's problem or concern, planning requires that goals be established. Client and nurse goals may differ,e.g., the client may want more information about sexuality or to learn techniques to improve sexual enjoyment; the nurse may want to help the client change his unrealistic expectations and, thus, decrease performance anxiety. It is important for the nurse and client to discuss their perceptions and to establish reasonable goals that will guide a self-care program.

At this point, nurses should assess their own knowledge and skills in the area of sexual health in order to recognize what problems they feel competent in working with and which problems should be referred to a sex counselor or therapist. This phase in planning may entail simply making a referral.

Clients should be referred to a sex therapist or sex counselor when the problem cannot be resolved with limited information or simple suggestions. There has been a tendency to refer people with sexual problems to psychiatrists, however, very few psychiatrists have had much success in the treatment of sexual dysfunction. This is probably due to the lack of sexual information in the medical school curriculum. Psychiatrists are more effective in treating depression, which may be an underlying cause of sexual dysfunction. The American Association of Sex Educators, Counselors, and Therapists publishes a list of certified counselors, educators, and therapists in every state and some foreign countries. Quite often sex counselors are listed under the marriage counselors heading in the telephone book. When making a referral, nurses should know to whom they are referring, what kind of training that person has had, and if a license is required to practice. Even a person who has a Marriage, Family, and Child Counseling license is not particularly prepared to do sex counseling unless he has had specialized training. Sex counselors provide the intensive therapy needed, as opposed to the brief therapy of permission, limited information, and specific suggestions that could be provided by nurses based on their knowledge and comfort with the topic.

Planning should take into consideration what the client has already tried and may consist of making a list of referral possibilities for different concerns or education. For example, planning may include suggesting appropriate reading for the client. There are many self-help books on the market that are excellent for sexual self-care, such as Barbach's (1975) *For Yourself: the Fulfillment of Female Sexuality*, Zilbergeld's (1978) *Male Sexuality*, and Nowinski's (1979) *Becoming Satisfied: A Man's Guide to Sexual Fulfillment*. Other resources include family planning clinics or self-help groups, e.g., a group for pre-orgasmic women, to which clients can be referred.

Implementation depends on the client's problem and whether or not the nurse has the knowledge, comfort, and experience to deal with sexual concerns. However, giving limited information and asking clients to look at their expectations and their performance anxiety will often go a long way to help them deal with their concerns or to solve their own problems.

An example of limited information might be telling an older male client about the need for increased tactile stimulation to produce erection with increasing age. Limited information may take the form of preoperative teaching or counseling, anticipatory education for developmental life stages, prevention of pregnancy or sexually transmitted diseases, or simply general facts about sexual anatomy or physiology.

The nurse may give specific suggestions for self-care based on the sexual problem history or on the Inventory for Self-Evaluation. For example, clients who have difficulty receiving pleasure from another might try taking a massage class with their partner and concentrate only on learning to enjoy non-sexual skin contact for a specified period of time.

If planning and implementation involve referral to a sex counselor or therapist, the nurse should be aware that certain sexual dysfunctions are easier to treat than others. There are three different phases of the sexual response cycle—desire phase, arousal phase, and orgasm (Kaplan 1979). Sexual dysfunctions that occur during the orgasmic phase are easier to treat than those that occur in the arousal stage. Such problems can often be helped by behavior therapy techniques and minimal psychotherapy. Examples of orgasm phase problems are:

- Premature ejaculation and delayed ejaculation for men

- No orgasm or orgasm only under certain circumstances for women

Dysfunctions that occur in the desire stage are often more difficult to treat than those in the arousal phase; however, behavioral therapy with some psychotherapy is quite useful. Examples of arousal phase problems are:

- Erection difficulties for men

- Lack of lubrication for women

The most difficult problems are those in the desire phase. Behavioral therapy is not very helpful in these cases because quite often the relationship needs help. There may be great amounts of resentment or anger with which to deal and the prognosis is less hopeful than for difficulties existing in the other two phases.

Evaluation

Evaluation of the self-care activities designed to promote sexual health is based on the extent to which the goals are met. If simple interventions by the nurse and client are not effective for meeting the client's needs, then the client should be referred to a sex therapist. Important criteria for evaluation are client satisfaction and the mutual agreement between nurse and client that the goals have been met. The self-evaluation inventory (page 246) could be used again in the interest of evaluating the self-care plan and implementation. This tool focuses attention on areas in which an individual may want to continue to improve or on areas on which mastery has been gained.

SUMMARY

Individuals can do a great deal for themselves to increase their own self-awareness, change their attitudes, and learn better techniques in the area of sexual health. At times minimal intervention by the nurse can serve as a catalyst to promote significant growth in the client. It is important to remember that sex, like any other skill, is learned. If there has been some faulty learning, new ways of expressing sexuality can be learned. It is important for the nurse and client always to be aware of the idea that in sexuality, there are no failures, only learning experiences.

CASE EXAMPLE

Fred is a 65-year-old male who came to the clinic for a well-health check. As part of the history, the nurse asked Fred if he is still sexually active. Fred complained that he cannot have erections anymore. The nurse told Fred that many older men have similar erection concerns (permission) and that quite often the problem can be helped. The nurse asked Fred if he was interested in exploring the problem further, to assess what factors could be contributing to the problem, and to plan for resolution. Fred agreed and said that he had always been sexually active in a mutually satisfying relationship with his wife. In their relationship, he had always initiated sex and gleaned a great deal of pleasure from caressing and fondling his wife. He stated that he believes that men do not need as much stimulation as women and, early in the marital relationship, expressed discomfort when his wife attempted to return his caresses. In addition, he stated that his wife, although very responsive to him, is also very shy and prefers the "old ways."

The nurse then considered what questions to pursue in order to establish an accurate diagnosis. She asked the following:

1. Does Fred ever wake up with a morning erection? Does he still masturbate and what are the results? (If Fred is having erections in either of the above situations, then there is probably no physical reason why Fred cannot have an erection.)
2. Have there been any ongoing or recent health problems? (The nurse would want to specifically look for evidence of diabetes, arteriosclerosis, bladder dysfunction or neuropathy, or circulatory problems.)
3. What medications has Fred been taking? (Some drugs cause erection problems, the antihypertensives, in particular. The nurse

should be prepared to check all medications in the *Physician's Desk Reference* for side effects that could impair sexual functioning.)

4. Has there been a recent stressful event in Fred's life, such as retirement, that might make him depressed, anxious or preoccupied? (It is difficult to be interested in sex when one is depressed; however, functioning may still be possible.)

5. Has Fred's wife had any health changes? (Fred may be trying to cope with his feelings about his wife's health status.)

6. What are Fred's beliefs regarding sexuality in people his age? (Often, beliefs become reality.)

7. What is the most recent sexual experience that Fred can remember? What specifically happened? Did he get a partial erection? Who initiated the experience? What are examples of the "old ways" that Fred's wife prefers?

Fred answered the nurse's questions. He said that he occasionally wakes up with morning erections but that he had stopped masturbating years ago. He did not know if he could have an erection that way. He has been in fairly good health except for some mild arthritis and a tendency towards high blood pressure and overweight. He has learned to control these problems with diet and exercise (walking) and has been able to avoid antihypertensive drugs so far. Fred retired three years ago and says he has adjusted pretty well. The only thing depressing him now is his inability to have intercourse. Fred said his wife is a healthy, active woman with no major health concerns except some skin cancers which have been removed and are being followed by a dermatologist. His wife's "old ways" are her beliefs about the man's role as sole initiator and provider of stimuation.

The nurse suspected that Fred's erection difficulties were probably due to insufficient penile stimulation. Contributing factors were:

1. He did not allow his wife to caress and fondle him.

2. He has established a pattern of sexual relating that may be hard to change.

3. He believes that men do not need penile stimulation.

4. Most important, the need for sufficient penile stimulation to cause an erection at his age is much greater than it has ever been.

The nurse discussed these factors with Fred and emphasized the need for increased tactile stimulation directly on the genitals as age increases (Limited Information). The nurse suggested that Fred try to stimulate himself, using fantasy or erotic literature if necessary, to see if he could successfully obtain and maintain an erection to the point of orgasm. Part of the plan was if that was possible, and Fred was willing to attempt intercourse, then the nurse would suggest that Fred stimulate himself before intercourse (Specific Suggestion). This would eliminate the need to immediately try to change his wife's behavior. Fred was told to practice the masturbation at least three times before he came back for a second appointment.

Fred returned in two weeks and seemed to be cautiously hopeful since he had had several successful masturbation experiences. This was a good indication that insufficient stimulation was a correct diagnosis. Fred was then instructed to stimulate himself with his wife present. The nurse suggested that he stimulate his wife first and then himself in order to have the penile stimulation timed just prior to intercourse.

Two weeks later, Fred called the nurse to say that he was quite happy with his results—he and his wife had been able to enjoy intercourse twice; he could now see for himself that direct penile stimulation was important and that he could not succeed merely by trying to "will" an erection. The nurse told Fred to call back if he needed further help.

CASE EXAMPLE

Betty is a 27-year-old woman who is coming back to the clinic for her six week post-partum checkup. She delivered her first baby, a girl, by vaginal delivery and has been breastfeeding successfully. Her husband was very supportive through her labor and delivery and now has indicated a desire to resume sex. In fact, her husband had been careful to comment on the subject that morning at breakfast when Betty reminded him she was going for her six week checkup. When the nurse asked Betty if she felt ready to resume sex, she looked completely overwhelmed and began to cry. Betty said that she used to enjoy sex with her husband, but she is so tired right now that she cannot imagine relaxing and enjoying it. The nurse told Betty that many new mothers feel this way and that she should not put a great deal of pressure on herself to resume sex (Permission).

Betty's examination reveals she is healing normally. The nurse suggested that Betty try to take all of life easier right now and not attempt to do all the housework she did before she had the baby. She helped Betty plan how she could nap more often and then discussed the changes that may occur when Betty does feel ready to resume sexual activity with her husband. She reminded Betty to proceed very slowly, and begin by having her husband insert one, two, then three fingers gently into her vagina to check for any pain that may occur with penetration (Specific Suggestion). Then the nurse mentioned that lack of lubrication occurs postpartum, particularly in breastfeeding women (Limited Information). The nurse suggested that Betty obtain bland salad oil, such as safflower oil, available at health food stores, because it lubricates longer than K-Y Jelly which is water soluble and tends to dry up very rapidly. The nurse explained that Betty will probably need this additional lubrication until her own lubrication capacity returns. The other problem that the nurse discusses is leaking of milk from Betty's breasts when she becomes aroused (Limited Information). The nurse suggests that Betty might want to wear her nursing bra with pads in the cups so that the bed does not get wet (Specific Suggestion). Betty is to come back in three weeks to see how things are going and, meanwhile, the nurse helps Betty choose a form of birth control that will be compatible with breastfeeding. Betty chooses foam and condoms. The nurse then talks to Betty about making some assertive statements to her husband regarding her requirements for resuming sex—that she rest as much as possible and that they proceed slowly.

At the next visit, Betty tearfully tells the nurse that it was still very painful when her husband tried to put his fingers in her vagina, even though they used safflower oil. She is worried that she will not be able to enjoy intercourse any more. The nurse finds out that the baby is not yet sleeping through the night, so that Betty is still quite tired most of the time. Betty's husband is not physically pressuring her to have intercourse but does refer to "the good old days" and makes frequent jokes about sex. The nurse asked Betty about what other kinds of sex play she and her husband have engaged in besides intercourse. Betty says that they used to touch each other with their hands and occasionally had oral sex. The nurse told Betty that it is very common for women to have painful intercourse for quite a while, maybe even as long as six months (Permission and Limited Information). The nurse suggested to Betty that she and her husband take a more realistic view of the situation in light of this fact—that intercourse is still painful and that they simply avoid trying to have intercourse and focus on other ways of mutual pleasuring (Specific Suggestion).

The nurse learns that Betty has not joined a support group for new mothers and suggests that such a group provides a setting in which to discuss her coping strategies with other new mothers and share common concerns about the resumption of intercourse. The nurse suggested that Betty allow herself plenty of time to heal further, sleep through the night, and feel like she is back in control of her life before she expect her sex life to return to "normal." She assured Betty that her sex life will naturally improve over time and that she will not improve anything by worrying about it. Betty makes an appointment for a six-month visit.

Betty seemed quite relaxed at her six-month visit. She decided to stop breastfeeding at five months, and she and her husband gradually attempted penetration in the last couple of weeks, and she was able to enjoy the experiences. She used a combination of condoms and foam and was ready to be fitted for a diaphragm. She said that the use of the safflower oil on the outer lips of her vagina helped when they were using manual stimulation on the outside. She thanked the nurse for her suggestions and said she was sure now that her sex life would continue to improve.

Discussion Questions

1. How do you assess your interest, knowledge, feelings, and comfort level regarding providing sexual health services to clients?
2. What services are available in your community that provide sexual health services? Who are the providers? What training do they have? What are the licensing laws?
3. List the barriers to providing sexual health services in the setting in which you practice.
4. Think about past clients to whom you have talked and try to recall hints that they wanted to discuss sexual topics. In what ways could you have encouraged these discussions?
5. In what ways could you increase the awareness of your colleagues for the need for further education and discussion of sexual concerns of clients?
6. What further information do you need in order to provide limited information and specific suggestions to clients who have diabetes, M.I., high blood pressure, spinal cord injury? Where would you begin to look for that information?

REFERENCES

Anderson T, Cole T: Sexual counseling of the physically disabled. Post Graduate Medicine, Vol 58, No 1, pp 117–123, 1975

Annon J: The Behavioral Treatment of Sexual Problems. In Brief Therapy, Vol 1, Harper and Row, New York, 1974

Barbach LG: For Yourself: The Fulfillment of Female Sexuality. Doubleday, Garden City, New York, 1972

Bohannon NJ, Zilbergeld B, Bullard DG, Stoklosa JM: Treatable impotence in diabetic patients. Western Journal of Medicine, Vol 136, No 1, pp 6–10, 1982

Brecher E: The Sex Researchers. Little, Brown and Company, Boston, Massachusetts, 1969

Capone MA, Good RS, Westie KS, Jacobson AF: Psychosocial rehabilitation of gynecologic oncology patients. Archives of Physical Medicine and Rehabilitation, Vol 61, No 3, pp 128–132, 1980

Fulton WC: Why the need for a sex information and education council of the United States as a new, separate organization. SIECUS Newsletter, Vol 1, No 1, 1965

Haeberle EJ: The Sex Atlas. Seabury Press, New York, 1978

Hite S: The Hite Report. Macmillan, New York, 1976

Kaplan H: Disorders of Sexual Desire. Brunner/Mazel, New York, 1979

Kinsey A, Gerhard P, Pomeroy W, Martin C: Sexual Behavior in the Human Female. W.B. Saunders, Philadelphia, Pennsylvania, 1953

Kinsey A, Pomeroy W, Martin C: Sexual Behavior in the Human Male. W.B. Saunders, Philadelphia, Pennsylvania, 1953

Kolodny R, Masters W, Johnson V: Textbook of Sexual Medicine. Little, Brown and Company, Boston, Massachusetts, 1979

Maddock J: Sexual health and health care. Post Graduate Medicine, Vol 58, No 1, pp 52–58, 1975

Masters W, Johnson V: Human Sexual Inadequacy. Little, Brown and Company, Boston, Massachusetts, 1970

Mims F, Swenson M: Sexuality: A Nursing Perspective. McGraw-Hill, New York, 1980

Nass G, Libby R, Fisher MP: Sexual Choices. Wadsworth, Monterey, California, 1981

Nowinski J: Becoming Satisfied: A Man's Guide to Sexual Fulfillment. Prentice-Hall Inc., Englewood Cliffs, New Jersey, 1979

Segraves RT: Pharmacological agents causing sexual dysfunction. Journal of Sex and Marital Therapy, Vol 3, No 3, pp 157–176, 1977

Woods, NF: Human Sexuality in Health and Illness, 3rd ed. The C.V. Mosby Company, St. Louis, Missouri, 1984

World Health Organization: Education and Treatment in Human Sexuality: The Training of Health Professionals. Report of a WHO Meeting, Technical Report Series No. 572. WHO, Geneva, 1975

Zilbergeld B: Male Sexuality. Bantam Books, New York, 1978

12 Social Support and Self-Help Groups

The influence that a person's supportive interactions with others has on health and well-being has received increasing attention from social scientists and clinicians during the past decade. The American Nurses' Association Statement of Research Priorities for the 1980s (1980) suggested that social support networks are examples of personal and environmental determinants of health functioning and are areas that need further study.

Social support has been defined by Caplan (1974) as "enduring interpersonal ties to people who can be relied upon to provide emotional support, help and reassurance in times of need." Cobb (1976) views social support as "information leading the subject to a belief that he is cared for, loved, esteemed, and a member of a network of mutual obligations". Kahn (1979) defines social support as interpersonal transactions that include one or more of the following:

- The expression of positive affect of one person toward the other
- The affirmation or endorsement of another person's behaviors, perceptions, or expressed views
- The giving of symbolic or material aid to another.

Self-help/mutual support groups are a type of social support system that has particular relevance for self-care. Self-help groups can be defined as small groups of peers who come together for mutual assistance to satisfy a common need or to overcome a common handicap or life experience. Such groups involve non-hierarchical, face-to-face interaction and depend on personal participation by all members. Groups are based on the premise that a person can best be helped by another who has been through or is currently experiencing a similar situation, through discussion of common feelings, information, and practical advice for coping with the situation on which the group is based.

This chapter discusses research and issues in the areas of social support and self-help groups, then describes clinical application of concepts, and concludes with examples of tools and techniques for use with individuals and families.

RESEARCH AND ISSUES

The terms social support, social support system, and social network are often used synonymously in the literature, although definitions differ to some extent. We use **social support** to mean *functions,* such as Kahn's "affect, affirmation, and aid;" **social network** refers to people, a set of relationships defined by the individuals who provide social support. Social networks can include family members, friends, neighbors, co-workers, and even professionals. **Social support system** is a more general term which includes specific networks of individuals as well as organized systems such as community programs, voluntary associations, churches, or peer self-help/mutual support groups.

Self-help groups are not analogous to informal social networks or professional systems, because they are "organizations usually composed of strangers, having a structure, and requiring those wishing to utilize their resources to spend effort and energy much as they would had they sought professional systems" (Borman 1979:4). The terms self-help group and mutual support group are used interchangeably in this chapter.

Social support Recent reviews of the literature demonstrate significant relationships between social support and the outcomes of crisis episodes, illness, and mortality. In a comprehensive review, Cobb stated that:

> *The conclusion that supportive interactions among people are important is hardly new. What is new is the assembling of hard evidence that adequate social support can protect people in crisis from a wide variety of pathological states: from low birth weight to death, from arthritis through tuberculosis to depression, alcoholism, and other psychiatric illness. Furthermore, social support can reduce the amount of medication required and accelerate recovery and facilitate compliance with prescribed medical regimens (1976:310).*

A classic study by Nuckolls, Cassel, and Kaplan (1972) measured the effects of life changes (stressors) and "psychosocial assets" among pregnant women. Following childbirth, an analysis of medical records revealed that 91% of women with a high life-change score and low psychosocial asset score that included social support measures had one or more complications of pregnancy or birth. In contrast, only 33% of women with equally high life change scores and high social support scores had complications. Another well-known study by Berkman and Syme (1979) followed a sample of 4,725 people over a nine-year period in order to trace the connection between their social support systems, and morbidity and mortality. Those with the strongest and most intimate types of social bonds, such as marriage and family and friends had the lowest mortality rates. This relationship held true for both sexes, all ethnic groups, and all socioeconomic classes.

How does social support work? According to Cassell (1976), social support acts to cushion or buffer the individual from the physiological or psychological consequences of exposure to the stressor situation. Pilisuk (1982) cites the work of Lazarus and colleagues who demonstrate that when a situation is *appraised* as stressful, a stress reaction is likely to follow. Pilisuk suggests that social support is protective in that other people can reaffirm the basic symbols of the individual's life and support that person's self-esteem and powers of coping, resulting in positive effects on restorative physiological and psychological capacities and, ultimately, the various immune systems of the body.

One important issue in the social support literature is that current popular notions of this concept promise too much. Norbeck (1982) suggests that just as it would be a mistake to ignore this important variable, it is equally dangerous to see social support as a panacea. Rather, individuals have different personality traits and needs for affiliation, and different subcultural groups have differing standards of what "support" is in various situations. The type and amount of available support is also influenced by the individual's social skills (social competence). For example, although cause and effect relationship between limited social support and mental illness cannot be determined, it is known that mentally ill patients have smaller, more restrictive social networks, receive less support, and have experienced more network disruption than the general population (Mueller 1980). It may be that people who have considerable social competence also have other strengths and coping mechanisms that buffer the effects of crisis or illness. Swift's (1979) prevention equation points out that social support is only one element in the prevention of illness:

$$\text{Incidence of dysfunction} = \frac{\text{stress} + \text{constitutional vulnerabilities}}{\text{social supports} + \text{coping skills} + \text{competence}}$$

However, this equation leaves out the importance of the environment in health promotion or prevention of illness. For example, Pilisuk points out that many of the consequences of poverty upon health are independent of supportive social ties:

All are affected at times by loneliness or by loss in the immunological protection offered by networks as people leave or die, and once-strong bonds fade and wither. But for the socially marginal individual, this state is chronic. *For many of the permanent poor, for some of the elderly, some disabled, and many minorities, the routine affronts from a noxious and sparse environment go beyond the buffering protection that a close group of family and friends might offer. It is worth noting again that those factors among the disadvantaged that are the course of high levels of life stress are also factors leading to the breakdown of supportive ties (1982:28).*

Peer Self-Help/Mutual Support Groups

Although well-known self-help groups such as Alcoholics Anonymous have existed since the 1930s, there has been an enormous expansion of both types and numbers of new groups in the past decade, with an estimate of at least 500,000 new groups in the United States, involving at least 15 million people (Evans 1979).

Gartner and Reissman (1977) attribute the recent growth in self-help groups to a need for the expansion and revitalization of human services, a breakdown of traditional authority and institutions, and a need for services that, in the past, have been performed by family, church, and neighborhood. The self-help movement has been powerfully affected by such values of the sixties as concern for personal autonomy, human potential, and quality of life, as well as by deprofessionalization and consumer rights. The growing emphasis on self-care in health was stimulated by these same social forces. Self-care is a strong theme in self-help groups related to health issues.

Self-help/support groups have been formed for people who have almost any conceivable medical condition, crisis, or addiction. Examples include Mended Hearts, Depressives Anonymous, Paralyzed Veterans of America, Torticollis Support Group, Parents Without Partners, Compassionate Friends, Parents of Prematures, Widow-to-Widow, and Gamblers Anonymous. Groups are categorized differently by different writers. Levy (1979) proposed a useful classification scheme comprised of four types:

1. Behavioral control or conduct reorganization groups, in which members want to eliminate or control some problematic behavior
2. Survival-oriented groups, composed of people society has discriminated against because of sex, sexual orientation, socioeconomic class, or race
3. Stress coping and support groups, composed of members who share a common status or predicament or health problem
4. Personal growth and actualization groups, composed of members whose common goal is enhanced effectiveness in all aspects of their lives.

Research on self-help/mutual support groups is relatively recent. Groups have been studied using various approaches, such as survey research, ethnography, clinical interviews, and outcome strategies. For an excellent discussion of the methodological issues facing self-help group researchers, we refer you to Lieberman and Bond (1979).

How do self-help groups work to help their members? Common to most groups are the functions of providing information, providing a setting for mutual emotional support, and providing a reference group and role models. Borkman (1976) suggests that the common basis for such groups is that members have "experiential knowledge and expertise" which is different from professional expertise. Gartner and Reissman (1977) suggest that the single most common denominator of various types of groups is the role of the person who has already lived through the experience— "the helper therapy role"—which is critical for helping newer group members. This function is one that cannot be fulfilled by professionals, family members, or friends—unless such people have also had the experience. Experiential knowledge shows others that one is not the only person who has experienced a particular problem or set of feelings, that another person has "been there" and learned to cope. In Levy's (1979) extensive survey of self-help groups, members identified 28 different help-giving activities that occur in groups. Levy named some of these activities— behavioral proscription and prescription, positive reinforcement, modeling, self-disclosure, sharing, confrontation, requesting and offering feedback, reassurance of competence, empathy, normalization, morale building, personal goal setting, explanation, and catharsis.

Although the purpose of this chapter precludes a detailed discussion of self-help groups (Evans 1979; Gartner and Reissman 1977; Katz and Bender 1976; Lieberman and Borman 1979), an important aspect of most self-help groups is their strong focus on self-care. Health self-help groups range from those that provide an alternative to standard professional health care (e.g., women's health collectives) to those that suggest self-care practices to those in which even group attendance is with "permission of your physician." Some groups divide their self-care information and practices between "lay" and "professional" realms, while others blur this distinction. For example, a breast-feeding support group that offers telephone counseling, advice, and information to nursing mothers covers such subjects as increasing milk supply, scheduling, the importance of relaxation and rest, which drugs to avoid while breast-feeding, choosing and using a breast pump, storing breast milk, nursing while working, nursing a premature baby, weaning, engorgement, and mastitis. While telephone counselors will describe symptoms of a breast infection to the caller, they insist she consult her physician for a diagnosis (Lipson 1983).

Another issue related to self-help groups is the fact that, although peer self-help/mutual support groups have helped countless people, they are not a panacea and they are not for everyone. Surveys of self-help groups show that they appeal mostly to the middle-class population and that marginal or disadvantaged populations are not utilizing some of the prominent national groups. Some barriers to self-help groups for low-income people are logistical—transportation, childcare, timing of meetings, and membership fees. Some ethnic group members are not comfortable in mostly white groups or with group discussion. For example, a black woman who attended one cesarean group meeting stated that she had learned a lot in the group but didn't feel she had enough in common with other group members to continue.

However, the fact that many American subcultures consider discussing intimate concerns with a group of strangers unthinkable is also a serious issue. Many groups believe that the only appropriate place to discuss one's problems is with family members or close friends. In addition, for some Asian and Middle Eastern populations, some conditions (e.g., mental illness) are heavily stigmatized. If a family member should attend a self-help group that focuses on a stigmatized situation, it would be perceived as publicly "bringing shame on the family."

CLINICAL APPLICATION

Social support and self-help groups have important roles to play in health promotion, illness prevention, and management. Norbeck (1982) outlines six key theoretical assumptions about social support that can be used to guide clinicians:

1. People need supportive relationships with others throughout the life span to manage the role demands of day-to-day living, as well as to cope with life transitions and stressors that may emerge.
2. Social support is given and received in the context of a network of relationships.
3. The relationships in the network have relative stability over time, especially those that comprise the inner circle or primary ties for the individual.
4. Supportive relationships are basically healthy, not pathological, in nature.
5. The type and amount of support needed is individually determined, based on individual differences and on characteristics of the situation.
6. The type and amount of support that is available also is determined by characteristics of the individual and of the situation.

It is vital that a description of the client's social support system be routinely included in the nursing assessment. A self-care emphasis suggests that clients should take the major role in assessing whether their social support system is adequate to meet current needs.

In addition to assessment, social support can be used as an intervention or treatment. For example, nurses often provide social support directly, and many clients consider health care professionals important members of their support systems. Consider mental health nurses who work with chronic clients in community settings—they are a strong source of support, perhaps the only people besides immediate family who provide support. See Table 12-1 for suggested social support interventions for psychiatric clients.

TABLE 12-1. TYPOLOGY OF DEFICIENCIES IN SOCIAL SUPPORT AND RECOMMENDED INTERVENTIONS

Deficiencies	*Interventions*
I. *Situational*	
1. Losses of network members	1. a. Assist client to deal with losses and provide temporary support
	b. Assist client to "repeople" the network
2. Crisis or problem exceeds network's capacity or experience	2. a. Influence key network member to provide support
	b. Volunteer linking
	c. Mutual aid groups
	d. Professional support
II. *Pathological*	
A. Person Deficiencies:	
3. Inadequate social skills	3. a. Training in social skill development
	b. Environmental manipulation to facilitate interaction
4. Negative network orientation	4. a. Assist client to decrease over-generalization from pathological relationships to other relationships
B. Network Deficiencies:	
5. Pathological relationships	5. a. Decrease face-to-face contact with key person
	b. Change attitudes and behavior of key person
6. Maladaptive network structure	6. a. Encourage non-kin contact
	b. Network therapy

From Norbeck JS: The use of social support in clinical practice. Journal of Psychosocial Nursing and Mental Health Services, Vol 20, No 12, PR 26, 1982 used with permission of Jane S. Norbeck, D.N.Sc., University of California, San Francisco.

More effective than providing direct social support is assisting clients to utilize their own natural helping systems or to enlarge their social networks when necessary. This emphasis is congruent with our self-care philosophy; it is a more efficient use of professional resouces, is less disruptive to daily living, does not foster dependence on professionals, and ensures that such support is available when needed. Professionals are usually unwilling to provide support without reimbursement, in the middle of the night, or for long periods of time. Although nurses "care for" their clients, they cannot "care about" them in the same way family members or close friends do. But most importantly, helping clients to use their own abilities and resources whenever possible is basic to self-care.

Besides helping clients to more effectively utilize their natural support systems, nurses can refer their clients to self-help groups or other organized support systems. Lay people have used self-help groups to help them cope with problem situations or illnesses for many years, but health professionals have not, until recently, recognized the strengths of such groups and their potential for clinical application. Systematic clinical research is needed in this area. It is important for nurses to be aware of such resources. In addition, an important role for nurses is helping to set up such resources or to work closely with existing resources. As described in *Medical Self-Care*, a physician who worked in a low income, primarily black housing project, realized there was an active network of lay health facilitators who provided advice and support. She set up a training program to help them increase their knowledge and resources. These natural helpers were consulted about a greater variety and number of problems than health professionals ever are, and such lay facilitators "are the most highly trained specialists we have in understanding the whole person" (Ferguson 1982:20).

It is important to consider the issue of how much professional involvement is appropriate in self-help groups. The stance taken by different groups toward professional involvement ranges from totally self-reliant and rejecting of professional "interference" to strong utilization of professionals in the group, as founders, facilitators, or advisory board members (see Table 12-2).

There are arguments against any professional involvement, the most important of which is that professionals may co-opt such groups and use them as extensions of professional services. Critics suggest that if self-help groups become "professionalized," they lose their unique self-empowering characteristics and their emphasis on self-care, and they also lose peer experience and expertise which make them so helpful to many people. Another problem is that many health professionals feel threatened by self-help groups encroaching on "their territory," particularly health self-help groups which emphasize self-care. Professionals may be unwilling to "give up control" or to acknowledge that such groups have information that is contrary to, or just as valuable as, current medical thought. In our impression, nurses are less threatened by self-help and self-care than are physicians; they are more willing to trust that their clients are capable of self-help and self-care, and cognizant that self and family responsibility is preferable to dependence on professionals in many health situations.

In this regard, we think that professional care and self-help groups are not substitutes for each other and that each has qualities that are different

TABLE 12-2. CONTINUUM OF PROFESSIONAL INVOLVEMENT

	Transition group model (e.g., divorce workshops, some mastectomy support groups)	*Intermediate model (e.g., Parents Anonymous, Epilepsy Concern, Recovery, Inc.)*	*"Classical" self-help group model (e.g., A.A., Gamblers Anonymous)*
Time	Limited (6–12 weeks)	Time limited or ongoing	ongoing
Leadership	Professional leader Members defer to leader for decisions on format of meeting	Professional facilitator or reliance on professional contact Mutual decision-making, leaders help members make decisions	Peer leader(s) or no leaders (no professionals) Group members make decisions in planning activities
Source of Support	Peer support, mutual aid, but only in group setting	Peer support, mutual aid in and outside of group setting	Peer support, mutual aid

from the other. Both are needed, as Gartner and Reissman (1977) suggest, "for complete human services." The most appropriate way for nurses to deal with the problem of "professionalizing" self-help groups is to help them strengthen the ways they relate to professionals, to interact through a partnership basis, and to play supportive roles. Professionals can collect and disseminate information, provide resources and facilities, promote public and professional awareness of self-help groups, and work with groups in whatever way group members desire. For example, one author, a member and researcher in a cesarean support group, coordinated inservice education sessions for maternity nurses taught by group members. She also disseminates information on self-help groups in general throughout schools of nursing and in hospitals in which she has consulted. The other author facilitated mastectomy self-help/support groups, helped a women's health center set up and acquire funds for a mastectomy group, and provides continuing education about self-help groups.

Before turning to tools and techniques, we will give some examples in which social support and self-help groups encourage self-care practices in health, illness, and chronic illness.

Self-Care Examples

Women's health self-help groups have been established because of dissatisfaction with existing health-care services as well as stimulation by the women's movement. Such groups originally focused on gynecological concerns but have expanded to cover all the information and skills needed for women to care for their own bodies (Kush-Goldberg 1979). Topics discussed in groups include birth control, abortion, nutrition, pregnancy, and rape; self-care skills taught include pelvic and breast examinations, rhythm birth control, herbal remedies, and menstrual extraction. If health professionals are involved, they have no special status in the group, although their skills are utilized as needed.

Another example of the use of social support in health care is a weight loss support group. Such groups are often time-limited, facilitated by a professional, and given in a workshop format. For example, a classified newspaper ad stated the following:

Eating support groups: Explore why you overeat with others who do the same. Learn how you can be in ultimate control without battling yourself through a combination of understanding your metabolism and guided imagery.

Self-awareness techniques used in such groups include keeping "food and mood" diaries and assigning buddies who support and are accountable to each other by telephone between meetings. However, there are some weight loss groups that adhere to a more classical self-help group format, such as TOPS (Take Off Pounds Sensibly) and Overeaters Anonymous. Support groups for professionals have recently developed. Examples are a Holistic Nurses special interest group in the American Nurses' Association and groups for impaired nurses (alcohol and drug abuse).

Readers are well aware of clients' needs for social support during acute illness—emotional support needs increase dramatically, as do needs for affirmation, the message that the ill person is important and needed. In these situations many people need material aid and help with usual tasks. Mothers of young children often state, "I can't get sick any more; if I do, I have to keep functioning, instead of going to bed to recover as I'd like to." Various cultural and ethnic groups utilize social support in different ways and have different expectations about what is proper help for the person who is ill. For example, hospitalized Middle Eastern patients are usually surrounded by numerous family members at almost all times; family members become distressed if staff attempt to interfere with what they see as their proper role, which is to be there to support the patient at all times and to do their best to obtain the best care for him. Such behavior is often perceived as "demanding" by hospital staff. However, in Middle Eastern cultural groups, the need for affiliation—to belong and be associated with and recognized by others— is very strong, with a strong emphasis on family interaction and dynamics in coping with day-to-day problems. Illness intensifies these needs (Meleis 1981).

While adequate social support can be a significant factor in recovery from acute illness, it is even more important when considering clients with chronic illness or long-term problems. Friends, relatives, and neighbors are often willing to help when a problem is acute but need to return to their other responsibilities when a crisis appears over. At this point, client and family must cope as best they can on their own. In addition, if a long-term situation or chronic condition is one which engenders discomfort in others or is stigmatized, individual and family social support may be difficult to establish and maintain. Self-help/mutual support groups are particularly useful for clients with chronic or long-term illness because they provide what may not be available from natural support systems. Consider the example of a "Spasmodic Torticollis Support Group," which meets for mutual support, allows members to share their experiences and help each other overcome self-consciousness and self-pity, and makes the public aware of this affliction. Spasmodic torticollis is characterized by abnormal contractions of the neck muscles, resulting in involuntary movements and postures of the head. Exercises are taught to members to help them strengthen their neck muscles. The group has developed a bibliography, a newsletter, and a national health referral system.

Families of individuals with chronic health problems are also in need of specific kinds of social support, such as that provided by such groups as Al-Anon or groups for families with a member who has had a stroke. Harris and Tarbutton (1983) describe a group for families of emotionally disabled children and older adults who are having problems with aging. In this group, the nurse leaders take an active role in using the group process to the advantage of group members and are knowledgeable about the problems of the identified clients. The dual role of the group is emphasized by the statement, "How do you care for this person in your life and also take care of yourself while caring?"

TOOLS AND TECHNIQUES

Before planning *how* to use social support and support systems in work with clients, it is important to assess clients' *needs* for support, and types of support that would be most appropriate. Again, think in terms of the nursing process—assessment, planning, implementation, and evaluation. These steps will be reviewed in the case examples at the end of the chapter.

While taking the nursing history, the client's social support system should be assessed; this can be done informally, or more formally, by using a tool such as Norbeck's Social Support Questionnaire (Norbeck, Lindsey, and Carrieri 1981). Although this is a research tool, the data can be used clinically as well, especially among clients in whom social support is a particular area of need. The actual questionnaire contains 24 questions and space to list 24 individuals. The example shown on page 269 is only a sampling of the actual form.

Considering the value of experiential expertise, a useful technique for supplementing social support during an illness or crisis is arranging for a client to have an opportunity to meet another who is experiencing a similar situation and who may give informal peer support. A maternity nurse might consider introducing two women who have had similar kinds of birth experiences to each other; it is likely that the two women will use the opportunity to share their experiences. Informal discussion sessions for cesarean mothers could be set up on the obstetrical unit, providing an opportunity for them to talk about their experiences and feelings. Another way of facilitating informal peer support is to ask a client who has experienced a certain situation or illness and who has learned to cope with it to telephone or visit an individual newly diagnosed or in crisis. Widow to Widow and Ostomy groups provide such role models on a regular basis, but there is no reason why nurses cannot arrange this informally. Those who are asked to help someone else are usually flattered to be seen as an "expert" whose help would be highly beneficial.

Resources. A more formal means of obtaining peer support for an individual is referral to a self-help/mutual support group. The first step is to find one, which may entail some work. The best way to begin is to contact a Self-Help Clearinghouse if one exists in the area; clearinghouses have lists of local self-help groups, with the name of a contact person and telephone number for each.

If a local clearinghouse is unavailable, nurses can write to the National Self-Help Clearinghouse, 33 West 42nd St., New York, New York, 10036. This organization has extensive information on national groups and their chapters all over the United States and also publishes detailed bibliographies and information of all kinds for professional and lay audiences. Frequently, health professionals are unaware of such resources. For example, one of us received a call from a community mental health nurse who was looking for a support group for the dying. She was surprised to learn that San Francisco had had a self-help clearinghouse for several years and eagerly alerted the rest of the staff to this valuable resource. One could also consult Gartner and Reissman (1979) or Evans (1979), which include listings of self-help groups and addresses all over the United States.

Another potential nursing role in the arena of social support is to help begin a self-help/support group. A good way to begin is to work with a lay individual who has experienced the situation or illness on which the group will be based or to use the dual perspective of the nurse who has experienced such a situation herself. Literature on how to set up a group is available from several sources. The Gartner and Reissman volume (1979) describes the role of the organizer, group processes, leadership, and suggestions for running a successful meeting, as well as giving advice to professionals who want to organize such groups. This advice includes a caution that the professional role must shift from organizer to gradual disengagement as natural leaders emerge from the group.

Some self-help groups prefer to work closely with professionals on an ongoing basis. However, most groups need the help of health professionals, at least as a referral source. Mastectomy and ostomy groups, for example, provide group members who visit patients pre-op and post-op in the hospital, and it takes awareness and cooperation of nurses to ensure that their patients are aware of such resources. However, nurses often plan a more active role in self-help/support groups, such as serving as facilitators in time-limited or ongoing groups—cancer groups, mastectomy groups, and parenting groups are examples. Nurses may also be invited to present specific information at a self-help group meeting.

SOCIAL SUPPORT QUESTIONNAIRE
PLEASE READ ALL DIRECTIONS
BEFORE STARTING.

Please list each significant person in your life on the right. Consider all the persons who provide personal support for you or who are important to you. Use only first names or initials, and then indicate the relationship, as in the following example:

Example:

First Name or Initials	Relationship
1.	
2.	
3.	
4.	
5.	
etc.	

Use the following list to help you think of the people important to you, and list as many people as apply in your case.

— spouse or partner   — health care providers
— family members or relatives — counselor or therapist
— friends   — minister/priest/rabbi
— work or school associates   — other
— neighbors

You do not have to use all 24 spaces. Use as many spaces as you have important persons in your life. For each person you listed, please answer the following questions by writing in the number that applies.

1 = not at all   4 = quite a bit
2 = a little   5 = a great deal
3 = moderately

Question 1:

How much does this person make you feel liked or loved?

1. _____
2. _____
3. _____
4. _____
5. _____
etc.

Question 2:

How much does this person make you feel respected or admired?

1. _____
2. _____
3. _____
4. _____
5. _____
etc.

Figure 12-1. A segment of the Norbeck Social Support Questionnaire, © 1980, revised 1982, used with permission of Jane S. Norbeck, D.N.Sc., University of California, San Francisco.

SUMMARY

Social support and self-help groups can be used in self-care in more numerous ways than have been described here. We hope that readers will use their creativity in thinking of additional ways to help their clients use social resources in self-care. The information presented in this chapter will be helpful for clients who are changing their own health behaviors. Previous chapters describe self-care strategies that have the potential to promote health in the biological and psychological realms, while this chapter focuses on the social realm. The final chapter in Part Three focuses most broadly in its consideration of the interaction of environmental factors and individuals and families and how such interaction affects personal safety and health.

CASE EXAMPLE

Carole is a 35-year-old, married physician who recently gave birth to her first child. She had been engaged full time in her career until the birth, and she and her physician-husband had an active social life and a number of interests, such as sailing. Following her delivery, she planned to take a six weeks leave, then return to work as a dermatologist in a health maintenance organization.

Following childbirth, Carole found that she was quite depressed and far more tired than she had anticipated. She was surprised at her ambivalent feelings about returning to work; she was reluctant to leave her baby, yet realized that she was unwilling to postpone or give up her career. She also felt that she knew very little about baby care—the couple's friends were childless, single, or had children nearing adolescence.

At her infant's two-week checkup, she voiced her confusion to the pediatrician; he suggested that she talk with the pediatric nurse practitioner, who had a special interest in the needs of new mothers. Carole and the nurse talked about Carole's feelings and about infant care. The nurse realized that Carole's major concerns had to do with her needs for a new type of social support. Despite a good relationship with her husband, their many friends, and her parents who lived nearby, Carole needed to talk with other women with infants and to make some arrangements for house and childcare. They discussed alternatives for childcare, and Carole decided to advertise in the newspaper for a live-in babysitter/housekeeper, because of the heavy demands of her work.

The nurse realized that Carole's feelings about her abilities as a mother were as important as arranging for childcare. Carole wondered if her depression was strictly the postpartum "blues" or if it had to do with the fact that she was the only person she knew having to learn to cope with a new baby at 35. Further assessment by Carole and the nurse revealed that Carole had no conflicts about combining career and motherhood but wondered if she would be adequate to both tasks.

Following the assessment process, the nurse suggested that Carole join a new parents' support group facilitated by a colleague, for at least a few weeks before she returned to work. They also discussed breast-feeding, and the nurse learned that Carole thought she must wean in order to return to work. As Carole was reluctant to begin bottlefeeding, the nurse gave her the telephone number of a breast-feeding support group that provides peer counseling by telephone. They agreed to talk again just before Carole returned to work to evaluate Carole's progress.

Carole attended her first support group meeting, which was attended by five other women and their new infants. Although she felt older than several of the women, she was delighted to find how much they all had in common. They spent the meeting talking about their birth experiences and what it was like with a new infant at home the first few weeks. Carole left the meeting in a positive frame of mind, the best she had felt since coming home from the hospital. It was a great comfort to learn that all the other women were "exhausted" and several others had experienced depression. In addition, two of the women were also professionals who planned to return to work relatively quickly.

Carole continued to attend the meetings until just before returning to work. She and the two other professional women met for lunch with their babies and enjoyed each other's company enough that they decided to continue to meet socially every few weeks once the group was over.

Two weeks before Carole was to return to work, she decided to begin pumping her breasts to save breastmilk for her baby. She phoned the nursing mothers' group for information on where to get a good breastpump and was referred to a counselor who had gone back to work after both her children were born. The counselor gave her advice about freezing milk and helped her think about scheduling her pumping sessions, and alternative ways she could choose to proceed—having the baby brought to her at lunch time or going home to feed the baby. She purchased an effective pump and began experimenting with the best times and circumstances in which to express breastmilk.

When Carole met again with the pediatric nurse practitioner, at her infant's two-month checkup, she had been at work for two weeks. She had found a competent babysitter/housekeeper. Carole and the nurse evaluated the self-care implementation in the area of social support. Carole was no longer depressed and was expressing breastmilk for her son while working; this helped to relieve some of her guilt about leaving him. She and the other women continued to get together weekly after the group ended and were deriving much mutual support and pleasure from their relationship. Her major problem was that she continued to be "exhausted", but she smiled at the nurse when she left and said, "I guess that will be a fact of life for a while."

CASE EXAMPLE

Brian is a 26-year-old, single, white male who lives with his parents in a small Midwestern city. He works as a salesman in the men's department of a department store about five miles from his home. Brian has had epilepsy since he was six years old. Although his grand mal seizures have been frequent during some periods in the past, they have been well controlled with anticonvulsants recently. Brian has only two to four seizures a month.

Brian's main problems are his poor self-esteem and social isolation. He spends his free time at home, working on his stamp collection, listening to music, or watching television. Although he would like to engage in outdoor activities, he is afraid to try because he never knows when he will have a seizure. His parents have been overprotective. Brian is bright but he did poorly academically because of missing school and his sensitivity to the ridicule of other children. When he graduated from high school, he began to work. He has had employment problems in the past, such as employers being unwilling to hire him when he was open about his epilepsy, being laid off by others whom he didn't tell following a seizure, and co-workers being reluctant to work with him; however, he has had his sales clerk job for two years now. His boss is understanding and his co-workers are cordial, although not seemingly interested in friendship.

On the way home from work one day, Brian had a seizure on the bus. Barbara, another passenger, who was a staff nurse on the neurology/ neurosurgery ward of a local hospital, assisted Brian, and stayed with him until he was oriented enough to get himself home. Barbara asked him how long he had had epilepsy and about the frequency of his seizures. She also asked him if he had heard of an epilepsy support group that had been formed in the area in the last year. One of Barbara's patients in the hospital was a middle-aged woman with epilepsy who had organized the group. Barbara told Brian that the group's purpose was for people with epilepsy to meet each other and to support each other in coping with their common problem. Barbara suggested that he call the organizer, whose name was in the telephone book.

Brian thought about what Barbara had said for the next week, feeling ambivalent about calling the woman. But he was fed up with his restricted life, bored, and didn't know how to change things, so he decided to call. The leader was very friendly on the phone and described what happened at meetings in such a way that Brian decided that attending one would not hurt him.

Brian's first epilepsy support group meeting was a revelation. He was surprised to see the variety of people who had epilepsy and how successful many of them seemed. Previously, his only contact with another person with epilepsy was a young man who was also mentally retarded. Some of the group members were married and had children, a dream that Brian thought he could never attain. He was quiet during the meeting but listened very carefully to what other members said about themselves, their lives, and how they coped with their epilepsy. He was particularly struck by a woman who described how she protected herself while sailing. She always sailed with a good friend who knew what to do should she have a seizure, and she wore a life jacket, and tethered herself to the mast. She said "I look like a three-year-old on a leash, but I don't care; sailing and being safe is more important." Brian could not quite believe that the woman was so nonchalant about what to him would be acutely embarrassing, but he was very impressed. He wondered if he could try some of the things he would so like to do.

Brian attended the next meeting and gradually became quite articulate and active in subsequent group meetings. He became close friends with a few other members who were single and in their 20s and 30s, and, together, they went hiking in the hills, horsebackriding, and to concerts. He also began to meet some of their friends who did not have epilepsy.

After about a year in the group, Brian thought about how he had changed as a result of the group. He had thought about Barbara several times but had never contacted her. He wrote to "Barbara ?, R.N., Neurology, Municipal Hospital" the following:

Dear Barbara,

I don't know whether you still work there, or whether you will remember the man you helped on the bus during a seizure a year ago. You told me about the epilepsy support group. You knew nothing about me, except that I had epilepsy. But then I had no friends, and spent all my time at home or work, and was bored and unhappy. I have been a member of the group since you told me about it, and it changed my life. I have several friends and we hike, picnic, horsebackride, and even ice skate. But the biggest change is my attitude about myself and my handicap. I now see myself as a person with epilepsy, rather than an epileptic. My epilepsy is only one part of me, and not the most important part. I have met others whose epilepsy is much worse than mine, but who do more with their lives. I can also help other people, which feels really good. In the group I have learned more about seizures and drug side effects, and, especially, what I can do for myself to prevent seizures. For example, we have learned stress reduction techniques in the group because many of us have more frequent seizures when we are tense.

I have wanted to write to you to thank you for taking the time to help me that day on the bus, and giving me the information that has changed my life. You deserve a place in Heaven.

Sincerely,
Brian

Discussion Questions

1. Discuss the difference between self-help and self-care.
2. How might social support patterns differ for the following—a Middle Eastern immigrant family, a nuclear middle-class family of Old American background, a single parent?
3. Discuss the importance of social support in changing health behaviors.
4. Describe the important elements that should be included when developing a support group for pregnant adolescents.

REFERENCES

American Nurses Association Commission on Nursing Research: Generating a scientific basis for nursing practice: Research priorities for the 1980's. Nursing Research, Vol 29, No 3, p 219, 1980

Berkman LF, Syme SL: Social networks, host resistance and mortality: A nine year follow-up of Alameda County residents. American Journal of Epidemiology, Vol 109, No 2, pp 186–205, 1979

Borman LD: Characteristics of development and growth. In Lieberman MA, Borman DD, and Associates: Self-Help Groups for Coping with Crisis. Jossey-Bass, San Francisco, California, 1979

Borkman T: Experiential knowledge: A new concept for the analysis of self-help groups. Social Service Review, Vol 50, No 3, pp 445–456, 1976

Caplan G: Support systems. In Caplan G (ed): Support Systems and Community Mental Health, Behavioral Publications, New York, 1974

Cassell J: The contribution of the social environment to host resistance. American Journal of Epidemiology, Vol 104, No 2, pp 107–123, 1976

Cobb S: Social support as a moderator of life stress. Psychosomatic Medicine, Vol 38, No 5, pp 300–314, 1976

Evans G (ed): The Family Circle Guide to Self-Help. Ballantine Books, New York, 1979

Ferguson I: Eva Salber on lay health facilitators. Medical Self-Care, pp 16–21, Winter 1982

Gartner A, Reissman F: Help: A Working Guide to Self-Help Groups. New Viewpoints-Vision Books, New York, 1980

Gartner A, Reissman F: Self Help in the Human Services. Jossey-Bass, San Francisco, California, 1977

Harris P, Tarbutton G: Support groups: The family connection. Free Association: A Forum for Psychiatric Nurses, Vol 10, No 2, pp 1–4, 1983

Kahn RL: Aging and social support. In Riley MW (ed): Aging from Birth to Death: Interdisciplinary Perspectives. Westview Press, Boulder, Colorado, 1979

Kush-Goldberg C: The health self-help group as an alternative source of health care for women. International Journal of Nursing Studies, Vol 16, No 3, pp 283–294, 1979

Levy LH: Processes and activities in groups. In Lieberman ML, Borman LD: Self-Help Groups for Coping with Crisis. Jossey-Bass, San Francisco, California, 1979

Lieberman ML, Borman LD: Self-Help Groups for Coping with Crisis. Jossey-Bass, San Francisco, California, 1979

Lipson JG: Cesarean support groups: Mutual help and education. Women and Health, Vol 6, No 3/4, pp 27–39, 1981

Lipson JG: Peer telephone counseling: Health care implications. Journal of the California Perinatal Association, Vol 3, No 1, pp 85–89, 1983

Meleis AI: The Arab American in the health care system. American Journal of Nursing, Vol 81, No 6, pp 1180–1183, 1981

Mueller DP: Social networks: A promising direction for research on the relationship of the social environment to psychiatric disorder. Social Science and Medicine, Vol 14A, No. 2, pp 147–161, 1980

Norbeck JS: The use of social support in clinical practice. Journal of Psychosocial Nursing and Mental Health Services, Vol 20, No 12, pp 22–29, 1982

Norbeck JS, Lindsey AM, Carrieri VL: The development of an instrument to measure social support. Nursing Research, Vol 30, No 5, pp 264–269, 1981

Nuckolls K, Cassel J, Kaplan B: Psychosocial assets, life crisis, and the prognosis of pregnancy. American Journal of Epidemiology, Vol 95, No 5, pp 431–441, 1972

Pilisuk M: Delivery of social support: The social inoculation. American Journal of Orthopsychiatry, Vol 52, No 1, pp 20–31, 1982

Swift C: The prevention equation and self-help groups. Self-Help Reporter, Vol 3, No 4, pp 1–2, 1979

13

Personal Safety and Environmental Awareness

Health and illness are as inextricably connected with environmental factors as they are to social and cultural factors. It has become more and more apparent in recent years that health hazards in the home, on the road, in the workplace, and in the broader environment have striking, if sometimes subtle, effects on health.

The theoretical orientation that underlies the following discussion is an ecological framework, which assumes that multiple factors in the environment have the potential to promote health or lead to disease. The environment includes such *inorganic* factors as climate, geography, geology (e.g., earthquakes, floods), such *organic* factors as disease pathogens, and human beings (e.g., overpopulation), and such *human-made* factors as urbanization, industrial pollution, and cultural health practices. Disease does not result merely from an accumulation of environmental factors but rather from their multiple interactions (Moore, Van Arsdale, Glittenberg, and Aldrich 1980). The nursing theorist who best exemplifies this perspective is Martha Rogers, who states that "Man is a unified whole, interacting with the environment. Man and the environment are continuously exchanging matter and energy with one another" (1970:54).

The purpose of this chapter is to alert nurses to the multitude of environmental factors that affect health and illness. The scope is so broad, however, that we can merely touch on a limited number of examples. Our intent is to stimulate readers to consider carefully other aspects of their environments in the interest of self-care for themselves and their clients. The self-care perspective assumes that individuals and families have the right to know about health risks in the environment. Based on such knowledge, the individual can choose to avoid health hazards or to minimize the risks. The nurse's role includes educating clients and encouraging them to educate themselves about environmental health hazards to clarify their values and make the choices that are best for them. In addition, we believe that nurses should function as role models by demonstrating environmental sensitivity.

PROBLEMS AND ISSUES

The subject of environmental health hazards, and particularly the human-made factors, is fraught with controversial issues, engendering strong feelings and questions about morals and ethics. Such subjects as pollution, crime, toxic waste disposal, and the nuclear arms race stimulate reactions that range from denial, e.g., "I've been working with this stuff for ten years and I'm not dead yet," to crippling fear, e.g., "I'm afraid to leave my house without a gas mask." Neither extreme is functional. McVeigh (1982) suggests that nuclear war is the number one health hazard in the world today and that we have all already been injured through psychic numbing, "We simply cease to feel anything about [nuclear weapons] because the possible consequences are too awful to imagine. Even if we could imagine them, our response would be unbearable" (1982:34).

However, there are many human-made factors over which people do have control, and such factors are the subject of this chapter. The following sections on toxic agent control, occupational safety and health, and accident prevention and injury control are excerpted from *Healthy People: the U.S. Surgeon General's Report on Health Promotion and Disease Prevention.* The purpose of this report is to encourage a second public health revolution in the United States. The first revolution was the successful struggle against infectious disease, while the second revolution must be aimed at major chronic diseases and accidents.

Toxic Agent Control

Toxic agents include natural and synthetic chemicals, dusts, minerals, and radiation which are thought to be precursors of acute or chronic illness. Such agents can be carcinogenic (cause cancer), mutagenic (cause gene alterations), or teratogenic (cause birth defects). Adverse effects also include systemic poisoning, growth impairment, infertility and other reproductive abnormalities, skin disorders, neurologic diseases, behavioral abnormalities, immunological damage, and chronic degenerative diseases involving the lungs, joints, vascular system, kidneys, liver, and endocrine organs.

Because of their potential for harm, these substances are regulated by the government in an attempt to control air and water emissions and effluents, hazardous waste disposal, transportation of hazardous materials, occupational exposure, products (food additives, pharmaceuticals, pesticides, consumer and industrial chemicals), and radiation exposure from medical devices. Despite national and local government regulations, however, control of environmental contaminants is hindered by strong competing interests, such as financial interests of industry and agriculture and ordinary people who are unwilling to change some aspects of their life-styles, e.g., reduced use of automobiles to decrease an important source of air pollution.

Another major problem is the rapid growth of synthetic chemicals in the last 25 years. More than 4 million chemical compounds are now recognized, with more than 60,000 commercially produced, and about 1,000 new ones are introduced each year (DHEW 1979). They make their way into food and water supplies, and some remain in the food chain for years. For example, 500 to 1000 pounds of the flame retardant PBB was accidentally added to dairy feed in Michigan in 1973, resulting in contamination of animals and human food products. Although banned because of its toxic effects, 97% of the Michigan population still showed measurable levels of the chemical five years later, including breastmilk (Reich 1983). In many cases, it takes at least 20 years to determine full effects of many new compounds on human health, and health problems caused by some chemicals now in use may not be known until the twenty first century.

Occupational Safety and Health

The National Institute for Occupational Safety and Health (NIOSH) estimates that 100,000 Americans die and almost 400,000 new cases of occupational disease are recognized each year. In 1977, more than 2.3 million workers experienced disabling injuries, 80,000 of which were permanently disabling. A broad range of health problems are associated with exposures to toxic chemicals, asbestos, coal dust, cotton fiber, ionizing radiation, physical hazards, excessive noise, and stress from routinized trivial tasks. Examples include cancers (see Table 13-1), lung and heart diseases, birth defects, sensory deficits, injuries, and psychological problems.

Occupational illnesses and injuries are of human origin and, thus, preventable. Hazards can be controlled by modifying the work environment, patterns of job performance, or both. However, there are many problems existing in occupational safety and health, such as inadequate data, that make it difficult to determine accurately the extent of health problems and to measure the effectiveness of prevention efforts. Because of long latency periods before disease develops, knowledge is lacking about the risks and hazards of new chemicals, their interactions, and route of exposure, e.g., inhalation, skin contact, ingestion.

Accident Prevention and Injury Control

More than 100,000 Americans lost their lives to accidental injuries in 1977, and 65 million people suffered non-fatal accidental injuries requir-

TABLE 13-1. COMMON OCCUPATIONAL CARCINOGENS

Agent	Organ Affected	Occupation
Wood	Nasal cavity and sinuses	Woodworkers
Leather	Nasal cavity and sinuses; urinary bladder	Leather and shoe workers
Iron oxide	Lung; larynx	Iron ore miners; metal grinders and polishers silver finishers; iron foundry workers
Nickel	Nasal sinuses; lung	Nickel smelters, mixers, and roasters; electrolysis workers
Arsenic	Skin; lung; liver	Miners; smelters; insecticide makers and sprayers; tanners; chemical workers; oil refiners; vintners
Chromium	Nasal cavity and sinuses; lung; larynx	Chromium producers, processers, and users; acetylene and aniline workers; bleachers; glass, pottery, and linoleum workers; battery makers
Asbestos	Lung (pleural and peritoneal mesothelioma)	Miners; millers; textile, insulation, and shipyard workers
Petroleum, petroleum coke, wax, creosote, anthracene, paraffin, shale, and mineral oils	Nasal cavity; larynx; lung; skin; scrotum	Contact with lubricating, cooling, paraffin or wax fuel oils or coke; rubber fillers; retort workers; textile weavers; diesel jet testers
Mustard gas	Larynx; lung; trachea; bronchi	Mustard gas workers
Vinyl chloride	Liver; brain	Plastic workers
Bis-chloromethyl ether, chloromethyl methyl ether	Lung	Chemical workers
Isopropyl oil	Nasal cavity	Isopropyl oil producers

Continued

TABLE 13-1. COMMON OCCUPATIONAL CARCINOGENS

Agent	Organ Affected	Occupation
Coal soot, coal tar, other products of coal combustion	Lung; larynx; skin; scrotum; urinary bladder	Gashouse workers, stokers, and producers; asphalt, coal tar, and pitch workers; coke oven workers; miners; still cleaners
Benzene	Bone marrow	Explosives, benzene, or rubber cement workers; distillers; dye users; painters; shoemakers
Auramine, benzidine, alpha-Naphthylamine, beta-Naphthylamine, magenta, 4-Amino-diphenyl, 4-Nitro-diphenyl	Urinary bladder	Dyestuffs manufacturers and users; rubber workers (pressmen, filtermen, laborers); textile dyers; paint manufacturers

From National Cancer Institute: Job, Safety, and Health, U.S. Department of Labor, July 1975 (*reprinted with permission of U.S. Department of Labor*)

ing medical treatment (see Table 13-2).

Unintentional injuries are the leading cause of death of people between one and 38 years old and a leading cause of disability. Accidental death and injury can be prevented and will be discussed below. Before turning to clinical application, we raise two issues important to environmental awareness and safety—the right to know and locus of responsibility.

TABLE 13-2. APPROXIMATE ANNUAL DEATH AND INJURY RATES

Cause	Deaths	Injuries
Motor vehicles	52,400	2 million
Falls	15,000	14 million
Burns	7,500	60,000 hospital admissions
Drownings	7,000	
Gunshot wounds	32,000	18,000–100,000
Poisoning	4,000	2 million ingestions

The Right to Know

Awareness of environmental, occupational, and safety hazards is basic to reducing health risks, preventing illness and injury, and promoting self-care. *Promoting Health/Preventing Disease* (DHEW 1980) states the following objectives:

> *By 1990, at least half of all adults should be able to accurately report an accessible source of information on toxic substances to which they may be exposed, including information on the interactions with other factors, such as smoking and medications.*

> *By 1990, at least half of all people ages 15 years and older should be able to identify the major categories of environmental threats to health and note some of the health consequences of those threats (DHEW 1980:35).*

California's "right-to-know" law (State of California 1980) requires that "Material Data Safety Sheets" (MSDS's) containing information accompany each hazardous substance that a manufacturer produces, and they must be provided to the employee, the union, and the employee's physician upon request. However, as of 1982, only three other states had passed right-to-know legislation (Stock 1982). In many areas, employees have no legal recourse when employers refuse to provide them with such information. Financial reasons undoubtedly underlie the reluctance of some employers to inform workers of the health risks associated with their work, as well as unwillingness to release "trade secrets" to the general public. Political reasons keep legislation to protect workers from being passed in some areas. Once the individual knows about potential hazards in the environment, is it then his responsibility to change the situation?

Whose Responsibility is it?

Federal and state laws require that employers maintain working conditions that are safe and healthy for workers. In California, the law specifies three levels of control for workplace hazards:

1. Engineering control, e.g., improved ventilation, providing hoists for lifting
2. Administrative control, e.g., changing work procedures, rotating workers to minimize risks
3. Personal protective equipment, e.g., dust masks, goggles, ear plugs.

The third level of control should be temporary until management redesigns the workplace or procedures to make the work environment healthier and safer (State of California 1980). However, in many industries, management focuses only on the third level of control and "blames the victim" when a worker becomes injured or ill as a result of not wearing personal protective devices (PPDs). PPDs are usually uncomfortable, can cause health or safety problems themselves, and may not be effective; further, they are made in limited sizes for men, and often fit poorly, especially when worn by women (Aufiero 1982). Should the worker or the employer assume the responsibility for a safe and healthy work environment?

In the larger sphere, individuals are encouraged to conserve energy and non-renewable resources through tax deductions for home improvements that reduce energy needs. Appliances and automobiles that are more energy efficient are being manufactured currently. But what about people who live in poverty and can barely meet their survival needs? And why must people use so many appliances and automobiles? How much power should government have to legislate and enforce energy conservation and environmental controls? Is it the government's responsibility to keep us from fouling the environment? Industry's? The individual's? We believe that this responsibility rests with everyone and needs all efforts from individual to worldwide to improve the health of our environment.

CLINICAL APPLICATION

At the most basic level, the process of self-care involves becoming aware of health and safety hazards in the environment and what can be done for protection. An important role of the nurse is educating and encouraging clients to avoid or minimize such hazards. Clients range from those who passively accept conditions as they are those who enthusiastically become change agents with new knowledge or encouragement. Although we favor the idea of the nurse acting as change agent, we realize that nurses also vary in their willingness to "rock the boat" in the interest of a healthier environment.

In terms of *nursing process*, consider Table 13-3. Assessment and implementation examples follow in four settings—the home, road and recreation, the workplace, and the broader environment.

The Home

Toxic substances in the home, such as cleaning agents, pesticides, and drugs, create particular hazards for children under the age of five. Each year, for example, ingestion or inhalation of lead leads to central nervous system damage or mental retardation in 6,000 children, as well as death for another 300 to 400. Lead poisoning is especially threatening for inner city children who live in housing where there is peeling paint on walls and

---

TABLE 13-3. THE NURSING PROCESS AND THE ENVIRONMENT

Assessment	Planning
• What are the risks in the environment? • What are particular risks for the individual? • What is the client's level of knowledge or awareness of risks?	• How can the individual best prevent injury or illness? • What is the best way to put distance between the individual/family and the hazard?
Implementation	*Evaluation*
• Can one remove self from the hazard? • How can one protect self from the hazard? • How can one remove the hazard? • How can one neutralize the hazard?	• Is the health hazard reduced or eliminated? • Are there fewer accidents or incidents occurring? • Is there a more widespread and higher level of knowledge?

---

lead is inhaled from automobile exhausts (DHEW 1979). Health assessment of children should include questions to parents related to such areas as accessibility of hazardous substances, knowledge about childproof cupboard locks and medication containers, the importance of having available emetics, and the telephone number of the local poison control center.

Less is known about potential carcinogenic and toxic effects of household products. One study found that housewives' mortality rate from cancer was twice the rate of women employed outside the home, implying that the household contains carcinogens to which the full-time housewife is more heavily exposed (White 1981). White suggests examining one's cupboards for products that contain such toxic chemicals as benzene, napthas, petroleum distillates, chromic acid, chlorinated hydrocarbons, and ammonium compounds; alternates such as baking soda, washing soda, and dishwashing detergent can be substituted. Other factors, however, may contribute to a higher cancer rate among housewives, such as exposure to low-level radiation from televisions and microwave ovens, or depression, which may contribute to smoking, overeating, excessive alcohol intake, and lack of exercise, all of which reduce resistance to illness (White 1981).

Pesticides are produced at the rate of 4 billion pounds a year, more than one pound for every person on this planet (Delehunty 1981), and can cause health problems. For example, some Northern Californians complained of discomfort following malathion spraying of fruit trees, despite the fact that this is a very mild, nontoxic pesticide. More toxic pesticides can be quite dangerous, and home use of insecticides/pesticides is a major factor. Consider the client who experienced three days of vomiting, diarrhea, and headaches after spraying her roses. Pesticides are used mainly on food crops. Although most have been washed off or dissipate into the air by the time food reaches the market, residues remain on the surface or within the tissues of the foods. A study of produce in Los Angeles revealed measurable amounts of 24 different pesticides on strawberries and 11 on lettuce (Delehunty 1981). Thus, the nursing assessment must include questions related to gardening and food preparation.

Cosmetics are also potential health hazards. Decker (1983) notes that the average North American uses 10 to 40 pounds of cosmetics, soaps, and toiletries annually, and that about 60,000 people, mostly women, suffer injuries from these products each year. The U.S. Food and Drug Administration (FDA) cannot require cosmetics manufacturers to inform the FDA of ingredients and cannot even ban hair dyes known to contain carcinogens (coal tars) from the market. NIOSH lists phenol, a coal tar derivative, as a potential carcinogen. It is so toxic that a one percent solution applied to the skin for several hours has been known to cause gangrene. Yet it is present in several skin care products and one brand of shaving cream. Decker (1983) lists products that contain suspected carcinogens, such as popular brands of toothpaste which contain carrageenan, or FD & C Blue #1. The nurse should encourage clients to read labels and to arm themselves with information about toxic substances.

The Road and Recreation

Recent legislation related to speed limits and public education campaigns about seat belts has decreased the rate and severity of injuries associated with automobile accidents. Despite clear evidence that seat belts reduce death rates and injuries, there are still many people who refuse to wear them. However, California now requires children under four years or weighing less than 40 pounds to be restrained in an approved car seat. New York has enacted a statute requiring the use of seat belts. Many other states will have laws in effect soon. In the Netherlands and Canada, police issue traffic citations to drivers not wearing seat belts.

Less reliance on the automobile would be beneficial in the interest of health. Travel by air, bus, or train is safer than car travel, and it is less polluting because the public vehicles carry more passengers. Many people are accustomed to using their cars for errands only two or three blocks away. It may be only a matter of encouraging clients to think about how they use their cars to stimulate them to walk or bicycle for short errands. See Chapter 8 for discussion of the health benefits of walking or bicycling.

In reference to safety, the nurse and client should discuss the importance of wearing reflective or white clothing and carrying a light when walking or cycling at dusk or dark. Cyclists decrease the likelihood of head injuries by wearing helmets. Clients should be asked about where they walk and ride, about lighting, and about traffic and crime patterns in the area.

Safety includes self-care measures to reduce the possibility of mugging or rape. The Gallup poll reported that an average of 23 percent of Americans were victimized by street crime at least once during 1981. Recent research shows that "muggable" people appear to walk and move differently than non-victims—their movements are not organized, they appear less comfortable in their bodies, and their eye movements, speed, or preoccupation invite attack (Grayson and Stein 1981). Although these findings are controversial, they suggest an area of self-care education (see tools and techniques).

Assessment of recreation safety should also include questions about what sports and hobbies the individual enjoys and the potential hazards associated with each. The nurse should alert the client who wants a suntan to the connection between excessive ultraviolet light and skin cancers. The Federal Trade Commission now requires that suntan lotions specify a "sun protection factor" on their labels; the factors range from 2 (minimum protection) to 15 (complete blockage of ultraviolet rays).

The Workplace

Nurses and their clients should be aware of different kinds of occupational hazards. Readers can consult such sources as *Occupational Health Nursing* and NIOSH publications for specific hazards associated with different occupations. We will discuss the office and the hospital in this chapter because we are convinced that nurses who are sensitized to their own work environments can better help their clients to become sensitized to theirs. Piller notes that "with the exception of farm workers, hospital workers sustain 40% more work-related injuries than those in any other industry" (1981:6). However, hospital workers include building/grounds workers, electricians, janitors, aides, and workers from many other industries.

The office. Headache and eye problems are common complaints among office workers and are often caused by glare from artificial light in office buildings with large expanses of white walls. Fluorescent light and ordinary lightbulbs emit only a limited spectrum, omitting ultraviolet and some red rays found in sunlight. The quality of light entering the eye can affect both physical and mental health; artificial light that does not have the right spectral distribution can contribute to irritability (Salinas 1982). The following self-care measures to employees who experience headache and eyestrain are suggested:

1. Examination by an ophthalmologist
2. Reduction of lighting in work areas to reduce glare
3. Using incandescent desk lamps
4. Leaving the building during lunch break
5. Organizing work to include distant vision to relax eye muscles (Salinas 1982:15).

If fluorescent lights are unavoidable, the tubes can be replaced with broad spectrum fluorescent tubes.

Videodisplay terminals have become common in offices and health care institutions; by 1985, a predicted 35 million people will use them either at work or at home. Although the FDA states that VDTs emit little or no harmful radiation under normal operating conditions (Frank 1983), this is another case in which the technology is too new to show long-term effects. See Table 13–4 for the health effects of VDTs and self-care measures.

Other hazards to clerical workers include exposure to photocopying machine chemicals, back and neck strain, secondary cigarette smoke, and such sociopolitical hazards as the effects of low pay, low status, and sexism.

The hospital. Nurses need to become more aware of many health hazards in hospital work (see Table 13-5). For example *chemical hazards* include anaesthetic agents, ethylene oxide, chemotherapeutic drugs, and others. Studies of women employees exposed to anaesthetic agents in operating room environments during the first trimester of pregnancy showed greater rates of spontaneous abortion, stillbirth, and birth defects in infants (Mattia 1983). California state health officials have recently issued a warning that ethylene oxide, used to sterilize heat sensitive medical supplies, has caused cancer mutations in laboratory animals. Workers in central supply and operating room nurses may be at risk of inhalation or direct skin contact when opening surgical supply packs in which gas may be trapped (Burgel 1982). Burgel suggests opening packs at arm's length out of the breathing zone and reporting capped or plugged tubing to central supply. It is not known whether nurses exposed to cytotoxic agents experience any chromosome damage. There is concern that nurses who care for patients undergoing chemotherapy sustain some exposure and should use at least minimal precautions of gloves and gowns when disposing of urine or excreta, followed by thorough hand-washing (Bartkowski-Dobbs 1983).

Ionizing radiation is a health risk that is frequently underestimated. Nurses must be aware that radiation is present in treated patients' bodies, secretions, and excreta. Self-care measures include limiting x-rays nurses receive as health care consumers, moving out of the vicinity when x-rays are taken, using lead shielding devices and monitoring devices, proper disposal of radioactive wastes, and becoming involved in the hospital health and safety committee (Henry 1982).

TABLE 13-4. HEALTH EFFECTS OF VIDEODISPLAY TERMINALS

Reported Problems	Possible Causes	Recommended Solutions
Musculo-Skeletal		
Back pain	Faulty work postures due to poorly	Adjustable office furniture
Shoulder and neck pain	designed furniture	Telephone head sets (if frequently use
Arm and leg pain	Faulty work postures due to poor sitting	phone at VDT)
Swollen muscles	habits	Regular breaks away from VDT
Hand cramps	Avoidance of distracting light sources	Exercises during rest breaks
Stiff/sore wrists	within visual field	Proper back care training
Visual		
Eyestrain	Direct glare from light source	Eliminate glare sources
Blurring, double vision	Reflected glare from work surfaces	Eliminate light background walls
Tearing	Excessive contrast between background	Use VDT's brightness control knob
Itching	and display screen	Properly adjust screen position
Stinging	Incorrect height of display screen	Alternate VDT work with other tasks
Temporary changes in color perception	Varying distances at which eye must	Regular rest breaks
Difficulty fixating on objects	focus between hard copy and screen	Conclude VDT work 15–30 minutes be-
Decrease in accommodation power	Flickering or fuzzy characters on screen	fore end of day
	Insufficiently corrected visual problems	Annual eye examinations
		Eye focusing exercises
		Service VDTs twice a year

Continued

TABLE 13-4. HEALTH EFFECTS OF VIDEODISPLAY TERMINALS (CONTINUED)

Reported Problems	Possible Causes	Recommended Solutions
Psychological		
Alienation	Routinized tasks	Task variation and adequate content
Anxiety	Speed ups	Regular rest breaks every 1–2 hours
Irritability	Monitoring by supervisor	Reasonable work rates
Depression	Delays in system response time	Elimination of monitoring
Sense of loss of control	Fear of job loss	Adequate training and employee participation in decision making
Isolation from peers		

From Frank C: Avoiding "terminal" illness. Healthline, The Robert A. McNeil Foundation for Health and Education, Vol. 2, No 4, P. 11, 1983

TABLE 13-5. OCCUPATIONAL HAZARDS IN THE HOSPITAL SETTING

Hazard	Examples
Physical hazards	Radiation, temperature (heat or cold), vibration, noise
Chemical	Formaldehyde, asbestos, chemotherapeutic agents, anaesthetic gases, ethylene oxide
Biological	Bacteria, viruses
Ergonomic	Back injuries, glare from video display units
Psychophysiological	Shift work, work stress, street crime in hospital locale
Unknown hazards	Radiation scatter

Among *biological hazards* are needle stick wounds, believed to be the main mode of transmission of Hepatitis B in hospital workers. Exposure to Hepatitis A, B, and Non A-Non B can also result from ingesting, being splashed in the eye, or allowing an open cut or abrasion to contact blood, saliva, or stool from hepatitis patients. Exposure should be reported to employee health service and the employee should receive gamma globulin. Hepatitis B vaccine is now available for those who are at high risk of exposure. But preventive measures such as thorough hand washing, proper isolation techniques and needle disposal, and careful blood drawing are best (Cantu 1982). Preventive self-care is also important for tuberculosis, which is on the rise in some areas of the country; isolation techniques, TB skin testing, and possible INH prophylaxis should be utilized. Biological hazards to pregnant woman employees include rubella and cytomegalic inclusion disease (CMV). All hospital employees, male and female, should have their rubella titers checked and should take the vaccine if the titer shows non-exposure. Hospital workers who are in the early state of pregnancy or attempting to become pregnant should avoid work with large numbers of small children to limit exposure to CMV (Burgel 1983).

An epidemic receiving much current attention is Acquired Immune Deficiency Syndrome (AIDS), found among previously healthy homosexual men, Haitian immigrants, IV drug users, and people who receive blood transfusions. AIDS is thought to be caused by a transmissible agent which severely impairs the body's ability to suppress disease-causing organisms and certain cancer cells, resulting in such life-threatening diseases as Kaposi's sarcoma and pneumocystis pneumonia. At the time of this writing, there is no known cure and a high mortality rate. AIDS researchers do not see any reason for panic among health care workers because AIDS seems to be transmitted only through intimate sexual contact and blood transfusions; 94% of the nation's diagnosed cases are in one of the four major risk groups. Until more is learned about the disease, however, clinical and laboratory staff are advised to take precautions suggested for hepatitis B (Center for Disease Control 1982).

Back injuries account for half of all worker compensation claims filed by hospital workers (Piller 1981). Although nursing personnel are usually taught to lift patients in a way that protects their backs, lack of staff, equipment, or time may reduce such precautions. The typical physical requirements of the staff nurse position in the hospital include 20 bed lifts and 5–10 transfer assists per shift.

Nuchols (1983:4) suggests the following for back safety:

1. ASSESS THE SIZE AND STABILITY OF WHAT YOU ARE LIFTING.
   - How probable is it that this patient could suddenly lose his strength or balance?
   - If the load is too heavy, bulky, or unstable, get a hoist or co-worker to help.
   - Be honest about what you feel comfortable lifting. Remember, it is better to wait and lift with help than jeopardize your back.
2. FACE THE LOAD.
   - Remember not to twist when you lift.
3. GET CLOSE TO THE LOAD.
   - Remember, never lift with your arms outstretched.
4. BEND YOUR KNEES.
   - Lift with your large leg and arm muscles, not your back.
   - Tighten your stomach muscles when lifting; this gives your back added support.
5. TEAM LIFT.
   - When you lift with a co-worker, have one of you give signals so you lift together.

Among *psychophysiological hazards* of hospital work are shiftwork and numerous sources of stress. Shiftwork can result in psychological problems that are more difficult to tolerate than physiological ones, such as social isolation, interference with family and social relationships, and sex-related problems. Other health effects of shiftwork include disturbed eating patterns, decreased appetite, and exacerbations in such conditions as diabetes mellitus and epilepsy, which are rhythmic in nature. Twenty percent of the working population cannot tolerate shiftwork, and people who live in noisy neighborhoods, or who have G.I. disorders, epilepsy, diabetes, or sleep problems should not be scheduled for rotating or night shifts (LaDou 1982). High intensity emotional work day after day, especially in understaffed settings, can result in physiological indications of prolonged stress or such psychosomatic problems as skin rashes, headaches, or ulcers. Snow lists the following emotional effects of stressful work conditions—anxiety, depression, boredom and fatigue, irritability, moodiness, emotional outbursts, and loneliness. Behavioral effects include excessive drinking, smoking, or eating (or loss of appetite), drug abuse, restlessness, impaired speech, nervous laughter, and trembling. Organizational effects include poor productivity, inability to concentrate, and decreased job dissatisfaction (Snow 1982).

Hutchinson (1983) suggests that nurses need to care for their professional selves, their emotional selves, and their physical selves, and offers the following self-care strategies:

1. Asserting behaviors (e.g., requesting help, confronting, setting limits)
2. Cultivating or encouraging good will (e.g., offering to help co-workers, socializing)
3. Catharsing (e.g., crying, using sarcasm or profanity, complaining)
4. Withdrawing physically or emotionally (e.g., floating, taking time out, intellectualizing)
5. Humor (e.g., laughing at oneself).

These techniques are applicable across all occupations.

TOOLS AND TECHNIQUES

In reference to environmental awareness and personal safety, self-care is an attitude and a framework for thinking about and avoiding health hazards. Environmental sensitivity can be a way of life (see case example) from choosing not to eat an apple until it is washed to forming an organization to support the nuclear weapons freeze. Readers should keep in mind the following questions for any environmental situation:

• What are the risks?
• Can I prevent the risk?
• What change will help most?
• Am I willing to make the change?
• What is preventing me from making the change?

Home and Road

Community health nursing texts provide references for assessing the home for health hazards. Table 13-6 is excerpted from a four page assessment guide used in one city health department. Clients with infants and toddlers should be encouraged to obtain such devices to prevent injuries as dummy plugs and childproof catches for cupboards and drawers. The nurse can suggest that a client spend some time crawling around the house at the eye and hand level of the young child "looking for trouble,"

TABLE 13-6. FAMILY ASSESSMENT GUIDE INSTRUCTIONS

I. Environmental
A. Housing

1. Size and adequacy for family

1	2	3
Very overcrowded:	Crowded:	Space abundant:
Many people sharing same bed or bedroom, with children sharing sleeping facilities inappropriately;	Sleeping arrangements adequate, with more than one child to a bedroom and/or infants sleeping in parents' bedroom;	Everyone has own bed or bedroom;
Home inappropriately large for older person(s);	Home slightly too large for reasonable maintenance by older person(s);	Home appropriate size for older person(s) to maintain
Play facilities for children insufficient or absent (in or outside the home);	Limited play facilities for children (in or outside the home);	Abundant play facilities for children (in and outside the home);
Opportunity for privacy of individuals either not provided for, or grossly insufficient.	Limited opportunity for privacy of individuals.	Abundant opportunity for privacy of individuals.

2. Condition of physical plant of dwelling

1	2	3
Structure fundamentally unsound and unsafe:	Structure sound, but beginning to show deterioration:	Structure sound:
Home does not provide protection from the elements; is condemned or does not meet local building standards;	Home provides moderate protection from the elements;	Home is safe from all but natural catastrophes;

TABLE 13-6. FAMILY ASSESSMENT GUIDE INSTRUCTIONS

I. Environmental
A. Housing

Inside paint peeling and/or plaster crumbling and is a danger to young children;	Inside walls are in relatively good condition, though some paint or repairs may be needed.	No repairs or paint needed;
No heating, ventilation or insulation.	Heating, ventilation or insulation minimal.	Home well-insulated, and heating and ventilating systems serviced regularly

Code: 1—potentially life destructive
2—life sustaining
3—life promoting

Adapted from Problem-oriented recording system. Reprinted with permission of Detroit Department of Health (CORE H_1)

e.g., what can the child pull off a table, get stuck in, fall off of or into, or eat?

People can take measures to avoid excessive ingestion of pesticides. Delehunty (1982) suggests that washing removes some pesticide residues, but fruits and vegetables treated with systemic pesticides may absorb some into their tissues, and the best protection is growing one's own food. For those who cannot, the suggestions listed below may help.

PROTECTION FOR PESTICIDES

- Wash all fruits and vegetables with biodegradable detergent.
- Soak produce in ¼ cup vinegar to one gallon water for five minutes, then rinse thoroughly with cold water.
- Peel root vegetables, e.g., carrots and turnips, before eating.
- Avoid produce from Mexico and Central America because many pesticides banned in the United States are used routinely there.
- Stay well-nourished and fit because people whose diets lack protein tend to accumulate more pesticides; dietary fiber may help to eliminate some pesticides.

Collective approaches to interpersonal safety and environmental awareness are making an impact in recent years. Neighborhood Watch programs, in which neighbors take responsibility for alerting law enforcement officials regarding strangers' unusual activity in a neighborhood, have deterred would-be burglars and muggers (King 1982). Parents have organized to pressure certain schools to close until asbestos is removed from ceilings. Mothers against Drunk Drivers (MADD) has had increasing media publicity for its activities in monitoring decisions by judges in court hearings of drunk drivers. The National Highway Traffic Safety Administration attributes some of the recent decline in traffic fatalities to national crusades against drunken driving launched by MADD and other organizations.

The Workplace

Self-awareness on the part of the nurse or client is the place to begin in assessing health hazards in the workplace. A yes to any of the following questions could indicate a job-related health problem (Stock 1982, III-1):

- Do you experience dizziness, headaches, or skin irritation while doing certain jobs?
- Do you have trouble breathing or a chronic cough?
- Do such symptoms as the above get better during your weekend or when you're away from work for a while?
- Do you consider the rates of cancer, heart disease, emotional

illness, or other chronic diseases to be high among your co-workers?
● Have you or your co-workers had difficulty in conceiving children or carrying them to term?

Occupational history questions should be added to the nursing history, such as Becker's (1982) recommendations, listed in Table 13-7.

In addition to assessing the employee, it is important to assess the workplace. Interested employees or health and safety committee members can conduct a survey to locate all detectable hazards. Keep in mind the following points:*

● Suspect everything (consider all substances as potentially toxic until proven otherwise).
● Keep written records of all hazards spotted during inspection.
● Diagram the workplace to locate workers, hazards, and controls
● Followup: Recheck problem areas to ensure corrections have been made, and keep records of repeat problems.

Nurses can raise questions to help assess safety in the hospital environment in reference to fire protection, electrical equipment, anaesthesizing locations, storage of medical gas, flammable liquids and radioactive materials, housekeeping, maintenance, and potential safety hazards in such departments as the kitchen, x-ray, laundry, and pharmacy (Stellman 1982).

Employees can request help from federal or state agencies if they have questions about the employer's obligation to protect employees' health and safety on the job. One should call the nearest state office of the Division of Occupational Safety and Health, as procedures vary from state to state.

Some states have consultation services that provide free on-site consultation by safety engineers and industrial hygienists, professionals who concentrate on hazards related to the work environment. Some large companies employ their own staff of health and safety professionals, such as occupational health nurses, physicians, and safety engineers. If the workplace does not have these resources, or if one desires an outside opinion, professional societies will provide names of members in the area. A discussion of how to request a health hazard evaluation begins on page 297.

Another source of information is written materials available through state and national occupational health agencies. The National Institute of

---

*Adapted from Stock L (ed): Community Right to Know: A Workbook on Toxic Substance Disclosure, Conference Manual. Governor's Office, State of California, and Labor Occupational Health Program, University of California, Berkeley, February 1982

TABLE 13-7. KEY POINTS OF AN OCCUPATIONAL/ ENVIRONMENTAL HISTORY

Present Illness (for each element of problem list)

Symptoms related to work
Other employees similarly affected
Current exposure to dusts, fumes, chemicals, biologic
    hazards
Prior first report of work injury

Work History

Describe—all prior jobs
      —typical work day
      —change in work process
Worksite—ventilation, medical and industrial hygiene
    surveillance, employment exams, protective
    measures
Union health and safety
"Moonlighting"
Days missed work last year. Why?
Prior worker compensation claims

Past History

Exposure to noise, vibration, radiation, chemicals,
    asbestos

Environmental History

Present and prior home and work locations
Jobs of "significant others"
Hazardous wastes/spills exposure
Air pollution
Hobbies: painting, sculpture, welding, woodworking
Home insulation-heating
Home and work cleaning agents
Pesticide exposure
Do you wear seat belts?
Do you have firearms in home or work?

Review of Systems

Specific emphasis: shift changes
              boredom
              reproductive history

From Becker CE: Key elements of the occupational history for the general physician. The Western Journal of Medicine, Vol 137, No 6, pp 581–582, 1982 (reprinted with permission of Western Journal of Medicine).

Occupational Safety and Health (NIOSH) has an extensive list of publications and booklets, which can be ordered from

NIOSH
Department of Health, Education, and Welfare
5600 Fishers Lane
Rockville, MD 20857

It is also important for the employee to locate other employees in the work setting who have similar concerns, both for mutual support and to consider how best to stimulate change for a healthier work environment. For example, a union can work together with management to institute a safety program in the workplace, or a group could get together to encourage a smoking ban in certain locations.

The Larger Environment

To protect the environment, individuals must do their part at home and work as well as alert their legislators about their concerns. However, making significant changes usually requires collective action and the interest of governing bodies. For example, when a chemical used in aerosol cans was suspected of damaging the atmosphere's ozone layer, a consumer's cooperative grocery store organization removed from its shelves aerosols containing fluorocarbons and launched an education campaign about the danger and substitutes for aerosol cans. Consumer boycotts of particular products are often useful in encouraging an industry to consider the safety of its products.

Organized citizen groups, such as the Sierra Club and Greenpeace (save the whales) have made headway in convincing some government bodies to consider banning environmentally hazardous practices. Letter writing campaigns and lobbying efforts do have an impact on legislators. Perhaps the growth and activity of nuclear weapons freeze groups will help to assure a safer future for the world.

HEALTH HAZARD EVALUATION

National Institute for Occupational Safety and Health
Hazard Evaluation and Technical Assistance Branch
4676 Columbia Parkway
Cincinnati, Ohio 45226

Is your job making you sick? Is your workplace unhealthy? If it is, you can request a health hazard evaluation

What. A Health Hazard Evaluation (HHE) is a study or investigation of a particular workplace that is done by National Institute for Occupational Safety and Health (NIOSH) to find out whether there is a health hazard to workers caused by exposure to chemicals or materials in the workplace. NIOSH, a federal agency in the Department of Health and Human Services, was founded by the OSHAct of 1970 (Public Law 91-596) and charged:

> *"To assure so far as possible every working man and woman in the Nation safe and healthful working conditions and to preserve our human resources."*

Who.

- WORKERS—An individual worker can request a Health Hazard Evaluation (HHE) on behalf of him or herself and two other workers.
- UNIONS—Any officer of a union which represents the workers for collective bargaining purposes can request an HHE.
- EMPLOYER—Any management official can request an HHE for the employer.

You may keep your name secret and NIOSH will not tell anyone who asked for the evaluation.

Also, the law forbids employers from punishing workers for making HHE requests or cooperating with NIOSH investigators.

Why. Heat, noise, stress (overtime, shift work, job design, etc), chemicals, dust, fumes, and radiation can affect your health. Substances in the workplace may cause cancer, lung or heart disease, nervous disorders, skin disease, and even damage a person's ability to produce healthy children. Some of these substances can even be brought home and produce these same diseases in children, husbands, and wives. Yet, many occupationally related diseases are not recognized as being related to the workplace.

Cost. It is free to you.

How.

1. WHAT YOU DO—fill out the request form contained with this fact sheet. Send it to the address on the form.

2. WHAT NIOSH WILL DO depends on the types of hazards where you work.

   A. If you ask about substances whose hazards are already well known, NIOSH may be able to give you the information you need without visiting your workplace. NIOSH may also suggest that you contact OSHA or MSHA about a regulatory inspection.

   B. Even if the hazard is well known, NIOSH may still need to know how serious it is at your particular workplace. In such cases, the agency may send an expert to measure the levels of exposure and then make recommendations to you and your employer for controlling the hazard.

C. If the hazard involves substances whose effects on health need further study, NIOSH may send staff members to conduct a more complete investigation. In some cases, this study later may be expanded to include other workplaces in the same industry or workplaces which have the same hazards.

3. THE INVESTIGATION—The NIOSH experts who investigate your workplace may be industrial hygienists, doctors, engineers, or scientists such as epidemiologists. Under the law, they may enter the workplace and take whatever steps are necessary to find out about the hazards. For example, they may:

A. Measure the amounts of toxic substances or other hazards to which workers are being exposed

B. Give medical examinations to workers who want them to check for health damage

C. Examine employers health and safety records of workers

D. Talk privately with any worker about the possible hazards

E. Take photographs to show the hazards

YOU CAN TAKE PART

You as well as your employer have the right to have someone accompany NIOSH staff during a visit to your workplace. More than one worker can go along if that is necessary for an effective and thorough investigation. NIOSH can also allow a union staff person to take part in the workplace study.

4. THE RESULTS OF THE INVESTIGATION—After the study is completed, NIOSH writes a report telling what hazards were found and recommending ways to reduce them. The report is given to a representative of the workers, to the employer, and to the federal or state safety enforcement agency which covers that workplace.

If during the investigation NIOSH finds an imminent danger—one that should be corrected immediately, NIOSH will report it to the employer, the workers, and the responsible federal or state inspection agency. AND REMEMBER NIOSH standards are frequently more protective than OSHA standards. You or your union may be able to use NIOSH recommendations to protect you when OSHA would not.

5. BUT—NIOSH has no power to force your employer to correct hazards. It is not an enforcement agency like OSHA or MSHA. So, you may have to work with your employer, file a grievance, alter your contract language, enlist the help of the press or others, or seek alternative methods to correct a hazard.

SUMMARY

The health of people is dependent on the health of the environment—the home, the workplace, and the larger world. Self-care is making the effort to obtain knowledge of health and safety hazards and taking responsibility for making changes that will reduce such hazards, rather than burying one's head in the sand.

CASE EXAMPLE

The Kingstons are a middle-class family of four who live in Northern California. They have been Sierra Club members for many years and are environmentalists at heart, although not active politically. They act on their beliefs in the way they organize their household.

During the drought of 1976, the family used only one quarter of their water allotment per month. They did not plant a vegetable garden or water outdoor plants, although they grew some vegetables in containers. Water being run to heat up for a shower or dishwashing was collected in watering pots to water the plants; bathtub water was similarly used. Showers were limited to five minutes at a time, with water shut off while soaping, using a water-saving shower head provided by the water department. Because toilets are large consumers of water, the Kingstons flushed their toilets only when they contained bowel movements; toilet paper from urine was placed in the trash can.

Even though water is not a problem at this time, the Kingstons are still careful not to waste. They do not have a lawn or elaborate landscaping that needs constant watering, but use water for their large vegetable garden. Laundry is done with warm or cold water to save gas, and they have recently purchased an energy efficient hot water heater, furnace, and refrigerator, as well as having replaced a broken toilet with a "water-saver" toilet. They maintain their house at 65 degrees during the day, and 55 degrees at night, and do not use an air conditioner during the summer, although a small fan cools the boys' room at night when it reaches 90°. The clothes dryer is used during rainy days or the few months of the winter when the sun is not high enough to reach the clothesline. The pilot lights on their gas stove are turned off, and burners are lit with matches; however, the oven pilot is left on for safety.

The Kingstons are careful of the garbage they put into the environment. They recycle cans, glass, and newspapers. They save all vegetable wastes for a compost pile for their garden. When their children were infants, they refused to use disposable diapers because they did not want to put more plastic into the environment. They prefer beverages in returnable bottles, reuse their grocery bags, and buy dried beans, grains, and herbs in bulk rather than in plastic packaging.

Because the Kingstons are concerned about pesticides, they grow their own vegetables and have berry vines and fruit trees. They do not use pesticides and put up with some waste from insects. When slugs eat their vegetables, they kill them by hand. Tree trimmings and foliage are ground up for mulch and soil conditioner. They dry fruits and vegetables in their dehydrator or can and freeze vegetables to use during the year. They wash fruits and vegetables carefully that are bought from the market.

These techniques have become such a way of life for the Kingstons that Mrs. Kingston will retrieve and recycle bottles or cans thrown by guests into her trash. Guests are sometimes annoyed or amused, but the Kingstons are pleased that they do what they can on a daily basis to protect the environment.

CASE EXAMPLE

In a medical unit, one of the residents had inserted a CVP line into a patient. As Annette, the patient's nurse, was removing the tray, she recapped a needle and inadvertently stuck herself. Because she had always been careful, thinking she was even "too cautious" about such things, she felt badly about the needle stick. She went to the employee health service to report the injury and also checked on the hepatitis status of the patient. The employee health nurse mentioned to her that an increasing number of needle stick injuries had occurred recently. Not only had nurses been stuck, but aides who were changing beds had been stuck, and also needles had been found in the laundry.

Annette and the employee health nurse talked about why there might now be more such injuries. Was it the result of having a new set of interns who had just arrived in July? Could it be due to the distance of the needle disposal units from individual patients' rooms?

When Annette went back to the unit, she talked to some of her fellow staff nurses about her injury. At the next staff meeting, she told the others about the needle stick and her discussion with the occupational health nurse, and stated that she wanted to do something about the problem. Others agreed, and during the meeting, they formed an ad hoc task group to investigate needle stick injuries. Annette volunteered to be a liaison between the unit and the employee health service and infection control nurse. Another nurse at the meeting stated that she had concerns about radiation and wondered if the ad hoc task group could focus on this issue after they had dealt with the needle stick problem.

Case contributed by Barbara J. Burgel, R.N., M.S., Assistant Clinical Professor, University of California, San Francisco

---

Discussion Questions

1. Discuss the occupational risks of surgical nursing.
2. What strategies would you suggest to parents to protect their children from accidents or injuries?
3. Discuss the implications of state regulations for motorcycle helmets and seat belts. Whose responsibility is it?
4. What recommendations would you make to the office worker who complains of headache and low back pain?

REFERENCES

Aufiero B: Personal protective equipment: Design and availability considerations. Occupational Health Nursing, pp 33–37, October 1982

Bartkowski-Dodds L: Chemotherapy hazard. California Nurse, May 1983

Becker CE: Key elements of the occupational history for the general physician. The Western Journal of Medicine, Vol 137, No 6, pp 581–582, 1982

Burgel B: State warning on ethylene oxide. California Nurse, September/October 1983

Cantu B: Controlling rubella and hepatitis, California Nurse, December 1982

Castleman M: How to prevent mugging and rape (most of the time). Medical Self-Care, pp 10–15, Summer 1982

Centers for Disease Control: Morbidity and Mortality Weekly Report, Vol 31, No 43, November 5, 1982

Decker R: The not-so-pretty risks of cosmetics. Medical Self-Care, pp 25–31, Summer 1983

Delehunty H: How to avoid pesticides (sometimes). Medical Self-Care, pp 20–25, Fall 1981

Frank C: Avoiding "terminal" illness. Healthline, Vol 2, No 4, pp 10–18, 1983

Grayson B, Stein M: Attracting assault: Victims' nonverbal cues. Journal of Communication, Vol 31, No 1, p 68, 1981

Henry T: Radiation exposure and margins of safety. California Nurse, November 1982

Hutchinson S: Nurses and self-care: Resource management and strategy utilization. Paper presented at the Society for Applied Anthropology annual meeting, San Diego, California, March 1983

King J: Creative crime control alternatives. Medical Self-Care, pp 26–29 Summer 1982

LaDou J: Health effects of shift work. The Western Journal of Medicine, Vol 137, No 6, pp 525–530, 1982

Mattia M: Hazards in the hospital environment.: Anaesthesia gases and methylmethacrylate. American Journal of Nursing, Vol 83, No 1, pp 73–77, 1983

Moore L, Van Arsdale P, Glittenberg J, Aldrich R: The Biocultural Basis of Health, The C.V. Mosby Company, St. Louis, Missouri, 1980

McVeigh K: Nuclear war: The last epidemic. Medical Self-Care, pp 32–36 Summer 1982

Nuchols B: Keeping your back healthy. California Nurse, March/April 1983

Piller C: Staying healthy at work. Medical Self-Care, pp 6–13 Summer 1981

Reich M: Environmental politics and science: The case of PBB contamination in Michigan. American Journal of Public Health, Vol 73, No 3, pp 302–313, 1983

Rogers M: An Introduction to the Theoretical Basis of Nursing. F.A. Davis, Philadelphia, Pennsylvania, 1970

Salinas J: Artificial light and occupational health. Occupational Health Nursing, pp 13–15, February 1982

Snow B: Safety hazards as occupational stressors: A neglected issue. Occupational Health Nursing, pp 38–41, October 1982

State of California, Department of Industrial Relations, CAL/OSHA Communications Unit: How to Protect Your Health and Safety on the Job: A Worker's Guide. S-20, December 1980

Stellman J: Safety in the health care industry. Occupational Health Nursing, pp 18–21 October 1982

Stock L (ed): Community Right to Know: A Workbook on Toxic Substance Disclosure. Conference manual, Governor's Office, State of California, and Labor Occupational Health Program, University of California, Berkeley, February 1982

United States Department of Health, Education, and Welfare: Healthy People: The Surgeon General's Report on Health Promotion and Disease Prevention. DHEW/PHS, 1979

United States Department of Health, Education, and Welfare: Promoting Health/Preventing Disease: Objectives for the Nation. DHEW/PHS, 1980

United States Department of Labor: Job, Health and Safety. July 1975

White R: Cancer: The hazard of housework? Medical Self-Care, p 11 Summer 1981

14

Self-Care: Implications for Nursing Education, Practice, and Research

Self-care is very important to the health of human groups. In this light it would seem that health professionals and government agencies would view it with high regard. This chapter discusses broader implications of the self-care themes and practices described in earlier chapters, with some suggestions for the future. Some ways in which self-care can be implemented most effectively into nursing education, nursing practice, and nursing research will be described. Because education, practice, and research are interrelated, recommendations for change in one area affect the other categories.

THE NURSE AS MODEL

Despite longstanding attempts of nurse theorists and leaders to base the foundation of nursing on the concept of *health*, nursing students, educators, and hospital administrators continue to expect that students learn and use the disease-oriented medical model. In this context, it is difficult to convince nursing students of the importance of health promotion and sound health practices to themselves, their clients, and society. The public looks to health professionals for guidance in how best to stay well. The implication is that nurses have the potential for being powerful models of health promotion and self-care. However, nurses as a group have not appreciated this important point.

One does not become a model of health just because one chooses nursing as a profession. Even if one enters nursing school convinced of the importance of health promotion and self-care, it is not unlikely that these ideals will get lost in the face of the dominant medical model. Convictions about self-care must be continually reinforced and supported, especially in acute care settings filled with people who are sick. Nursing faculty need to help students integrate such ideas into all phases of the educational program and all clinical settings and, indeed, should serve as role models themselves.

Practicing nurses have an important role in modeling health for their clients and their colleagues, especially in work environments that are often unhealthy. Modeling health does not imply being perfectly healthy or self-righteous about health practices. It does mean that we strive toward positive health behaviors on an ongoing basis and that we be as caring of ourselves as we are of our clients.

It is difficult to expect nurses to maintain good health practices in unsupportive or poor psychological environments. In our experience, academic pressures on students and faculty often interfere with self-care and sound health practices. While we believe strongly in quality education, there must be a way to achieve it without interfering with the health of students and faculty. In the broader view, academic nursing itself should provide a supportive context for the individuals engaged in it.

Within the educational setting, services and facilities that encourage individual self-care behaviors should be provided. The environment must be safe and pleasant. For example, incidents of rape on campus may make it difficult to focus on work and can interfere with psychological well-being. In addition, provision of comfortable lounges, places to rest and relax, alone or with others, can help people reduce stress and encourage interaction apart from purely academic pursuits. Educational settings should also provide facilities and areas in which people can exercise or participate in other physical or cultural activities.

In addition to striving for a safe and pleasant environment, it is important to consider social and emotional support services that encourage self-care. For example, students and faculty who are also parents are often given very little support in academic settings. Their own needs become secondary to the demands of their educational programs, their families, and sometimes their jobs as well; they often do not have time or give themselves "permission" for self-care. How can we expect these students to become good role models in the clinical setting if there is little opportunity to practice self-care as they pursue their professional education. Financial support, while important for many students, is especially important to those who are parents and those who must work to support themselves and their families. Opportunities for part-time study would be helpful to such students.

Health care settings should be places in which students, clients, and staff can maintain and promote their health. They need to have nutritious foods available. In academic and institutional settings, food is usually high in fats and carbohydrates, it is overcooked, and fresh fruits and vegetables are scarce. In some settings, vending machines stocked with fast foods, "junk foods," and cigarettes are heavily relied on. Cafeterias may be crowded, noisy, and smoky, and schedules allow too little time to enjoy a meal.

Health care settings are notoriously stress-producing environments. Nurses cannot utilize self-care effectively or encourage their clients to do so when their own stress level is too high.

Nurses should not have to call in sick because they need a day off; they should be able to assess their stress levels and needs for a break daily and request paid time off when necessary. Rather than providing nurses with a set number of allowable sick days, vacation days, and holidays per year, a combined number of paid days off per year should be allowed. Nurses should be able to use these days at their discretion and not be forced to become sick or pretend to be sick in order to take a day off when they think one is needed. If we expect nurses to be good self-care role models, they need the latitude to assess their own state of well-being and intervene when necessary.

SELF-CARE CONTENT IN NURSING EDUCATION

With the exception of nursing education programs that utilize Orem's self-care model, many programs do not emphasize self-care as an approach to nursing. Even when self-care is taught, there is no guarantee that it will be practiced in clinical settings. Nursing models are often difficult to apply in clinical practice.

It is essential for curricula to include content on self-care, but we think that self-care should be taught as an approach to nursing in general, rather than as a specific type of theory or nursing intervention. The content should be integrated into every course as well as offered in specific courses, giving students multiple opportunities to translate theory and concepts into practice. Self-care content should not be directed only to clients and their families but to nursing students themselves.

In order for students to learn personal self-care effectively, it must be included in such a way that allows time and a setting in which to practice. Self-paced learning modules on self-care are a good way of providing content to individual students. Study groups help students to understand and apply self-care concepts as well as providing a supportive environment for personal change. For example, students can help each other by making contracts to change health behaviors.

SELF-CARE AS A BASIS FOR PRACTICE

Self-care can be a powerful philosophical basis for nursing practice in a variety of health care settings. Self-care teaching units are currently being set up in some hospitals and are well established in others. For example, some kidney dialysis units teach their clients to participate in their care to the greatest extent possible—from simple tasks as weighing themselves and noting their weight on the chart to more complex ones such as setting up the dialysis machine and inserting their own needles. The Loeb Center at Montefiore Hospital in New York is an example of an entire hospital based on self-care, with graduated units from partial self-care to total self-care. Nurses should recognize that there are missed opportunities in every hospital for patients and employees to practice self-care.

Economic and public policy issues pose a number of implications for nursing and self-care. People have debated for years whether health care is a right or privilege, how best to provide access to care, and who is responsible for providing and paying for services. One effect of rising health care costs has been that people are not seeking health care as early as might be necessary. By seeking professional care later or not at all, they lose the opportunity to learn how to better care for themselves. The advantages of prevention and early detection are available only to those who can afford health care services. When less fortunate people finally do seek care, often they will be more seriously ill and will encounter long-term complications and higher costs.

Escalating health care costs over the last two decades have defied efforts to contain costs (Fagin 1982). The federal and state governments are responding to such escalation of costs with a program of prospective reimbursements by diagnosis related groups (DRGs). Hospitals will be reimbursed a flat fee for the care of a client based on his diagnosis, rather than for the actual cost of his care in the hospital. As DRG reimbursement is phased in, length of hospital stays will continue to be reduced. In the future, it will be in the hospital's best interest to teach hospitalized patients to participate more effectively in their own care, during hospitalization as well as through early discharge. Although teaching self-care in and of itself is important, soon it will become economically mandatory; hospitals and clients alike will need to take a new look at the implications of self-care education. Self-care teaching focused on health promotion and disease prevention appears to have a greater effect on cost savings than do highly technological interventions (Luginbuhl 1981).

Nurses are in a key position to help clients prevent hospitalization and facilitate early discharge from acute care settings by providing clients with knowledge and skills needed to care for themselves. In addition, nursing is the backbone of community services such as outpatient departments and home health agencies. A philosphy of self-care is essential in these settings; the goal of nursing should be to help clients increase their ability to take care of themselves. In addition to the clinical services they currently offer, outpatient clinics, home health and community health agencies, and nursing centers can provide teaching services in self-care. For example, the recent and large increase in the elderly population dictates the need for expanded health care services. Not all will be sick or in need of hospitalization, but many will need monitoring and assistance for a variety of chronic conditions. Conway (1981) suggests a social model of care that encourages care of the elderly in their own homes or homelike group living facilities. This model is an opportunity for expansion of the nurse's role and a natural arena for self-care teaching and supervision.

Self-care teaching should also be provided in specific locations within outpatient and acute care settings. An example of this is in place in a number of Kaiser-Permanente medical centers, which are health maintenance organizations. All Kaiser outpatient clinics have health education materials readily available in clinic waiting rooms and excellent lending libraries. Health educators are available to assist clients with their specific learning needs, individually or in groups. In another example, at Cooperative Care at New York University Medical Center, clients can practice specific self-care skills under the supervision of a health care professional; for example, a newly diagnosed diabetic can learn to make food choices from a cafeteria line under the supervision of a dietician.

These and other innovative ideas could be utilized and improved upon in many health care settings. It is a challenge to nursing to develop creative ideas to promote self-care and increase the utilization in the health care system. Self-care teaching might be the greatest contribution that the nursing profession can make to the health of society and to cost containment in health care.

SELF-CARE AS A FOCUS FOR NURSING RESEARCH

Much more nursing research in the area of self-care is needed. Studies have examined lay participation in self-care including self-medication (Dunnell and Cartwright 1972; Harper 1984), the extent to which self-care activities were performed prior to seeking professional health care (Elliot-Binns 1973), the self-care practices of women (Freer 1980), cost effectiveness and other benefits of self-care (Avery 1980; Brownlea, Taylor, Landbeck, Wishart, Nadler, and Behan 1980; Estabrook 1979; Fireman, Friday, Gira, Vierthaler, and Michaels 1981, Goodwin 1979; Irish and Taylor 1980; Voineskos, Butler, Bullock, and El-Gaaly 1975; Zapka and Averill 1979); consumer attitudes toward self-care (Green and Moore 1980; Krantz, Baum, and Wideman 1980; Kubricht 1984), physicians' attitudes toward self-care (Linn and Lewis, 1979) and nurses' attitudes toward self-care (Kurzek 1982). However, no studies have focused specifically on the nurse's role in promoting self-care. We currently operate under many unexamined assumptions regarding nursing and self-care; it will be a challenge for nurse researchers to gather the necessary data to test our assumptions about self-care and the nurse's role in it.

We consider the following to be some areas of importance in future nursing research.

Nurses' Attitudes Toward Self-Care

We assume that nurses generally have positive attitudes toward self-care, health teaching, and health promotion, but data to support that assumption are lacking. The following research questions might guide nurse researchers

1. What are nurses' attitudes about self-care?
2. Does the educational preparation of the nurse influence the nurse's attitude about self-care?
3. Does a positive attitude on the part of the nurse influence nursing practice and promotion of self-care?
4. Do personal self-care practices on the part of the nurse influence nursing practice and promotion of clients' self-care?

The cost of providing nursing services has not been considered in previous attempts to contain health care costs (Fagin 1982). In fact, we do not yet have specific data on the cost of nursing care by either intensity of nursing care required or by diagnosis of client. Previously, nursing care costs have been embedded in such general costs as hospital room rates or outpatient services (Walker 1983). With very few exceptions, such as teaching or counseling, nurses are not reimbursed on a fee-for-service basis. We need studies that address the cost of specific kinds of nursing interventions, as well as for specific types of patients. We know that nursing care has an impact on client outcomes in and out of the hospital, but additional studies are needed to document the outcome of nursing interventions (Barham and Steiger 1984). Runyan (1975) showed dramatic improvements in objective measurements in hypertensive and diabetic clients. Can we assume that part of that improvement resulted from nurses providing self-care teaching?

Cost Effectiveness of Self-Care

Many argue that health teaching is too expensive for hospitals and other health care settings to provide. Others argue that health is responsibility and that with responsibility comes the task of learning to care for oneself. More data are needed to document the cost and the outcome of health teaching and self-care nursing interventions. The following questions might guide researchers:

1. Does the self-care and health teaching influence hospital admission or length of hospital stay?
2. How much does it cost to teach clients to care for themselves or to participate more effectively in health care? Clients could be categorized by need for prevention, detection, or management of illness.
3. What methods and settings are most cost-effective for teaching clients about their health?

4. Will economic incentives such as decreased cost of health insurance influence self-care behaviors?

In addition to gathering data on cost effectiveness, we need clinical research that demonstrates the most effective ways of teaching and motivating clients to participate actively in self-care. More information is needed on what methods are most effective (e.g., group or individual teaching, use of written materials, or a combination of methods), when self-care is most effectively encouraged, and how long effects of self-care teaching last over time.

At present, there is a small body of research on self-care. In the face of cost-containment efforts in health care, nurses will need to document the effectiveness of their self-care and health teaching. Not only must nurses take an active role in generating research about self-care, they must also participate in decision-making in professional education, clinical practice, and wider public issues related to health and illness care.

SUMMARY

The suggestions offered in this chapter and throughout the book are just a beginning in suggesting the potential for implementing self-care as a foundation for all aspects of nursing. Self-care has strong roots throughout history and is a powerful approach for health promotion today. Socially and politically, the time is right for nurses to take the lead in encouraging health care consumers to actively participate in health promotion, health maintenance, disease prevention, disease detection, and disease management. Our conviction that our clients have the *right* and the *ability* to participate in most aspects of health care and to make sound health decisions if they have been given accurate information and self-care tools is the philosophy on which this book is based. Nurses can improve individuals' and families' use of the health care system by helping them to use it only for what they cannot do for themselves.

Discussion Questions

1. Discuss ways to improve the quality and quantity of self-care practices among nursing students and nursing faculty.
2. Compare the influences that faculty self-care practices have on nursing student self-care practices, and those staff nurse self-care practices have on their clients' self-care practice.
3. Why it is important for nursing students and staff nurses to practice self-care?
4. What creative ideas can you think of to facilitate early hospital discharge?
5. What data need to be collected to support self-care?

REFERENCES

Avery CH, March J, Brook RH: An assessment of the adequacy of self-care by adult asthmatics. Journal of Community Health, Vol 5, No 3, pp 167–180, 1980

Barham V, Steiger N: H.M.O.'s: The Kaiser experience. In Aiken L (ed): Nursing in the eighties: Crises, Opportunities, Challenges. American Academy of Nursing, J.P. Lippincott, Philadelphia, Pennsylvania, 1982

Brownlea A, Taylor C, Landbeck M, Wishart R, Nadler G, Behan S: Participatory health care: An experimental self-helping project in a less advantaged community. Social Science and Medicine, Vol 14, No 2, pp 139–146. 1980

Conway ME: The impact of changing resources on health care of the future. In The Impact of Changing Resources on Health Policy, American Academy of Nursing, 1981

Dunnell K, Cartwright A: Medicine Takers, Prescribers, and Hoarders. Routledge and Kegan Paul, London, 1972

Elliott-Binnes CP: An analysis of lay medicine. Journal of the Royal College of General Practitioners, Vol 23, No 120, pp 255–264, 1973

Estabrook B: Consumer impact of a cold self-care center in a prepaid ambulatory care setting. Medical Care, Vol 17, No 11, pp 1139–1145, 1979

Fagin CM: Nursing as an alternative to high-cost care. American Journal of Nursing, Vol 82, No 1, pp 56–60, 1982

Fireman P, Friday GA, Gira C, Vierthaler WA, Michaels L: Teaching self-management skills to asthmatic children and to their parents in an ambulatory care setting. Pediatrics, Vol 68, No 3, pp 341–348, 1981

Freer CB: Self-care: A health diary study. Medical Care, Vol 18, No 8, pp 853–861, 1980

Goodwin JO: Programmed instruction for self-care following pulmonary surgery. International Journal of Nursing Studies, Vol 16, No 1, pp 29–40, 1979

Green KE, Moore SH: Attitudes toward self-care. A consumer study. Medical Care, Vol 18, No 8, pp 872–877, 1980

Irish EM, Taylor JM: A course in self-care for rural residents. Nursing Outlook, Vol 28, No 7, pp 421–423, 1980

Krantz DS, Baum A, Wideman MV: Assessment of preferences for self-treatment and information in health care. Journal of Personality and Social Psychology, Vol 39, No 5, pp 977–990, 1980

Kubricht DW: Therapeutic self-care demands expressed by outpatients receiving external radiation therapy. Cancer Nursing, February 1984

Kurzek G: Attitudes Among Nurses Toward Self-Care Practices. Unpublished master's thesis, Unviersity of California, San Francisco, School of Nursing, 1982

Linn L, Lewis C: Attitudes toward self-care among practicing physicians. Medical Care, Vol 17, No 2, pp 183–190, 1979

Luginbuhl WH, et al: Prevention and rehabilitation as a means of cost containment: The example of myocardial infarction. Journal of Public Health Policy, Vol 2, pp 103–116, 1981

Runyan JW: The Memphis chronic disease program: Comparisons in outcome and the nurse's extended role. Journal of the American Medical Association, Vol 231, No 3, pp 264–267, 1975

Walker D: The cost of nursing care in hospitals. Journal of Nursing Administration, Vol XIII, No 3, pp 13–18, 1983

Voineskos G, Butler JA, Bullock LJ, El-Gaaly A: Self-care program for inpatients in a mental hospital. Canadian Medical Association Journal, Vol 112, No 2, pp 177–180, 1975

Zapka J, Averill BW: Self-care for colds: A cost-effective alternative to upper respiratory infection management. American Journal of Public Health, Vol 69, No 8, pp 814–816, 1979

INDEX

313

reduction, 149
see also Health behavior
Behavior contract, for dietary changes, 146
Behavior modeling, 116
Behavior styles, comparisons of, 200t
Behavioral objectives
  for psychological and spiritual well-being, 223
  in teaching plan, 105, 111
Behavioral science theories, see Social and behavioral science theories
Behavioral therapy, for sexual problems, 249
Belief(s)
  healing and remission and, 215
  relationship to attitudes and health, 215
  see also Personal beliefs
Benefit of treatment, questioning of client on, 39
Beverages, caffeine content of, 140
Bioenergetics, 226t
Biofeedback, 226t
  basic operations, 199
  for stress management, 198, 199
  autonomic processes controlled by, 198
Biological hazards, in hospital setting, 289t, 289
Birth, religious customs related to, 214
Bladder infections, prevention and management, 149
Blumer, Herbert, symbolic interactionism theory, 26, 28, 32
Body, connection to mind and spirit, 209, 210f, 210
Body discipline therapies, 226t
Body-mind awareness therapies, 224, 226t
Body size, perception of health and illness and, 130–131, 132–133
Body weight, ideal, 130, 135, 136t
  see also Weight loss
"Botanical movement," 6
Brain, limbic system, 210
Breathing techniques, for stress management, 195
  see also Deep breathing
Burnout, 217
  prevention and interruption of, 217–218

Caffeine, 137
  content in common beverages and drugs, 138t
  control, 145
  stress and, 193
Calisthenics, 164
Calories, consumption of, calculation of, 147f
Carbohydrates, 131–132, 133–134

complex, see Complex carbohydrates
Carcinogens
  in cosmetics, 284
  in home, 283
  occupational, 279t–280t
Cardiac rehabilitation, self-care for, case example, 92–99
Cardiac symptoms, in stress, 192t
Cardiorespiratory exercises, 174
Cardiovascular conditions
  related to stress, 185t
  Risk Appraisal Form, 44–45
Cardiovascular function
  exercise and, 165, 169, 170
  subdivisions, 169–170
Cardiovascular system, benefit of exercise on, 165
Catheterization, self-catheterization teaching strategies, case example, 124
Central supply nurse, health hazards, 286
Checklists, in teaching plan, 113, 114f
Chemical hazards, in hospitals, 286, 289t
Chemotherapy, teaching strategies in, case example, 122–124
Chief complaint, 35, 37
  problem list of, 48
Childbirth
  role changes following, anxiety over, case example, 70–74
  sexual problems following, case example, 252–253
  working following, social support for, case example, 270-271
  see also Pregnancy
Children
  adult learning theory and, 30, 115
  health assessment of, 283
Chinese medicine, ancient, 4
Cholesterol, 132–133
  control, 144
Chronic illness, 78
  detection of, 81
  exercise for, 167–168
  management of, 82, 83t
  preventive behaviors, 79
  utilization of social support, 266–267
Client
  adjustment to illness and treatment, 102
  attitudes toward discussion of sexual functioning, 241–243
  explanatory model of illness, 29–30
  health, self-assessment of, 64–65
  participation in care and cure, 102, 310
  perception of illness, 84
  relationship with health care professional, 15
  see also Nurse-client relationship
Clinical category of health, 55, 57
Clinical research on self-care, 310

dressing change, 107
Hickman Catheter Educational Record,
  107–108, 109–110
  items to learn, 106
Hierarchy of needs (Maslow), 59, 61
Hippocrates, 4–5
"High blood," 119
High-calorie-density foods, control,
  145–146
"High-level wellness," 11, 57
"High status" foods, 130
History, sexual problem, 245
  see also Health History, Nursing history,
    Sexual history
History of self-care, 4, 16
  American, 5–8
  ancient and early European, 4–5
  present day, 8–11
"Holistic health," 11
  defined, 12
Holistic health movement, 57, 59, 210
Home
  health hazards in, assessment for,
    291–294
  toxic substances in, 282, 283–284
Homeopathy, 6–7
Hope, 215
  effect on physical response, 215
  loss of, 214, 215
Hope behaviors, compared to despair
  behaviors, 215, 216t–217t
Hospital, health hazards in, 286,
  289t–291
Hospital stays, reduction of, 307
Hospitalization, prevention of, 307
Household products, carcinogenic and
  toxic effects of, 284
Housewives, cancer rate, 283
Human body, perception of, historical
  perspective, 5
Human conduct, values about, 118
Hydrotherapy, 6
Hygiene, 6
Hyperplasia obesity, 135
Hypertension, 133
  stress-related, treatment, case
    examples, 202–203
Hypertrophic obesity, 135
Hypnosis
  with deep relaxation, physiological
    changes from, 196t
  Eriksonian, 229t

Illness
  adjustment to, 102
  choices of care, 85t
  coexistence with health, 58, 58f
  connection to health and religious faith,
    211
  cultural perception of, 232–233

definitions of, 58, 59
explanatory models of, 29–30, 32
  client's, 218, 219
  communication and, 119
nursing process, 84–85
  assessment, 85–86
  decision-making and responsibility,
    84–85
  planning, implementation and
    evaluation, 87–88
  setting goals, 86–87
perceptions of, 84
  fatalistic view, 214
  historical perspective, 5, 8
  self-care and, 214
related to sexuality, 242–243
self care in, 78, 88
  case examples, 88–89
  components of, see Components of
    self-care in illness
  detection, 81
  nursing process, see Illness, nursing
    process
  sexual dysfunction and, 247
  social support and, 257, 258, 266
Immune system, effect of stress on, 185
Implementation, in nursing process, see
  Planning and implementation
Impotence, 240–241
  case example, 250–252
Indigenous medicine, 84t
Information
  collection of, for assessment, 34–35
  for decision-making, 102
  need for, assessment of, 103–104
  related to sexual health, 239, 248, 249
Initial insomnia, 161
Injury
  control, 277, 278, 280
  from exercise, 166
  rates, from accidents, 280t
Inorganic factors, in environment, 276
Insomnia, 161
  types of, 161
Integumentary conditions, related to
  stress, 105t
"Intensive journal," 224–225
Intermittent insomnia, 161
"Internals," 214
Interpersonal relationships, 220
Intrinsic motivation, 115
Ionizing radiation, health hazards from,
  286
Isokinetic muscle contraction, 163
Isometric muscle contraction, 162–163
Isometrics, 164
Isotonic muscle contraction, 163

Journal, for psychological and spiritual
  well-being, 224–225, 231

DATE DUE
